COMMUNICATION
FOR THE
SPEECHLESS

COMMUNICATION FOR THE SPEECHLESS

An Introduction
to Nonvocal Communication Systems
for the Severely Communicatively Handicapped

Franklin H. Silverman

Marquette University

PRENTICE-HALL, INC., Englewood Cliffs, N.J. 07632

Library of Congress Cataloging in Publication Data

Silverman, Franklin H.
  Communication for the speechless.

  Bibliography: p.
  Includes index.
  1. Speech, Disorders of. 2. Communication devices for the disabled.
3. Handicapped--Means of communication. I. Title.
RC423.S518   616.8'55'06   79-13985
ISBN 0-13-153361-4

To James Viggiano, Rick Hoyt, and others
who as consumers have demonstrated
the efficacy of nonvocal communication systems.

Printed in the United States of America

10 9 8 7 6 5 4 3 2 1

Editorial/production supervision
and interior design by Scott Amerman
Cover design by Jayne Conte
Manufacturing buyer: Harry P. Baisley

PRENTICE-HALL INTERNATIONAL, INC., *London*
PRENTICE-HALL OF AUSTRALIA PTY. LIMITED, *Sydney*
PRENTICE-HALL OF CANADA, LTD., *Toronto*
PRENTICE-HALL OF INDIA PRIVATE LIMITED, *New Delhi*
PRENTICE-HALL OF JAPAN, INC., *Tokyo*
PRENTICE-HALL OF SOUTHEAST ASIA PTE. LTD., Singapore
WHITEHALL BOOKS LIMITED, *Wellington, New Zealand*

Contents

Preface   ix

I

Introduction   1

1
Need for Nonspeech Communication Modes 3

    Definition of Nonspeech Communications Modes, 3
    Conditions Which May Necessitate
    the Use of Nonspeech Communication Modes, 4
    Role of the Speech Pathologist
    in the Habilitation and Rehabilitation of the
    Speechless, 11
    References, 21

2
Impacts of Nonspeech Communication Modes
on Behavior 29

    Impact on Communication, 30
    Impact on Speech, 39
    Other Impacts on Users, 45
    Acceptance by Users and Others, 46
    Investment Required, 46
    Long-Term Impact, 47
    References, 48

II
Nonspeech Communication Modes   53

3
Classification of Nonspeech Communications Modes   55

Gestural Modes, 55
Gestural-assisted Modes, 58
Neuro-assisted Modes, 60
References, 61

4
Gestural Modes   63

American Sign Language (Ameslan), 63
American Indian Sign Language (Amerind), 67
Other Gestural Communication Modes, 72
Which System to Use? 81
References, 82

5
Gestural-assisted Modes   85

Symbol System, 86
Nonelectronic Gestural-assisted Communication
Systems, 113
Electronic Gestural-assisted Communication
 Systems, 127
References, 157

6
Neuro-assisted Modes   162

Use of Muscle Action Potentials
 for Controlling Communication Systems, 163
Use of Brain Wave Patterns
 for Controlling Communication Systems, 170
References, 170

III
Clinical Considerations   173

7
Selecting a Nonspeech Communication Mode
(or Modes)   175

What is the Cause of the Person's
   Communicative Disorder?   176
How Does the Person Communicate at Present?   177
What Are His Communication Needs?   179
What Is His Inner, Receptive,
   and Expressive Language Status?   180
Of the Existing Nonspeech Communication Systems,
   Which Would it be Possible for Him to Use?   182
Of the Systems He Could Use, Which Would be
   Optimal for Meeting His Communication Needs?   204
References,   205

8
Intervention Strategies
for Nonspeech Communication Modes   207

Gaining Acceptance for a System
   from Potential Users and Those with
   Whom They Communicate,   208
Generating Motivation for Communication,   210
Increasing Awareness of the Nature of
   Communication,   212
Periodically Reassessing Communication Needs,   215
Funding Communication System Components,   216
Gaining Administrative Support
   for the Use of Nonspeech Intervention Programs,   217
Training Persons in a User's Environment
   to Interpret Messages Transmitted
   by Nonspeech Communication Systems,   217
Assessing the Impact
   of Nonspeech Intervention Programs on Users,   218
Preventive Maintenance for Components
   of Gestural-assisted and Neuro-assisted
   Communication Systems,   219
Utilizing Gestural-assisted Electronic Systems
   and Neuro-assisted Systems
   for Environmental Control,   220
References,   220

Appendix A
Comprehensive Bibliography Relevant to
Nonspeech Communication Modes   223

Gestural Modes, 223
Gestural-assisted Modes, 232
Neuro-assisted Modes, 249

Appendix B
Sources of Materials for Teaching the Use
of Nonspeech Communication Modes   250

Appendix C
Sources of Components for Gestural-assisted
and Neuro-assisted Nonspeech
Communication Systems   252

Appendix D
Construction Details for Several Inexpensive
Displays and Other Components   254

Voice Operated Switch, 254
Scanning Encoding Aid Number 1, 254
Scanning Encoding Aid Number 2, 258
Lever Microswitch Switching Mechanism, 265
Etran Charts, 265
Radio Control Device for Interfacing Switching
   Mechanisms with Displays, 267
Device for Determining Optimal Positioning in Space for
   Communication Boards and Switching Mechanisms, 269

Appendix E
Form for Summarizing an Evaluation for Selecting
the Optimal Nonspeech Communication Mode
for Speechless Persons   271

Subject Index   279

Author Index   286

Preface

There are a number of children and adults with essentially normal hearing who are "locked in" in the sense that their speech is unlikely ever to be adequate for their communicative purposes. This poor prognosis for speech communication could result from one of several conditions including severe dysarthria, severe verbal apraxia, aphasia, glossectomy, severe mental retardation, or childhood autism. During the past few years there has been considerable work on developing nonspeech (nonvocal) communication modes, or systems, for such persons. Members of several professions have been involved, including the professions of speech pathology, special education (particularly the aspect dealing with teaching severely retarded and autistic children), occupational therapy, physical medicine, biomedical engineering, and electrical engineering. Based on reports in the literature, it would be difficult to conceive of a child or adult who is so severely impaired that there would be no nonspeech communication system that he or she could use.

This book is intended to acquaint the advanced undergraduate and masters-level graduate student in speech pathology as well as the professional speech pathologist and professionals in related fields (such as special education for autistic and severely retarded children, engineering, nursing, physical medicine, and occupational therapy) with the various modes of nonvocal communication that have been developed. Persons in these fields will be provided with the information necessary to select the most advantageous mode of nonvocal communication for a particular client and will be instructed on how to teach him or her to use it. The book also may be useful for acquainting the families of speech- less children and adults with available systems and for providing such persons with information about fabricating them.

Communication for the Speechless is divided into three parts. In the first, or introductory, part (which consists of the first two chapters) I describe what is meant by a nonspeech communication mode; indicate how such modes

x   *Preface*

have been used with several clinical populations; describe the need for a "communication" rather than a "speech" orientation when dealing with persons from these populations; and summarize the outcome literature relevant to the "impacts" of intervention with these systems on speechless children and adults. In the second part of the book (which includes chapters three through six) I describe and evaluate the various gestural, gestural-assisted, and neuro-assisted communication systems that have been developed. And in part three (which includes chapters seven and eight) I describe an evaluation procedure that can be used for selecting the "optimal" communication system (or combination of systems) for a client and indicate a number of considerations in developing an intervention program for any child or adult who could profit from such a system.

The book contains a comprehensive bibliography of books and articles (both published and unpublished) relevant to nonspeech communications modes (Appendix A); a list of sources of materials for teaching the use of these modes (Appendix B); a list of sources of "components" for gestural-assisted and neuro-assisted systems (Appendix C); and construction details for several inexpensive displays and other components (Appendix D).

It is impossible to give credit to the many sources from which the concepts presented in this book have been drawn. This book is the result of years of reading and hundreds of hours of conversation with students and colleagues in the areas of communicative disorders, occupational therapy, special education, and electrical engineering. Thus, I cannot credit this or that concept to a specific person, but I can say "thank you" to all who have helped, particularly my graduate students at Marquette University whose questions and criticisms through the years have helped me to clarify my own ideas.

Some special thanks are due to Dr. Gregg Vanderheiden of the University of Wisconsin-Madison—Director of the Trace Research and Development Center for the Severely Communicatively Handicapped—for input on gestural-assisted communication systems and Dr. Madge Skelly of the St. Louis Veterans Administration Hospital for input on gestural communication systems (particularly Amerind Sign). Some special thanks are also due to Dean Alfred Sokolnicki of the Marquette University College of Speech for making the arrangements necessary for my Sabbatical during the 1977-1978 Academic Year to facilitate the writing of this book. And last, but certainly not least, I wish to thank my wife Ellen-Marie for her patience, wisdom, and love, without which this book couldn't have been written.

Franklin H. Silverman

I

INTRODUCTION

1 Need for Nonspeech Communication Modes

There are several populations of persons who are not deaf but whose members frequently lack adequate speech for their communicative purposes. Such persons may derive benefit from one or more nonspeech communication modes. My objective in this chapter is to indicate how nonspeech communication modes can be used in the habilitation and rehabilitation of such persons. To accomplish this end I will (1) describe what is meant by a nonspeech communication mode, (2) indicate conditions that might necessitate the use of such a mode, and (3) demonstrate why it would be both appropriate and advantageous for speech pathologists to assume responsibility for selecting and teaching the use of such communication modes—that is, demonstrate why it would be advantageous for them to function as *communication* therapists rather than as *speech* therapists.

Definition of Nonspeech Communication Modes

Nonspeech communication modes can be defined operationally (Bridgman, 1927) as *procedures for encoding and transmitting messages without their being directly encoded into phonemes by the vocal tract.* Thus, any approach to encoding and transmitting messages that does not require a person to *directly* produce speech sounds would be classifiable by this definition as a nonspeech communication mode. The word "directly" is italicized because with some such approaches it is possible to *indirectly* encode a message into phonemes and transmit it as speech. With one approach of this type (Machine turns handwriting into sound, 1976) the user writes the message he or she wishes to communicate with a special pen that is attached to a computer. As each word is entered, the computer's memory is scanned to identify it. If the computer locates the word in its memory, it will activate a phoneme generator that will record the phonemes in the word on audiotape in the appropriate sequence. The recording could be played over a loud speaker or telephone. The time required for the computer to recognize a word and translate it into phonemes usually would be less than a second. Thus, words could be encoded and transmitted as speech almost as quickly as they could be written.

More than 100 systems for encoding and transmitting messages have been developed that could be classified by this definition as nonspeech communication modes. There is considerable variation in the level of refinement of these systems. While some have been tested and refined to the point where they can be regarded as both practical and dependable, others would have to be regarded as highly experimental. An example of the first type would be American Sign Language—the manual communication system used by the deaf (This system is described in Chapter 4). The second type would include systems which use muscle action potentials to control typewriters and other electronic displays (Combs, 1969; Torok, 1974). These systems are described in Chapter 6.

Conditions Which May Necessitate the Use of Nonspeech Communication Modes

Children and adults who have speech that is inadequate for their communicative purposes for a variety of reasons have benefited from nonspeech communication modes. The conditions that may necessitate the use of such a communication mode (either temporarily or permanently) are described briefly in this section. These include (1) dysarthria, (2) verbal apraxia, (3) aphasia, (4) glossectomy, (5) dysphonia, including laryngectomy, (6) mental retardation, (7) childhood autism, and (8) deafness. Representative reports describing the use of nonspeech communication modes with persons having each of these conditions also are indicated.

Dysarthria

The term *dysarthria* refers to an impairment in the functioning of the musculature of respiration, phonation, and articulation due to a lesion (or lesions) in the peripheral nervous system, central nervous system, or both. The degree of impairment can be so minimal that dysarthria would be difficult to detect during normal conversational speech, or the degree of impairment can be so severe that any speech produced is completely unintelligible.

The impact of dysarthria on speech is a function of several factors, including (1) the specific muscle groups affected and (2) the extent to which the functioning of each affected muscle group is impaired. While there is a negative relationship between the number of muscle groups affected and speech intelligibility (i.e., the more muscle groups affected, the poorer speech intelligibility), the relationship is not perfect. An impairment in the functioning of only a few muscle groups (e.g., the adductors of the vocal folds bilaterally) can result in unintelligible speech. (If the adductors of the vocal folds were paralyzed bilaterally and the abductors were unimpaired, the vocal folds would be fixed in the "open" position and phonation probably would be impossible.)

The *extent* to which the functioning of individual muscle groups is impaired also influences the impact of dysarthria on speech. Extent of impairment can range from being able to produce a desired muscle gesture (or movement), but at a slower rate than normal, to being completely unable to produce that gesture. While there is a negative relationship between the degree of impairment of muscle groups and speech intelligibility (i.e., the greater the degree of impairment, the poorer speech intelligibility), the relationship is not perfect. Relatively mild involvement of certain parts of the speech musculature (e.g., that of the tongue) can more adversely effect speech intelligibility than can moderate involvement of other parts of this musculature (e.g., that of the lips).

Specific deficits in muscle functioning are determined by the location of the lesion (or lesions) in the nervous system and its magnitude, rather than by what produced it. A lesion of a given magnitude at a given point in the nervous system resulting from trauma, a tumor, or a degenerative disease process will produce the same deficit. If the lesion is in the lower motor neurons, the result will be flaccidity. If it is in the upper motor neurons, the result will be spasticity. If it is in the basal ganglia, the result will be involuntary movement. And if it is in the cerebellar system, the result will be dysmetria and other symptoms of ataxia. (For a discussion of dysarthria, see Darley, Aronson, & Brown, 1975.) Thus, persons who have cerebral palsy can have the same neuromuscular deficits as those who have had a stroke.

Most dysarthrias result in some reduction in speech intelligibility. In some cases this reduction is so great that speech is inadequate for most interpersonal communication. Nonspeech communication modes can be used in such cases as a substitute for or an adjunct to speech.

Involvement of certain of the muscle groups that control the vocal tract is particularly likely to result in speech which is not sufficiently intelligible to successfully transmit most messages. These muscle groups include those that control the tongue, the velum, and the vocal folds (particularly the adductors).

There are a number of neurological conditions and neuromuscular disorders that frequently have a severe enough dysarthria associated with them to warrant the use of nonspeech communication modes. These include cerebral palsy, amyotrophic lateral sclerosis, bulbar palsy, pseudobulbar palsy, cerebellar ataxia, Parkinsonism, dystonia, chorea, stroke (CVA), brain tumors, and trauma (for a description of these conditions, see Darley, Aronson, & Brown, 1975).

Several types of nonspeech communication modes have been used with children and adults who are dysarthric. These include *manual sign languages* (Chen, 1971; Egan, Anthony, & Honke, 1976; Fenn & Rowe, 1975; Peters, 1973), gestural Morse code (Adams, 1966), *nonelectronic communication, or conversation, boards* (Cohen, 1976; Goldberg & Fenton, 1960; Handicapped youth "talks" with eyes, 1974; Kladde, 1974; McDonald & Schultz, 1973; McNaughton, 1976b; Sayre, 1963; Vanderheiden, 1976; Vicker, 1974), *electronic communication systems* (Bullock, Dalrymple, & Danca, 1975; Burnside, 1974; Butler & Fouldes, 1974; Carlson, 1976; Charbonneau, Cote, & Roy, 1974; Clappe *et al,* 1973; Combs, 1969; Computerized device speaks for handicapped youngsters, 1976; Copeland, 1974; Hagen, Porter, & Brink, 1973; Harmon, 1974; Harris-Vanderheiden, 1976b; He puffs past his handicap, 1974; Hill *et al,* 1968; Jack H. Eichler: Builds communication device, 1973; Lavoy, 1957; Maling & Clarkson, 1963; Perron, 1965; Shane & Melrose, 1975; Vanderheiden, 1976; Vanderheiden, Lamers, Volk, & Geisler, 1975; Vasa & Lywood, 1976; Wendt, Sprague, & Marquis, 1975; White, 1974), and *Blissymbolics* (Australian News and Information Bureau, 1973; Hartley, 1974; Kates & McNaughton, no date; McNaughton, 1976a, 1976b; Vanderheiden, Brown, MacKenzie, Reinen, & Scheibel, 1975). Blissymbolics, strictly speaking, is not a nonspeech communication mode, but a symbol system that can be used with electronic and nonelectronic communication devices.

Verbal Apraxia

Verbal apraxia is a condition which prevents a person from normally producing the muscle gestures required for speech on a voluntary level. A person who has this condition is able to produce them normally, however, on a vegetative, or involuntary, level. This differentiates apraxics from dysarthrics since the latter have some degree of motor deficit on *both* voluntary and involuntary levels.

Nonspeech communication modes have been used for two purposes with verbal apraxics: (1) facilitating communication and (2) facilitating speech. They serve to facilitate communication by providing the apraxic with an additional channel (or additional channels) for encoding and transmitting messages. They thus supplement the two channels usually used for this purpose: speech and normal nonverbal communication. Nonspeech communication modes also have been used for a second purpose with oral apraxics—that is, for facilitating speech. There is some evidence (Skelly *et al.,* 1974) that teaching verbal apraxics a nonspeech communication mode is likely to result in an increase in their attempts at speech. (The effect of teaching a nonspeech communication mode on subsequent attempts at verbalization is dealt with further in Chapter 2.) Thus, teaching verbal apraxics a nonspeech communication mode may improve both their ability to speak and their ability to communicate.

Several nonspeech communication modes have been used with verbal apraxics. These include *pantomime* (Schlanger, 1976), *manual sign languages* (Chen, 1968, 1971; Eagleson, 1970; Goldojarb, 1976; Goldstein & Cameron, 1952; Hanson, 1976; Helfrich, 1976; Skelly, Schinsky, Smith, & Fust, 1974), *nonelectronic communication,* or *conversation, boards* (Cohen, 1976; Nuffer, no date; Sklar & Bennett, 1956), and *electronic communication systems* (Copeland, 1974; Perron, 1965).

Manual sign language appears to have been used more often with these patients than other nonspeech communication modes. The relatively frequent use of this mode may be at least partially due to the fact that many verbal apraxics are only hemiplegic. Since hemiplegics have one upper extremity that is normal motorically, it would be relatively simple for them to learn a one-hand manual sign language.

Aphasia

Aphasia is a neurological condition in which there is a deficit in one or more aspects of symbolic formulation and expression (Head, 1926). It is thought to result from a lesion (or lesions) in the cerebral cortex or related subcortical structures. The aspects of language behavior in which there may be a deficit include speech comprehension, speaking, reading, writing, and computation. Also included may be the ability to comprehend and use gestures for communicative purposes (Duffy, Duffy, & Pearson, 1975). The degree of deficit for a given language ability may be so mild that it only can be detected by a sensitive testing instrument or so severe that it appears to be completely, or almost completely, absent. Also, the degree of impairment of a given language ability may not remain constant over time: it may intensify (if the cause, for example, is a tumor) or become less severe (by spontaneous recovery, the effects of therapies, or both). The condition described in the previous section—verbal apraxia—is classified by some authors as an aphasic disturbance. (For additional information of the symptomatology and etiology of aphasia, see Head, 1926; Penfield & Roberts, 1959; Eisenson, 1972, 1973.)

Nonspeech communication modes can be used with aphasics on a temporary or permanent basis to facilitate communication. Those with moderate to severe deficits in speech comprehension, speaking, reading, and writing may be able to communicate basic needs to persons taking care of them by pointing to pictures on a communication board, by pantomiming, or by using manual sign language. The need for such communication modes may only be temporary—perhaps during the first few months post-trauma— because speech comprehension, speaking, reading, and writing may improve sufficiently through spontaneous recovery and speech therapy to again be adequate for the person's communicative purposes. There is some evidence, incidently, which suggests that the use of a nonspeech communication mode during the post-trauma period may facilitate the language-recovery process (see Chapter 2).

Several nonspeech communication modes have been used with aphasics. These include *pantomime* (Schlanger, 1976), *manual sign languages* (Chen, 1968, 1971; Eagleson, Vaughn, & Knudson, 1970; Gardner, Zurif, Berry, & Baker, 1976; Goldojarb, 1976; Goldstein & Cameron, 1952; Hanson, 1976; Skelly, Schinsky, Smith, Donaldson, & Griffin, 1975), *manipulatable symbols* (Glass, Gazzaniga, & Premack, 1973), *nonelectronic communication,* or *conversation, boards* (Cohen, 1976; Nuffer, no date; Sklar & Bennett, 1956), and *electronic communication systems* (Copeland, 1974; Perron, 1965).

Glossectomy

The term *glossectomy* refers to surgical excision, or removal, of all or part of the tongue, usually because of cancer. The amount of tissue removed may preclude the post-surgical learning of intelligible speech. Using a nonspeech communication mode would obviously facilitate communication in such instances. (For further information on glossectomy and its impact on communication, see Skelly, Donaldson, & Fust, 1973.)

All of the nonspeech communication modes described in this book could be used by glossectomy patients. The only one, however, that appears to have been used extensively with this population is *American Indian Sign Language,* or *Amerind* (Skelly, Schinsky, Smith, Donaldson, & Griffin, 1975).

Dysphonia (Including Laryngectomy)

Dysphonias are voice disorders. They often result from anatomical or physiological anomalies of the larynx that make normal phonation impossible. Such anomalies include (1) absence of the vocal folds following laryngectomy, (2) bilateral flaccid paralysis of the adductors of the vocal folds (which prevents them from approximating), and (3) lesions on the vocal folds, such as vocal nodules. (For additional information on the symptomatology and etiology of dysphonias, see Boone, 1977.)

Nonspeech communication modes have been used for several purposes with children and adults who have voice problems. They have been used, for example, as a *temporary* communication mode for patients who are on vocal rest because of a lesion (or lesions) on their vocal folds (e.g., vocal nodules) resulting from vocal abuse. They also have been used as a *permanent* communication mode for patients who have permanently lost the ability to phonate, such as laryngectomies who are poor candidates for an electrolarynx or esophageal speech (included in this group would be persons who have had both laryngectomies and glossectomies). In addition, they have been used as a *temporary* communication mode for persons who have had laryngectomies, until they acquire adequate esophageal speech for their communicative purposes. They can provide such persons, for example, with a means of transmitting emergency and other messages over a telephone.

All of the nonspeech communication modes described in this book could be used by dysphonic patients. The only type, however, that appears to have been used extensively with this population is manual sign language (Skelly, Schinsky, Smith, Donaldson, & Griffin, 1975).

Mental Retardation

Mental retardation is a condition that is presumed to result at least partially from organically based slowness in cognitive development—that is, slowness in the ability to solve problems and see relationships. Because this ability influences all aspects of functioning, the overall development of persons with this condition would be expected to be slow, including their use of speech for intrapersonal and interpersonal communication. The degree of slowness in cognitive development can be so little that it is unlikely to have a significant impact on a person's ability to cope with his or her environment or so great that a person can only cope with a highly structured institutional environment that would make almost no demands on him. The cognitive development of persons with this condition rarely, if ever, catches up to that of normal persons. (For further information on the symptomatology, phenomenology, and etiology of mental retardation see Stevens & Heber, 1964.)

Some children and adults who are diagnosed mentally retarded (particularly those who are diagnosed severely mentally retarded) do not appear to be able to acquire enough speech for their communicative purposes. They usually attempt to communicate primarily by crying (or screaming or producing other noises), pointing, and/or using very concrete gestures. These behaviors often are not perceived as messages; or if they are perceived as such, not appropriately interpreted. There is considerable clinical evidence (see papers cited in the next paragraph) that nonspeech communication modes can not only improve the abilities of such persons to communicate, but can facilitate their acquisition of speech. (The impact of learning nonspeech communication modes on the verbal output of mentally retarded children and adults is discussed in Chapter 2.)

Several types of nonspeech communication modes have been used with mentally retarded children and adults. These include *mime* (Balick, Spiegel, & Greene, 1976; Levett, 1969, 1971), *manual sign languages* (Bicker, 1972; Brookner & Murphy, 1975; Grecco, 1972; Green, 1975; Lake, 1976; Hoffmeister & Farmer, 1972; Kent, 1974; Kimble, 1975; Kopchick and Lloyd,

1976; Kopchick, Romback, & Smilovitz, 1975; Larson, 1971; Lebeis & Lebeis, 1975; Peters, 1973; Richardson, 1975; Shaffer & Geohl, 1974; Sutherland & Beckett, 1969; Topper, 1975; Van Hook & Stohr, 1973; Wilson, 1974a, 1974b; Wilson, Goodman, & Wood, 1975), *manipulatable symbols* (Carrier, 1974a, 1974b, 1976; Carrier & Peak, 1975; Premack & Premack, 1974), and *Blissymbolics* (Australian News and Information Bureau, 1973; Harris-Vanderheiden, 1976a; McNaughton, 1976a, 1976b; Vanderheiden, Brown, MacKenzie, Reinen, & Scheibel, 1975). For nonspeech communication modes that have been used with cerebral palsied and other physically handicapped mentally retarded children and adults, see the papers cited in the *dysarthria* section under the subheadings "nonelectric communication, or conversation, boards" and "electronic communication systems."

Childhood Autism

Autism is a condition that appears to begin early in childhood. A child with this condition is presumed to be in less than normal contact with his or her total external sensory environment, since children diagnosed as having this condition do not tend to respond normally to most, if not all, forms of external sensory stimulation (Myklebust, 1954). There does not appear to be general agreement on the etiology of childhood autism—whether it is a learned response pattern, the result of abnormal functioning of some structure (or structures) within the central nervous system, both of these, or something else. (For additional information on childhood autism see Myklebust, 1954 and recent volumes of the *Journal of Autism and Childhood Schizophrenia.*)

Autistic children typically make little, if any, attempt to use speech for communicating with persons in their environments. Such children, in fact, are reported to make little, if any, use of vocalization or gesture for this purpose (Myklebust, 1954). Also, they typically do not respond normally to speech directed to them, and for this reason are sometimes misdiagnosed as having a hearing loss (Myklebust, 1954).

There is some evidence (see the papers cited in the next paragraph) that the interpersonal communication of autistic children can be facilitated in two ways by teaching them a nonspeech communication mode. First, at least some such children will attempt to communicate with persons in their environment more while using the mode than they did previously. And second, at least a few will begin to use speech for interpersonal communication. (The impact of teaching autistic children a nonspeech communication mode on their verbal output is dealt with in Chapter 2.)

Several types of nonspeech communication modes have been used with autistic children, including *manual sign languages* (Bonvillian & Nelson, 1976; Creedon, 1975; Fulwiler & Fouts, 1976; Haight, 1975; Hollander &

Juhrs, 1974; Konstantareas, Oxman, Webster, Fischer, & Miller, 1975; Leibl, Pettet, & Webster, 1974; Lucas & Dean, 1976; Menyuk, 1974; Miller & Miller, 1973; Offir, 1976; Ricks & Wing, 1975; Schaeffer, Kolinzas, Musil, & McDowell, 1975; Smith, 1975; Tatman & Webster, 1973; Webster, McPherson, Sloman, Evans, & Kuchar, 1973) and *nonelectronic conversation, or communication, boards* (Ratusnik & Ratusnik, 1974;1976).

Deafness

The term deafness usually is used to designate a profound hearing loss. Persons with this condition receive little or no information necessary to understand speech through the auditory channel. (They may, however, receive such information through the visual channel by speechreading.) Because they have both a profound interpersonal and intrapersonal hearing deficit for speech, the deaf usually do not learn to talk without special training. Even with such training, their speech may not become sufficiently intelligible for at least some communicative purposes. Many deaf persons, therefore, rely on nonspeech communication as either a supplement to or substitute for speech.

The nonspeech communication mode that is used most often by the deaf is a manual gestural system known as American Sign Language, or Ameslan (Moores, 1974; this system is described in Chapter 4). Ameslan is used by the deaf in two ways. The first is as a supplement to speech: messages are encoded and transmitted *simultaneously* in manual sign and speech (this approach to communication for the deaf is referred to in the literature as "total communication"). The second is as a substitute for speech: messages are encoded and transmitted in manual sign.

While almost all the nonspeech communication modes that have been used with the deaf are described in this book, their use with members of this population is not treated in depth, for several reasons. First, there is already a very large literature describing the use of them, particularly Ameslan, with this population (representative bibliographies of this literature can be obtained from the Gallaudet College Bookstore, Washington, D.C.). And second, a systematic review of this literature would not have been possible within the length restrictions established for this book.

Role of the Speech Pathologist in the Habilitation and Rehabilitation of the Speechless

An attempt has been made in this chapter to establish the need for nonspeech communication modes (1) by indicating that there are children and adults who are functionally speechless temporarily or permanently because of one or more of several conditions and (2) by providing evidence that nonspeech communication modes can make functional communication possible for such persons. Assuming that a need for such communication modes has been established, who should have the primary responsibility for selecting and teaching the use of them? This section will present the point of view that the person who should assume this responsibility is the speech pathologist. It also presents the point of view that speech pathologists, to successfully discharge this responsibility, have to function as *communication* therapists rather than *speech* therapists and consult when necessary with other professionals such as physical therapists, occupational therapists, engineers (electrical or biomedical), nurses, and teachers.

Professional Responsibility of the Speech Pathologist to the Communicatively Handicapped

The speech pathologist is responsible for diagnosing and treating (nonmedically) all communicative disorders except those arising from hearing loss. (The diagnosis and nonmedical treatment of communicative disorders resulting from hearing loss is the responsibility of the audiologist.) The speech pathologist assesses the communicative status of his or her clients and then develops therapy strategies that will hopefully improve their ability to communicate. In most cases, such therapy strategies are intended to improve their ability to speak to the point where, if it is not within normal limits, it is adequate for their communicative purposes.

Speech pathologists following an assessment of their clients' communicative status sometimes are forced to conclude that the prognosis for speech ever being adequate for their communicative purposes is extremely poor. Or they are forced to conclude that, though the prognosis for their clients developing speech that will be adequate for their communicative purposes is good for some future time, their speech probably will not be adequate for their communicative needs for the immediate future. Under either of these circumstances, speech pathologists have a responsibility to help their clients develop nonspeech communication strategies (i.e., strategies for encoding and transmitting messages) for meeting their communication needs. This responsibility has several aspects:

1.   selecting the nonspeech communication mode (or modes) that will be most likely to meet the client's communication needs;
2.   securing necessary "hardware" and "software";
3.   teaching the client how to use the mode (or modes) selected for encoding and transmitting messages; and
4.   periodically reassessing the client's cognitive, motor, and sensory abilities and communication needs to insure that the modes he uses continue to permit him to meet his communication needs.

The first aspect of the speech pathologist's responsibility to the non-vocal patient is selecting an optimum nonspeech communication mode (or combination of nonspeech communication modes) for meeting his or her communication needs. The speech pathologist first determines which nonspeech communication modes the client has the motor, sensory, and cognitive abilities to use, and then selects from this subset of nonspeech modes the one (or possible combination of several) that would be optimum for meeting the client's communication needs. (An approach that can be used for these purposes is described in Chapter 7.)

Once the nonspeech communication mode (or modes) has been selected for a client, the speech pathologist is responsible for securing any necessary *hardware* or *software*. The concepts "hardware" and "software" are adopted from computer terminology: hardware refers to the instrumentation in a computer system, and software to the programs that are necessary for it to perform its functions; thus, hardware refers to instrumentation, and software to the symbol system (or systems) required for it to perform its function. Figure 1.1 illustrates the application of these concepts to nonspeech communication modes. The device pictured is a simple conversation, or communication, board. The hardware component of this device would be a piece of plywood, cardboard, Masonite, plastic, or other material of the desired size and shape and the software component would be the symbols (in this case words) attached to it or printed on it. (The construction of communication boards is described in Chapter 5.) Both the hardware and software components of nonspeech communication modes often are considerably more complex than those illustrated in Figure 1.1. (The types of hardware and software components in nonspeech communication devices are described in Chapters 5 and 6.)

After the mode (or combination of modes) has been selected and any necessary hardware and software has been secured, the speech pathologist is responsible for teaching the client how to use it (or them) for encoding and transmitting messages. For some client-mode combinations, such instruction would only take a few minutes, and for others it could take a year or longer. An example of one that would probably only take a few minutes is

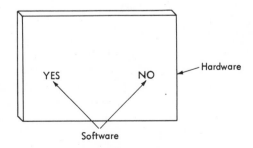

FIGURE 1.1. *Hardware and software components of a nonspeech communication device.*

teaching a glossectomy patient to use a simple picture communication board. An example of one that could take a year or longer is teaching a spastic quadriplegic to use a sophisticated electronic Blissymbol communication system. (Considerations in teaching the use of nonspeech communication modes are discussed in Chapter 8.)

The final aspect of the responsibility of the speech pathologist to nonvoca clients is periodically reassessing their cognitive, motor, and sensory abilities and communication needs to insure that the modes they use continue to permit them to meet their needs. This aspect of responsibility includes (1) making certain that the modes used by clients continue to be optimum for them; (2) helping clients maintain hardware and software; and (3) counseling clients and those with whom they communicate if problems arise effecting the use of the mode or combination of modes.

It is not usually safe to assume that what appears to be an optimum communication mode (or combination of modes) when a client is first seen will be optimum permanently. There are several reasons. First, clients, communication needs may vary over time. An expressive aphasic, for example, immediately following the stroke that caused his aphasia may be able to communicate necessary messages to hospital personnel by means of a relatively simple conversation board. After he is discharged from the hospital and returns home, however, this conversation board may be inadequate for transmitting the messages he needs to communicate in this environment.

Another reason why it is not safe to assume that a given nonspeech mode (or combination of such modes) will be optimum permanently is that a client's sensory, cognitive, and motor abilities may not remain constant. They tend to become worse, for example, as some neurological conditions and diseases progress. Persons who have such a condition or disease may become unable at some point during the course of its development to effectively use a nonspeech communication mode that they could previously employ. It is necessary, therefore, that speech pathologists periodically reassess their nonvocal clients who have degenerative diseases or conditions, and modify their nonspeech communication modes when necessitated by changes in their sensory, cognitive, or motoric status.

Nonvocal clients who are using nonspeech communication modes also have to be reassessed periodically because there may be some improvement in their motor, sensory, or cognitive abilities. If there is improvement in any of these abilities, they may be able to use a more efficient and/or flexible mode. A child who has cerebral palsy, for example, may improve in his cognitive, motor, and sensory abilities as he grows older. Thus, a combination mode (or combination of communication modes) that would be optimum for such a child at age three may not be optimum for him at age nine.

A second reason why it is necessary for speech pathologists to periodically contact nonvocal clients is to help them maintain the hardware and software components in their communication systems. Such contact is particularly important if their communication systems contain electronic components. Even the simplest electronic component is likely to malfunction if it is used frequently or for a long period of time. Obviously, any malfunction will interfere to some extent with the client's ability to encode and transmit messages. It is important, therefore, for the speech pathologist both to periodically check clients' communication systems and to arrange to have them repaired when notified that they have malfunctioned.

A third reason why it is important for speech pathologists to periodically contact their nonvocal clients is to provide necessary counseling. The attitudes of the client and those with whom he or she communicates toward a nonspeech communication mode can influence the effectiveness of that mode. If these attitudes are positive, the effectiveness of the mode is likely to be enhanced. However, if they are negative for either the client or those with whom he or she communicates, its effectiveness as a channel for encoding and transmitting messages is likely to be reduced. While a client and his family may initially accept his communicating in a nonspeech mode, their attitude may change with time, particularly if they rightly or wrongly regarded the mode as only temporary until speech became adequate for communicative purposes. This is apt to happen with adults who have a severe oral apraxia. Immediately following their stroke (or whatever was responsible for the lesion that precipitated the apraxia) they may have a positive attitude toward using a nonspeech communication mode because it provides them with a way to communicate. If their speech does not return after a few months, however, and they sense they may have to continue using the mode on a long-term or permanent basis, their attitude toward the mode may change from acceptance to rejection. There obviously would be a need for counseling in such a case. (Considerations in counseling users of nonspeech communication modes and their families are dealt with in Chapter 8.)

The Speech Pathologist as Communication Pathologist

Speech pathologists would best serve their clients if their orientation were that of a *communication* pathologist rather than a *speech* pathologist. Having a *communication orientation* could influence their clinical functioning in several ways including their goals for therapy—and consequently their termination criteria and their criteria for evaluating both therapy outcome and the adequacy of their own clinical performance.

From the *speech* orientation, the ultimate goal of therapy is either normal speech or speech that is adequate for the client's communicative purposes. (The latter would tend to be the ultimate goal for persons in the clinical populations that were mentioned earlier in this chapter.) The emphasis in therapy is on improving speech. Improving speech tends to be regarded as an end in itself rather than as a means to an end. Therapy usually is terminated when further improvement in speech seems unlikely. Therapy outcome is assessed primarily in regard to speech status, and clinicians tend to base judgments of the adequacy of their clinical performance on the amount their clients improved their speech.

From the *communication* orientation, on the other hand, the ultimate goal of therapy would be developing the ability to communicate to a level adequate to meet communication needs. Since speech is almost universally regarded as the most flexible and efficient mode for encoding and transmitting messages, attempts would be made to improve speech as much as possible. Improving speech from this orientation, however, would tend to be regarded as a means to an end (i.e., achieving adequate ability to communicate) rather than as an end in itself.

The emphasis in therapy from a communication orientation would be on developing adequate ability to communicate. Several channels for encoding and transmitting messages may be developed, *including speech.* The client may be encouraged to combine speech and nonspeech modes while communicating (particularly if the nonspeech mode is a gestural mode). This approach to the rehabilitation of hearing clients is similar to the "total communication" approach used by teachers of the deaf.

Therapy would be terminated from a communication orientation when it appeared that further significant improvement in *communication* was unlikely. The point at which therapy would be terminated from this orientation sometimes would differ from the other. The discharge criteria used by a clinician having a communication orientation would include the following: no further significant improvement likely *at this time* in the client's ability to encode and transmit messages. Obviously, the possibility of there being further significant improvement at some future time cannot be eliminated. This aspect of the discharge criteria for clinicians having a speech orientation would tend to be more limited: no further significant improvement likely at this time in the client's ability to encode and transmit messages *through speech.*

Therapy outcome from a communication orientation is assessed primarily in regard to *communication* status. The closer clients' communication abilities come to meeting their communication needs, the better the therapy outcome is judged to be. Clients' speech status, of course, is considered when assessing therapy outcome from this perspective.

Clinicians who have a communication orientation tend to base judgments about the adequacy of their clinical performance on the amount their clients improve their ability to communicate. While such clinicians would attempt to improve their clients speech as much as possible, and would judge their clinical performance positively if they were able to significantly improve their clients' speech, they would not necessarily judge their clinical performance negatively if they were unsuccessful in helping them improve their speech. Since their goal for therapy is the improved ability to communicate, they would tend to judge the adequacy of their clinical performance positively if their clients significantly improved their abilities to encode and transmit messages, regardless of the contribution of speech to their clients' improved communication abilities. Because for most nonvocal clients the prognosis for developing adequate speech for communicative purposes tends to be poorer than that for developing adequate ability to communicate by non-speech means, clinicians are more likely to assess the adequacy of their clinical performances positively when working with such clients if they have a communication orientation than if they have a speech orientation.

Another way by which clinicians' orientations (i.e., speech versus communication) can influence their clinical functioning is the impact it can have on their attitudes toward the role of nonspeech communication modes in the habilitation and rehabilitation of children and adults who have inadequate speech for their communicative purposes. From the speech orientation, nonspeech communication modes would tend to be regarded as "last resorts." They usually would not be introduced before attempts had been made to develop adequate speech for communicative purposes. Only after it became obvious that further speech therapy would be unlikely to facilitate adequate speech for a client's communicative purposes would a nonspeech communication mode tend to be considered. In some cases, a nonspeech communication mode would not be considered even then. The speech pathologist may not consider developing and teaching the use of nonspeech communication modes to be a part of his or her professional responsibility. A speech pathologist is particularly likely to have this attitude if a client requires a nonspeech mode more sophisticated than a simple nonelectronic communication board (e.g., one that uses an electronic switching mechanism to control an electric typewriter).

In some cases, when a speech pathologist does not assume the responsibility for developing and teaching a client to use a nonspeech communication mode, someone else will (e.g., an occupational therapist or an electrical engineer). In others, no one will assume this responsibility, and the client will remain unable to communicate adequately. This is unfortunate since there are currently nonspeech modes available through which the communication ability of almost any speechless child or adult can be enhanced. (These modes are described in Chapters 4, 5, and 6.)

From a communication orientation, nonspeech communication modes are not viewed as "last resorts," but as techniques that can assist a clinician in achieving his or her ultimate goal—adequate ability to communicate. They may be introduced at the beginning of therapy before a reliable prognosis can be made about the likelihood of the client developing adequate speech for

TABLE 1.1. Summary of differences between the speech and communication orientations.

Speech Orientation	*Communication Orientation*
The ultimate goal in therapy is developing either normal speech or adequate speech for communicative purposes.	The ultimate goal of therapy is developing the ability to communicate at a level adequate to meet communication needs.
Improvement of speech is regarded as an end in itself.	Improvement of speech is regarded as a means to an end (i.e., achieving adequate ability to communicate).
The primary emphasis in therapy is on improving speech.	The primary emphasis in therapy is on developing adequate ability to communicate.
Therapy usually is terminated when it appears that further significant improvement in speech is unlikely.	Therapy usually is terminated when it appears that further significant improvement in communication is unlikely.
Therapy outcome is assessed primarily in regard to speech status.	Therapy outcome is assessed primarily in regard to communication status.
Clinicians tend to base judgments of the adequacy of their clinical performance on the amounts their clients improve their speech.	Clinicians tend to base judgments of the adequacy of their clinical performance on the amounts their clients improve their abilities to communicate.
Clinicians tend to regard nonspeech communication modes as "last resorts"—that is, they only tend to introduce them after attempts to improve speech have failed.	Clinicians tend to regard nonspeech communication modes as useful temporary or permanent techniques for achieving their goal—that is, adequate ability to communicate.

communicative purposes. When they are introduced at this stage of the habilitation or rehabilitation process, they may be regarded merely as temporary. Whether they are viewed as temporary or permanent at this stage of therapy, they do permit the clinician's ultimate goal to be achieved, usually in a relatively short period of time.

If it appears at a later stage of therapy that *speech alone* is unlikely to ever be adequate for a client's communicative purposes, a speech pathologist who has a communication orientation will attempt to select and teach the client to use the optimum mode or modes which alone or in combination with speech will allow him or her to communicate adequately. This mode or combination of modes is likely to be more sophisticated than that used by the client initially. One reason why a more sophisticated mode or combination of modes might be recommended is a client's communication needs becoming more complex. Once stroke patients return home from the hospital, for example, they are apt to find that the messages they need to communicate are both greater in number and more complex than those which it was necessary for them to transmit in the hospital. The main point here is that clinicians with the communication orientation will introduce nonspeech communication modes during the course of therapy whenever they feel such communication modes are necessary for their clients to communicate adequately.

The differences between the two orientations that were discussed here are summarized in Table 1.1. These differences, obviously, should not be regarded as the only ones.

The Speech Pathologist as a Team Member

While speech pathologists with communication orientations would assume the primary responsibility for helping "speechless" patients communicate adequately, to discharge this responsibility they would frequently find it necessary to consult with and utilize the services of other professionals. Such professionals can include physical therapists, occupational therapists, engineers (electrical or biomedical), nurses (registered and practical), and teachers.

Physical and occupational therapists can contribute in several ways to the communication habilitation or rehabilitation of speechless patients. First, they can provide an assessment of muscle function in the extremities and other parts of the body. This information would be needed when selecting a switching mechanism for a client and the muscle group (or muscle groups) to activate it. (Switching mechanisms are dealt with in Chapters 3 and 5.) This information also would be needed when selecting a pointing mode (e.g., finger, eye, or head) that would make it possible for a client to indicate message components on a communication board. (Pointing modes that can be used for this purpose are described in Chapter 5.)

A second way in which physical and occupational therapists can contribute to the habilitation or rehabilitation of speechless patients is by helping them to develop or refine muscle gestures that are to be used for activating switching mechanisms or for indicating message components on a communication board. The more quickly and accurately the person is able to make these muscle gestures, the more flexible and efficient the communication system she or he will be able to use.

A third way in which physical and occupational therapists can contribute here is by assisting in the design and construction of hardware components for communication systems, including:

> switching mechanisms,
> headsticks and other indicating devices for use with communication boards,
> braces for stabilizing an extremity or part of an extremity to permit the muscle gesture (or muscle gestures) required to activate a switching mechanism or point to message components on a communication board, and
> hardware components of communication boards and the frames for supporting them.
> (These components of communication systems are described in Chapter 5.)

Biomedical and electrical engineers also can contribute in several ways to the communication habilitation or rehabilitation of speechless patients. First, they can recommend switching mechanisms that would be within the limits of the physical abilities of such patients to activate. Second, they can design an electronic communication system that can be controlled by the switching mechanism they recommend. Third, they can construct, or arrange to have constructed, the components of the communication system that they design. And fourth, they can service, or arrange to have serviced, the electronic components of the system when they malfunction. (Components of electronic communication systems are described in Chapters 3, 5, and 6.)

Another professional group that can contribute in several ways to the communication habilitation or rehabilitation of speechless patients while they are under their care are registered and practical nurses. First, they can suggest messages or message components that it would be important for a patient to be able to communicate to them. Such message components might include "doctor," "bed pan," "medication," "food," "water," and "nurse." Second, they can make it possible for such patients to use their communication systems whenever they wish to communicate. This involves, for example, making certain that a patient who is using a communication board has the board available and positioned so that he can indicate message components on it. It also involves making certain, if he is using a headpointer to indicate message components, that the device is in place whenever he wishes to communicate. For a patient who is using a switching mechanism to control a display, this responsibility would involve making certain that he can activate the switching mechanism whenever he wishes to communicate. Third, nurses can positively reinforce patients' use of their nonspeech modes for communication.

A fourth professional group that can contribute to the communication habilitation and rehabilitation of speechless persons, particularly children, are teachers. The ways in which they can contribute are similar to those indicated for nurses.

REFERENCES

ADAMS, M.R. Communication aids for patients with amyotrophic lateral sclerosis. *Journal of Speech and Hearing Disorders, 31,* 274-275 (1966).

Australian News and Information Bureau. Blissymbolics. *Hearing and Speech News, 41* (5), 6-7 (1973).

BALICK, S., SPIEGEL, D., & GREENE, G. Mime in language therapy and clinician training. *Archives of Physical Medicine and Rehabilitation, 57,* 35-38 (1976).

BICKER, D.D. Imitative sign training as a facilitator of word-object association with low-functioning children. *American Journal of Mental Deficiency, 76,* 509-516 (1972).

BONVILLIAN, J.D., & NELSON, K.E. Sign language acquisition in a mute autistic boy. *Journal of Speech and Hearing Disorders, 41,* 339-347 (1976).

BOONE, D.R. *The Voice and Voice Therapy* (2nd ed.). Englewood Cliffs, N.J.: Prentice-Hall (1977).

BRIDGMAN, P.W. *The Logic of Modern Physics.* New York: The Macmillan Company (1927).

BROOKNER, S.P., & MURPHY, N.O. The use of a total communication approach with a nondeaf child: A case study. *Language, Speech, and Hearing Services in Schools, 6,* 131-137 (1975).

BULLOCK, A., DALRYMPLE, G.F., & DANCA, J.M. The Auto-Com at Kennedy Memorial Hospital: Rapid and accurate communication by a multi-handicapped student. *American Journal of Occupational Therapy, 29,* 150-152 (1975).

BURNSIDE, S. All he could do was breathe—It's enough to run computer. *Miami Herald* (March 21, 1974).

BUTLER, O., & FOULDES, J. Typing aid remote controlled (TARC). In Keith Copeland (Ed.), *Aids for the Severely Handicapped,* New York: Grune & Stratton, pp. 83-88 (1974).

CARLSON, F.L. *An adapted communication project for a nonspeaking child.* Paper presented at the 51st annual meeting of the American Speech and Hearing Association, Houston (1976).

CARRIER, Jr., J.K., Application of functional analysis and a non-speech response mode to teaching language. In L.V. McReynolds (Ed.), *Developing Systematic Procedures for Training Children's Language,* ASHA Monographs No. 18 (1974a).

————. Application of a nonspeech language system with the severely language handicapped. In Lyle L. Lloyd (Ed.), *Communication Assessment and Intervention Strategies.* Baltimore: University Park Press, pp. 523-547 (1976).

————. Nonspeech noun usage training with severely and profoundly retarded children. *Journal of Speech and Hearing Research, 17,* 510-517 (1974b).

CARRIER, Jr., J.K., & PEAK, T. *Program Manual for Non-SLIP (Non-Speech Language Initiation Program).* Lawrence, Kansas: H & H Enterprises, Inc. (1975).

CHARBONNEAU, J.R., COTE, C., & ROY, O.Z. *NRC's "Comhandi" communication system technical description and application at the Ottawa Crippled Children's Treatment Center.* Paper presented at the seminar "Electronic Controls for the Severely Physically Handicapped," Vancouver, British Columbia (1974).

CHEN, L.Y. Manual communication by combined alphabet and gestures. *Archives of Physical Medicine and Rehabilitation, 52,* 381-384 (1971).

————. "Talking hands" for aphasic patients. *Geriatrics, 23,* 145-148 (1968).

CLAPPE, C., GRANT, M., HAZARD, G., LANG, J., & TOMLINSON, R. *The Morse code visual translator—A means of communication for the anarthric patient.* Paper presented at the 48th annual convention of the American Speech and Hearing Association, Detroit (1973).

COHEN, L.K. *Communication Aids for the Brain Damaged Adult.* Minneapolis: Sister Kenny Institute (1976).

COMBS, R.G., Myocom: Communication for non-verbal handicapped. *Transactions of the Missouri Academy of Science, 3,* 102 (1969).

Computerized device speaks for handicapped youngsters. *Journal of the Acoustical Society of America, 59,* 1520-1521 (1976).

COPELAND, K. (Ed.), *Aids for the Severely Handicapped.* New York: Grune & Stratton (1974).

CREEDON, M.P. (Ed.), *Appropriate Behavior through Communication: A New Program in Simultaneous Language.* Chicago: Dysfunctioning Child Center (1975).

DARLEY, F.L., ARONSON, A.E., & BROWN, J.R. *Motor Speech Disorders.* Philadelphia: W.B. Saunders (1975).

DUFFY, R.J., DUFFY, J.R., & PEARSON, K.L. Pantomime recognition in aphasics. *Journal of Speech and Hearing Research, 18,* 115-132 (1975).

EAGLESON, H.M., VAUGHN, G.R., & KNUDSON, A.B. Hand signals for dysphasia. *Archives of Physical Medicine and Rehabilitation, 51,* 111-113 (1970).

EGAN, J.J., ANTHONY, G.M., & HONKE, L.E. *Joan: A case study of manual communication with a severe cerebral palsied dysarthric.* Paper presented at the 51st annual meeting of the American Speech and Hearing Association, Houston (1976).

EISENSON, J. *Adult Aphasia.* New York: Appleton-Century-Crofts (1973).

————. *Aphasia in Children.* New York: Harper & Row (1972).

FENN, G., & ROWE, J.A. An experiment in manual communication. *British Journal of Disorders of Communication, 10,* 3-16 (1975).

FULWILER, R.L., & FOUTS, R.S. Acquistion of American Sign Language by a noncommunicating autistic child. *Journal of Autism and Childhood Schizophrenia, 6,* 43-51 (1976).

GARDNER, H., ZURIF, E.B., BERRY, T., & BAKER, E. Visual communication in aphasia. *Neuropsychologia, 14,* 275-292 (1976).

GLASS, A.V., GAZZANIGA, M.S., & PREMACK, D. Artificial language training in global aphasics. *Neuropsychologia, 11,* 95-103 (1973).

GOLDBERG, H.R., & FENTON, J. *Aphonic Communication for those with Cerebral Palsy: Guide to the Development and Use of a Conversation Board.* New York: United Cerebral Palsy of New York State (1960).

GOLDOJARB, M.F. *The use of video confrontation in teaching AMERIND to aphasic adults.* Videotape presented at the 51st annual meeting of the American Speech and Hearing Association, Houston (1976).

GOLDSTEIN, H., & CAMERON, H. A new method of communication for the aphasic patient. *Arizona Medicine, 8,* 17-21, (1952).

GRECCO, R., *Manual Language Program.* Can be obtained from the Mansfield Training School, Mansfield Depot, Connecticut (1972).

GREEN, L.C. *Acquisition of words versus signs in receptive language therapy with severely retarded, institutionalized children.* Paper presented at the 50th annual meeting of the American Speech and Hearing Association, Washington, D.C. (1975).

HAGEN, C., PORTER, W., & BRINK, J. Nonverbal communication: An alternative mode of communication for the child with severe cerebral palsy. *Journal of Speech and Hearing Disorders, 38,* 448-455 (1973).

HAIGHT, C. Modification of signs to maximize the learning of concepts. In M.P. Creedon (Ed.), *Appropriate Behavior through Communication: A New Program in Simultaneous Language,* Chicago: Dysfunctioning Child Center, pp. 74-84 (1975).

Handicapped youth "talks" with eyes. *News Journal* (Mansfield, Ohio) (October 22, 1974).

HANSON, W.R. *Measuring gestural communication in a brain-injured adult.* Videotape presented at the 51st annual meeting of the American Speech and Hearing Association, Houston (1976).

HARMON, G.M. He'll huff and puff, turn his TV set on, thanks to space device. *Times-Picayune* (New Orleans, Louisiana) (March 21, 1974).

HARRIS-VANDERHEIDEN, D. Blissymbols and the mentally retarded. In Gregg C. Vanderheiden and Kate Grilly (Eds.), *Non-vocal Communication Techniques and Aids for the Severely Physically Handicapped,* Baltimore: University Park Press, pp. 120-131 (1976a).

————— . Field evaluation of the Auto-Com. In Gregg C. Vanderheiden & Kate Grilley (Eds.), *Non-vocal Communication Techniques and*

Aids for the Severely Physically Handicapped, Baltimore: University Park Press, pp. 144-151 (1976b).

HARTLEY, N. Symbols for diplomats used for children. *Special Education Canada, 48*(2), 5-7 (1974).

He puffs past his handicap. *The News and Observer* (Raleigh, North Carolina) (March 21, 1974).

HEAD, H. *Aphasia and Kindred Disorders of Speech* (2 volumes). New York: Macmillan (1926).

HELFRICH, K.R. *Total communication with an oral apractic child.* Videotape presented at the 51st annual meeting of the American Speech and Hearing Association, Houston (1976).

HILL, S.D., CAMPAGNA, J., LONG, D., MUNCH, J., & NAECHER, S. An explanation of the use of two response keyboard as a means of communication for the severely handicapped child. *Perceptual and Motor Skills, 26,* 699-704 (1968).

HOFFMEISTER, R.J., & FARMER, A. The development of manual sign language in mentally retarded deaf individuals. *Journal of Rehabilitation of the Deaf, 6,* 19-26 (1972).

HOLLANDER, F.M., & JUHRS, P.D. Orff-Schulwerk, an effective treatment tool for autistic children. *Journal of Music Therapy, 11,* 1-12 (1974).

JACK H. EICHLER: Builds communication device. *Case Alumnus* (Publication of Case Institute of Technology Alumni Association, Cleveland, Ohio) (June, 1973).

KATES, B., & MCNAUGHTON, S. The first application of Blissymbolics as a communication medium for non-speaking children: History and development, 1971-1974. Distributed by Blissymbolics Communication Foundation, 862 Eglinton Avenue East, Toronto, Ontario, Canada (no date).

KENT, L. *Language Acquisition Program for the Severely Retarded.* Champaign, Illinois: Research Press (1974).

KIMBLE, S.L. *A language teaching technique with totally nonverbal, severely mentally retarded adolescents.* Paper presented at the 50th annual meeting of the American Speech and Hearing Association, Washington, D.C. (1975).

KLADDE, A.G. Nonoral communication techniques: Project summary #1, August, 1967. In Beverly Vicker (Ed.), *Nonoral Communication System Project 1964/1973,* Iowa City: The University of Iowa, pp. 57-104 (1974).

KONSTANTAREAS, M., OXMAN, J., WEBSTER, C., FISCHER, H., & MILLER, K. *A five week simultaneous communication programme for severely dysfunctional children: Outcome and implications for future research.* Toronto: Clarke Institute of Psychiatry (1975).

KOPCHICK JR., G.A., & LLOYD, L.L. Total communication programming for the severely language impaired—A 24-hour approach. In Lyle L. Lloyd (Ed.), *Communication Assessment and Intervention Strategies.* Baltimore: University Park Press, pp. 501-521 (1976).

KOPCHICK, G.A., JR., ROMBACK, D.W., & SMILOVITZ, R. A total communication environment in an institution. *Mental Retardation, 13*(3), 22-23 (1975).

LAKE, S.J. *The Hand-Book.* Tucson, Arizona: Communication Skill Builders (1976).

LARSON, T. Communications for the nonverbal child. *Academic Therapy Quarterly, 6,* 305-312 (1971).

LAVOY, R.W. Ricks communicator. *Exceptional Child, 23,* 338-340 (1957).

LEBEIS, S., & LEBEIS, R.F. The use of signed communication with the normal-hearing, nonverbal mentally retarded. *Bureau Memorandum* (Wisconsin Department of Public Instruction), *17*(1), 28-30 (1975).

LEIBEL, J., PETTET, A., & WEBSTER, C.D. *Two behavior modification approaches to the treatment of autistic children: Simultaneous communications vs. vocal imitation* (Substudy 74-7) Toronto: Clarke Institute of Psychiatry (1974).

LEVETT, L.M. A method of communication for non-speaking, severely subnormal children. *British Journal of Disorders of Communication, 4,* 64-66 (1969).

——— . A method of communication for nonspeaking, severely abnormal children—Trial results. *British Journal of Disorders of Communication, 6,* 125-128 (1971).

LUCAS, E.V., & DEAN, M.B. *An alternative approach to oral communication for an autistic child.* Videotape presented at the 51st annual meeting of the American Speech and Hearing Association, Houston (1976).

Machine turns handwriting into sound. *The Milwaukee Journal* (December 1, 1976).

MALING, R.G., & CLARKSON, D.C. Electronic controls for the tetraplegic (Possum) (Patient Operated Selector Mechanism—P.O.S.M.). *Paraplegia, 1,* 161-174 (1963).

McDONALD, E.T., & SCHULTZ, A.R. Communication boards for cerebral palsied children. *Journal of Speech and Hearing Disorders, 38,* 73-78 (1973).

McNAUGHTON, S. Blissymbolics—An alternative symbol system for the non-vocal pre-reading child. In Gregg C. Vanderheiden & Kate Grilley (Eds.), *Non-vocal Communication Techniques and Aids for the Severely Physically Handicapped,* Baltimore: University Park Press, pp. 85-104 (1976a).

――――― . Symbol Communication Programme at OCCC. In Gregg C. Vanderheiden & Kate Grilley (Eds.), *Non-vocal Communication Techniques and Aids for the Severely Physically Handicapped,* Baltimore: University Park Press, pp. 132-143 (1976b).

MENYUK, P. The bases of language acquisition: Some questions. *Journal of Autism and Childhood Schizophrenia, 4,* 325-345 (1974).

MILLER, A., & MILLER, E.E. Cognitive-developmental training with elevated boards and sign language. *Journal of Autism and Childhood Schizophrenia, 3,* 65-85 (1973).

MOORES, D.F. Nonvocal systems of verbal communication. In Richard L. Schiefelbusch & Lyle L. Lloyd (Eds.), *Language Perspectives-Acquisition, Retardation, and Intervention,* Baltimore: University Park Press, pp. 377-417 (1974).

MYKLEBUST, H.R. *Auditory Disorders in Children.* New York: Grune & Stratton (1954).

NUFFER, P.S. *Communication Bracelet Manual.* Distributed by Ideas, P.O. Box 741, Tempe, Arizona (no date).

OFFIR, C.W. Visual speech: Their fingers do the talking. *Psychology Today, 10*(1), 72-78 (June, 1976).

PENFIELD, W., & ROBERTS, L. *Speech and Brain Mechanisms.* Princeton, New Jersey: Princeton University Press (1959).

PERRON, J.V. Typewriter control for an aphasic quadriplegic patient. *Canadian Medical Association Journal, 92,* 557 (1965).

PETERS, L. Sign language stimulus in vocabulary learning of a brain-injured child. *Sign Language Studies, 3,* 116-118 (1973).

PREMACK, D., & PREMACK, A.J. Teaching visual language to apes and language-deficient persons. In Richard L. Schiefelbusch & Lyle L. Lloyd (Eds.), *Language Perspectives—Acquisition, Retardation, and Intervention,* Baltimore: University Park Press, pp. 347-376 (1974).

RATUSNIK, C.M., & RATUSNIK, D.L. A comprehensive communication approach for a ten-year-old nonverbal autistic child. *American Journal of Orthopsychiatry, 44,* 396-403 (1974).

――――― .*A comprehensive communication approach for a ten-year old autistic child.* Paper presented at the 51st annual meeting of the American Speech and Hearing Association, Houston (1976).

RICHARDSON, T. Sign language for SMR and PMR. *Mental Retardation, 13* (3), 17 (1975).

RICKS, D.M., & WING, L. Language, communication, and use of symbols in normal and autistic children. *Journal of Autism and Childhood Schizophrenia, 5,* 191-221 (1975).

SAYRE, J.M. Communication for the non-verbal cerebral palsied. *CP Review, 24,* 3-8 (November/December, 1963).

SCHAEFFER, B., KOLLINZAS, G., MUSIL, A., & McDOWELL, P., *Signed Speech: A new treatment for autism.* Paper presented at the annual meeting of the National Society for Autistic Children, San Diego (1975).

SCHLANGER, P.H. *Training the adult aphasic to pantomime.* Paper presented at the 51st annual meeting of the American Speech and Hearing Association, Houston (1976).

SCHLANGER, P.H., GEFFNER, D.S., & DiCARRADO, C. *A comparison of gestural communication with aphasics: Pre- and Post-therapy.* Paper presented at the 49th annual meeting of the American Speech and Hearg Association, Las Vegas (1974).

SHAFFER, T.R., & GOEHL, H. The alinguistic child. *Mental Retardation, 12* (2), 3-6 (1974).

SHANE, H., & MELROSE, J. *An electronic conversation board and an accompanying training program for aphonic expressive communication.* Paper presented at the 50th annual meeting of the American Speech and Hearing Association, Washington, D.C. (1975).

SKELLY, M., DONALDSON, R. C., and FUST, R. S., Glossectomee Speech Rehabilitation. Springfield, Illinois: Charles C. Thomas (1973).

SKELLY, M., SCHINSKY, L., SMITH, R., DONALDSON, R., & GRIFFIN, J. American Indian Sign: A gestural communication system for the speechless. *Archives of Physical Medicine and Rehabilitation, 56,* 156-160 (1975).

SKELLY, M., SCHINSKY, L., SMITH, R.W., & FUST, R.S. American Indian Sign (AMERIND) as a facilitator of verbalization for the oral verbal apraxic. *Journal of Speech and Hearing Disorders, 39,* 445-456 (1974).

SKLAR, M., & BENNETT, D.N. Initial communication chart for aphasics. *Journal of the Association of Physical and Mental Rehabilitation, 10,* 43-53 (1956).

SMITH, C.H. Total communication utilizing the simultaneous method. In M.P. Creedon (Ed.), *Appropriate Behavior through Communication: A New Program in Simultaneous Language,* Chicago: Dysfunctioning Child Center, pp. 45-74 (1975).

STEVENS, H.A., & HEBER, R. (Eds.) *Mental Retardation: A Review of Research.* Chicago: University of Chicago Press (1964).

SUTHERLAND, G.F., & BECKETT, J.W. Teaching the mentally retarded sign language. *Journal of Rehabilitation of the Deaf, 2,* 56-60 (1969).

TATMAN, T., & WEBSTER, C.D. *Teaching autistic-retarded children through simultaneous (gestural and verbal) communications* (15-minute black and white moving film). Distributed by Clarke Institute of Psychiatry, Toronto, Ontario, Canada (1973).

TOPPER, S.T. Gesture language for a non-verbal severely retarded male. *Mental Retardation, 13*(1), 30-31 (1975).

TOROK, Z. A typewriter operated by electromyographic potentials (GMMI). In Keith Copeland (Ed.), *Aids for the Severely Handicapped,* New York: Grune & Stratton, pp. 77-82 (1974).

VANDERHEIDEN, D.H., BROWN, W.P., MACKENZIE, P., REINEN, S., &
SCHEIBEL, C. Symbol communication for the mentally handicapped.
Mental Retardation, 13, 34-37 (1975).

VANDERHEIDEN, G.C. Providing the child with a means to indicate. In Gregg
C. Vanderheiden & Kate Grilley (Eds.), *Non-vocal Communication
Techniques and Aids for the Severely Physically Handicapped,* Balti-
more: University Park Press, pp. 20-76 (1976).

VANDERHEIDEN, G.C., & GRILLEY, K. (Eds.), *Non-vocal Communication
Techniques and Aids for the Severely Physically Handicapped.* Baltimore: University Park Press (1976).

VANDERHEIDEN, G.C., LAMERS, D.F., VOLK, A.M., & GEISLER, C.D. *A portable non-vocal communication prosthesis for the severely physically
handicapped.* Distributed by the Trace Research and Development
Center for the Severely Communicatively Handicapped, University of
Wisconsin, Madison, Wisconsin (1975).

VANHOOK, K.E., & STOHR, P.G. *The development of manual communication
in a profoundly retarded hearing population.* Paper presented at the
48th annual meeting of the American Speech and Hearing Association,
Detroit (1973).

VASA, J.J., & LYWOOD, D.W. High-speed communication aid for quadriplegics. *Medical and Biological Engineering, 14,* 445-450 (1976).

VICKER, B. (Ed.) *Nonoral Communication System Project 1964/1973.*
Distributed by Campus Stores, The University of Iowa, Iowa City,
Iowa (1974).

WEBSTER, C.D., MCPHERSON, H., SLOMAN, L., EVANS, M.A., & KUCHAR, E.
Communicating with an autistic boy by gestures. *Journal of Autism and
Childhood Schizophrenia, 3,* 337-346 (1973).

WENDT, E., SPRAGUE, M.J., & MARQUIS, J. Communication without speech.
Teaching Exceptional Children, 38-42 (Fall, 1975).

WHITE, S.D. A modular communication device for paralyzed patients.
Archives of Physical Medicine and Rehabilitation, 55, 94-95 (1974).

WILSON, P.S. *A manual language dialect for the retarded.* Paper presented
at the 49th annual meeting of the American Speech and Hearing
Association, Las Vegas (1974a).

————. *Sign language as a means of communication for the mentally
retarded.* Paper presented at the April meeting of the Eastern Psychological Association (1974b).

WILSON, P.S., GOODMAN, L., & WOOD, R.K. *Manual Language for the Child
Without Language.* Distributed by Paula Starks Wilson, Department
of Mental Retardation Developmental Team, 79 Elm Street, Hartford,
Connecticut (1975).

2 Impacts of Nonspeech Communication Modes on Behavior

The previous chapter dealt with the need for nonspeech communication modes. It was argued that they can make it possible for children and adults who have insufficient speech for their communicative purposes to transmit the messages they wish to transmit. Some support for this contention can be found in the papers that were cited in Chapter 1 describing the use of non-speech communication modes with dysarthric, apraxic, aphasic, dysphonic, glossectomized, mentally retarded, and autistic children and adults. This evidence is summarized in this chapter.

This chapter is concerned with the *impacts* of nonspeech communication modes on the behavior of children and adults who use them. It is necessary when evaluating any therapy strategy, method, or technique to be concerned about its total impact on a person, not just its impact on the particular behavior (or behaviors) it is intended to modify or facilitate. Determining these impacts involves answering a series of questions, including the following (Silverman, 1977b, pp. 250-251):

1. What are the effects of the therapy upon specific behaviors that contribute to a client's communicative disorder at given points in space-time?
2. What are the effects of the therapy upon other attributes of a client's communicative behavior at given points in space-time?
3. What are the effects of a therapy upon a client other than those directly related to communicative behavior?
4. What are the client's attitudes toward the therapy and its effects upon his communicative and other behaviors?
5. What are the attitudes of a client's clinician, family, friends, and others toward the therapy and toward its effects upon the client's communicative behavior and other attributes of behavior?
6. What investment is required of client and clinician?
7. What is the probability of relapse following termination of the therapy?

The remainder of this chapter presents tentative answers to these questions for nonspeech modes *in general*. The answers given must be regarded as tentative because the data available for answering all except possibly the first are insufficient or have levels of validity, reliability, and generality that are uncertain (for a discussion of validity, reliability, and generality in this context, see Silverman, 1977a, 1977b).

Impact on Communication

The first question deals with the impacts of a therapy strategy on a client's communicative disorder *per se* at various points in space-time. In the case of children and adults who lack adequate speech for their communicative purposes, this question would refer to the impact of the therapy strategy (i.e., a nonspeech communication mode or combination of such modes) on their ability to communicate. (This, of course, assumes that the clinician has a "communication" rather than a "speech" orientation.) The space-time concept is used here to indicate that the impact of a therapy strategy on a client cannot be assumed to be the same at all points in time and in all situations. A simple picture-communication board, for example, can allow an aphasic to communicate necessary messages to hospital personnel during the first few days following his stroke, but may not adequately meet his communication needs after he returns home. There is a need, then, to consider the space-time dimension when assessing the impacts of nonspeech communication modes on clients.

How likely are nonspeech communication modes to significantly improve a speechless client's ability to communicate—that is, to transmit messages? By "significantly improve" here is meant the presence of sufficient improvement that clients, their clinicians, and others (e.g., spouses and parents) judge that there has been real improvement in their abilities to transmit messages in their environments. Note that the emphasis here is on message transmission outside of the therapy room for the purpose of communication. A client would not be regarded as having demonstrated significant improvement if he only used his nonspeech mode within the therapy room.

Intervention with nonspeech communication modes seems quite likely to significantly improve a "speechless" client's ability to communicate regardless of the reason for his speech being inadequate for his communication needs. This conclusion is supported by a number of clinical case reports, representative examples of which are summarized in Table 2.1. While the reliability and generality of the data in most of these reports is uncertain, the fact that they all conclude that a high percentage of the clients improved their ability to communicate provides strong support for this conclusion. Of course, the probability of clients significantly improving their ability to communicate may not be quite as high as suggested by the data summarized in Table 2.1 because both clinicians and journals tend to be more likely to report "successes" than "failures."

While there seems to be little question that nonspeech communication modes can significantly improve the ability of almost any speechless child or adult to communicate, the amount of such improvement possible is not a constant. Some persons are reported to be able to transmit almost any message they wish to communicate through the use of such modes while others apparently are only able to learn to communicate a few basic needs with them.

There are a number of factors that appear to influence the amount of impact learning a nonspeech communication mode can have on a "speechless" child's or adult's ability to encode and transmit messages. Included are:

cognitive status;
motor status;
sensory status
receptive language status;
"inner" language status;
desire, or motivation, to communicate;
the specific communication mode (or combination of modes) used; and
attitudes toward the communication mode (or combination of such modes)
used.

Cognitive Status

The more normal the cognitive (i.e., intellectual) abilities of children and adults, the more impact learning and using a nonspeech communication mode is likely to have on their communication potential. Some support for this conclusion can be found in the papers cited in Table 2.1 dealing with the impact of nonspeech communication modes on the mentally retarded. More manual signs, for example, tend to be acquired by the moderately mentally retarded than by the severely mentally retarded (the severely mentally retarded, however, do appear to be able to acquire at least a few such signs).

The cognitive status of adults who were not diagnosed mentally retarded as children also influences the probable impact of using a nonspeech communication mode on them. Persons who have neurological conditions that can adversely effect cognitive functioning such as Huntington's chorea and cerebral arteriosclerosis may do less well with such communication modes than those with comparable motor and sensory abilities (or disabilities) who do not have a condition of this type. Of course, as the cognitive status of persons with these conditions deteriorates, the impact of any nonspeech mode on their communication ability is likely to be reduced.

TABLE 2.1. Impact of nonspeech communication modes on ability to communicate.

Reference	Number of Clients	Children or Adults	Diagnosis	Nonspeech Mode	Number Significantly Improving Communication Ability
Bonvillian & Nelson (1976)	1	Child	Autism	Ameslan Sign	1
Brookner & Murphy (1975)	1	Child	Mental Retardation	Total Communication	1
Bullock, Dalrymple, & Danca (1975)	1	Child	Cerebral Palsy	Auto-Com Communication Board	1
Carlson (1976)	1	Child	Cerebral Palsy	Gestural "yes" and "no signals; communication board; electronic direct-selection matrix device	1
Chen (1971)	26	Adults	19 Aphasics 5 Dysarthrics 2 Laryngectomies	Manual alphabet combined with manual sign gestures	7 Aphasics 4 Dysarthrics 2 Laryngectomies
Charbonneau, Cote, & Roy (1974)	5	Children	Cerebral Palsy	Comhandi electronic communication system	5
Clappe, Grant, Hazard, Lang, & Tomlinson (1973)	1	Adult	Dysarthria	Electronic device	1
Computerized device speaks for handicapped youngsters (1976)	6	5 Children 1 Adult	Cerebral Palsy	Electronic device	6*
Creedon (1975)	30	Children	Multiply-Handicapped	Total communication	30
Duncan & Silverman (1977)	32	Children	Mental Retardation	Amerind Sign	27
Eagleson, Vaughn, & Kundson (1970)	31	Adults	Expressive Aphasia	Hand signals	31

Reference	N	Age	Condition	Technique/Device	N
Egan, Anthony, & Honke (1976)	1	Adult	Cerebral Palsy	Manual sign language	1
Ellsworth & Kotkin (1975)	1	Child	Apraxia (?)	Manual sign language	1
Feallock (1958)	12	Children	Dysarthria	Communication boards	6
Fenn & Rowe (1975)	7	Children	Cerebral Palsy & Hearing Loss	Manual sign language	7
Fulwiler & Fouts (1976)	1	Child	Autism	Ameslan sign language	1
Fouts (1973) (Cited in Fulwiler & Fouts, 1976)	1	Child	Autism	Ameslan sign language	1
Gertenrich (1966)	1	Adult	Cerebral Palsy	Mouth-held writing device	1
Gitlis (1975)	1	Child	Cerebral Palsy	Total Communication	1
Glass et al (1973)	7	Adults	Global Aphasia	Premack manipulable symbols	All demonstrated "...some capacity for symbolization and primitive linguistic functions."
Goldberg & Fenton (1960)	5	Children	Cerebral Palsy	Conversation boards	At least 3
Goldstein & Cameron (1952)	?	Adults	Aphasia	Manual sign language	Most, if not all
Goodwin & Goodwin (1969)	2	Children	Aphasia	Edison Responsive Environment	2
Hagen, Porter, & Brink (1973)	4	Children	Cerebral Palsy	Morse code oscillator	3
Handicapped youth "talks" with eyes (1974)	1	Child	Cerebral Palsy	ETRAN chart	1
Harris-Vanderheiden (1976a)	5	Children	Cerebral Palsy & Mental Retardation	Blissymbolics	5
Harris-Vanderheiden (1976b)	7	Children	Cerebral Palsy	Auto-Com communication board	7

TABLE 2.1 *(Continued)*

Reference	Number of Clients	Children or Adults	Diagnosis	Nonspeech Mode	Number Significantly Improving Communication Ability
Helfrich (1976)	1	Child	Oral Apraxia	Total communication	1
Hill *et al* (1968)	1	Child	Cerebral Palsy	2 direct-selection aids	1
Hoffmeister & Farmer (1972)	16	8 Children 8 Adults	Mentally Retarded & Deaf	Ameslan	15
Jack H. Eichler: Builds Communication Device (1973)	1	Adult	Amyotropic Lateral Sclerosis	ETRAN chart	1
Jenkins (1967)	1	Child	Cerebral Palsy	Possum typewriter	1
Kates & McNaughton (no date)	19	Children	Cerebral Palsy	Blissymbolics	"Nearly all"
Kimble (1975)	4	Adolescents	Mental Retardation	Signed English	3
Kladde (1974)	3	Children	Cerebral Palsy	Communication board	3
Konstantareas *et al* (1975)	5	Children	Autism	Total communication	4
Lebeis and Lebeis (1975)	27	Children	Mental Retardation	Ameslan	24
Levett (1971)	12	Children	Cerebral Palsy	Mime	7
Lucas & Dean (1976)	1	Child	Autistic	Ameslan	1
McDonald & Schultz (1973)	1	Child	Cerebral Palsy	Communication board	1
Miller & Miller (1973)	19	Children	Autism	Total communication	19
Nicol (1972)	1	Child	Cerebral Palsy	P.O.S.M. controlled typewriter	1
Offir (1976)	30	Children	Autism	Ameslan	30

Study	Number	Population	Disorder	Technique/System	Number Improved
Ontario Crippled Children's Centre Symbol Communication Program (1974)	150	Children	Neuromuscular Disorder	Blissymbolics	122
Ratusnik & Ratusnik (1974)	1	Child	Autism	Communication board	1
Rice & Combs (1972)	6	4 Children 2 Adults	Cerebral Palsy	Myocom communication device	4 Children 1 Adult
Richardson (1975)	9	Children	Mental Retardation	Ameslan	9
Schlanger (1976)	5	Adults	Aphasia	Pantomime	5
Schaeffer et al (1976)	3	Children	Autism	Total communication	3
Skelly et al (1975)	1	Adult	Glossectomy	Amerind sign language	1
Skelly et al (1975)	12	Adults	Glossectomy, Dysarthria, Dysphonia, & Verbal Apraxia	Amerind sign language	12
Skelly et al (1974)	6	Adults	Verbal Apraxia	Amerind sign language	6
Topper (1975)	1	Adult	Mental Retardation	Ameslan	1
Vanderheiden et al (1975)	5	Children	Mental Retardation	Blissymbolics	5
Vanderheiden & Harris-Vanderheiden (1976)	9	Children & Adolescents	Cerebral Palsy	Auto-Com Communication Board	9*
Vicker (1974)	22	Children	Severe Dysarthria	Communication boards	Most, if not all
Vicker (1974)	1	Child	Cerebral Palsy	Communication board	1
Webster et al (1973)	1	Child	Autism	Ameslan	1
Wendt, Sprague, & Marquis (1975)	1	Child	Cerebral Palsy	Auto-Com communication board	1
Wilson (1974)	26	Children	Mental Retardation	Ameslan	26

*Report suggests, without directly stating so, that all subjects significantly improved their abilities to communicate.

35

Motor Status

The more normal the motor abilities of children and adults—particularly those of the upper extremities—the more impact learning and using a nonspeech communication mode is likely to have on their communication potential. Some levels of motor ability will support more flexible nonspeech communication systems than will others. A person whose upper extremities are normal motorically, for example, has the motor potential to use a highly flexible manual communication system such as American Sign Language (see Chapter 4). On the other hand, a person whose upper extremities are not normal motorically may have to use a more limited system such as a communication board (see Chapter 5). The range of messages that can be transmitted by the latter tends to be more restricted than that which can be transmitted by the former.

Sensory Status

The more normal the sensory abilities of children and adults, the more impact learning a nonspeech communication mode is likely to have on their communication potential. There are three sensory channels the functioning of which can influence this potential: *auditory, visual,* and *tactile-kinesthetic-proprioceptive.*

The presence of a peripheral hearing loss (conductive, sensori-neural, or mixed), central hearing loss, or auditory agnosia can reduce the communication potential of any speechless person because it may interfere with his or her ability to decode and thereby understand speech. Such a reduction in communication potential could occur regardless of the nonspeech mode the person used unless a nonauditory communication mode were also used for encoding and transmitting messages to him or her.

The presence of any deficit in visual acuity, a visual field disturbance, or a visual agnosia can reduce the communication potential of a speechless person if the encoding or transmission process being used has to be monitored visually. The use of a communication board, for example, can be impeded by any of these disturbances. If a person has a visual acuity problem, a visual field problem, or a visual agnosia, he or she may not be able to find and accurately indicate the desired message components.

Finally, a disturbance in tactile-kinesthetic-proprioceptive sensation, or feedback, can reduce the potential for the effective use of any nonspeech communication mode. Such a disturbance could, for example, interfere with the accurate production of manual gestures used in American Sign Language and in American Indian Sign Language (see Chapter 4). It also could interfere with indicating message components on communication boards and activating switching mechanisms in electronic communication schemes (see Chapter 5).

Receptive Language Status

The more normal the ability of a child or adult to comprehend speech, the more impact learning and using a nonspeech communication mode is likely to have on his or her communication potential. Obviously, if a person does not understand a question, he is unlikely to respond appropriately. Some degree of receptive-language deficit is likely to be manifested by aphasics and mentally retarded persons.

Inner Language Status

The term *inner language* is used here to refer to the use of language for thinking, or "talking to oneself" (Myklebust, 1954). If a person has a disturbance in inner language, he also will have a disturbance in receptive language, or speech comprehension (Myklebust, 1954). Hence, persons who have such a disturbance may not respond appropriately to questions regardless of the channel (i.e., speech or nonspeech) used to transmit messages to them.

Desire or Motivation to Communicate

The more highly motivated children and adults are to communicate, the more impact learning and using a nonspeech communication mode is likely to have on their communication potential. A person may become quite proficient at communicating with a nonspeech mode, but if he chooses not to communicate or to communicate only when absolutely necessary, it can have little impact upon him. There are several reasons why a child or adult may have limited desire or motivation to communicate, including those below.

1. Depression. People who are depressed usually are not highly motivated to communicate. A child or adult who has inadequate speech because of aphasia, apraxia, dysarthria, laryngectomy, or glossectomy is quite likely to be depressed, especially during the period immediately following the onset of the condition. Such depression is apt to result from several factors, one being loss of ability to communicate and its implications. Teaching a person who is depressed for this reason to communicate by a nonspeech mode may help to reduce the depression.

2. Little or No Need to Communicate. Persons who have little or no need to communicate obviously will not realize their communication potentials. Two of the most frequent reasons why persons tend to have little or no need to communicate are (1) their needs are anticipated by those with whom they would ordinarily have to communicate and (2) they have limited opportunity to communicate because they interact with very few people.

3. Lack of Positive Reinforcement for Communicating.   If a person does not regard communication as an enjoyable (or positively reinforcing) experience, his attempts at communication probably will be limited. Mentally retarded and autistic children, in particular, may not realize their communication potentials for this reason.

Communication Mode (or Modes) Used

Some nonspeech communication modes (or combinations of such modes) are likely to have greater impact on a "speechless" child's or adult's ability to encode and transmit messages than are others. Some, for example, are more portable than others: they are relatively small and light in weight; and if they are electrical, they can operate on batteries. The more portable the hardware and software components of a nonspeech mode, the more likely users are to have it available when they wish to communicate and, hence, the greater the impact it could have on them. Gestural modes such as manual sign language are, of course, the most portable of all since they require neither hardware nor software.

Some nonspeech systems can have greater impact than others because they are more *flexible*—that is, they allow a greater number of messages to be encoded and transmitted. American Sign Language (Ameslan), for example, can be used to encode and transmit a greater variety of messages than American Indian Sign Language (Amerind). (Both manual sign systems are described in Chapter 4.) Also, a communication board containing letters of the alphabet and numbers has the potential for encoding a greater variety of messages than one containing Blissymbolics or pictures (these symbol systems for communication boards are dealt with in Chapter 5).

Another variable that influences the relative impacts of nonspeech systems is *efficiency*. Some allow messages to be encoded and transmitted in less time and with less expenditure of energy than others. A system in which each letter, for example, has to be encoded and transmitted by Morse code is less efficient than one in which fingerspelling is used. The reason is that the former requires more than one gesture (e.g., activation of a switch) to transmit a letter while the latter requires only one. The more time-consuming and energy-consuming message transmission becomes, the fewer the messages that are likely to be transmitted; the fewer the messages that are likely to be transmitted, the less the impact that any nonspeech system is likely to have.

A fourth variable that is likely to influence the relative impact of a mode is the *symbol system* used. Some nonspeech systems allow one to communicate with a greater variety of people than do others. A communication board on which words are spelled out would not permit one to communicate with preschool children. And the use of American Sign Language would not permit one to communicate with as many people as would the use of American Indian Sign Language (the intelligibility of the manual signs in these systems is dealt with in Chapter 4).

Attitudes Toward the Communication Mode(s) Used

The attitudes of the user of a nonspeech communication mode and of those in his environment influence the impact that the mode is likely to have on his ability to communicate. The more positive these attitudes, the greater the probable impact. If a child or adult who could benefit from a nonspeech communication mode either refuses to use it or only uses it when absolutely necessary, its potential impact on communication will be reduced. Also, if the members of the person's family and others do not respond positively to the use of the mode, its frequency of use probably will be reduced. This is particularly likely to happen if members of the person's family feel that using the nonspeech mode is likely to reduce attempts at speech communication. (Research summarized in the next section of this chapter indicates that learning a nonspeech mode is highly unlikely to reduce verbal output.)

Impact on Speech

A second question that needs to be answered when assessing any therapy method is concerned with its impacts on aspects of communication behavior other than those it is intended to modify. A nonspeech communication mode, in addition to facilitating communication, may influence a person's communication behavior in other ways, either desirable or undesirable. Perhaps the most important aspect of communication behavior on which it would be necessary to determine the impact of using any nonspeech communication mode is verbal, or speech, output. Does learning and using a nonspeech communication mode appear to influence a person's attempts at speech communication? More specifically, does teaching a child or adult a nonspeech communication mode *reduce* his or her motivation for speech communication? If the answer to this latter question were yes, a clinician might justifiably hesitate to teach a client to use a nonspeech communication mode if there were any chance that he or she could learn to communicate by speech.

Teaching a person to use a nonspeech communication mode does not appear to reduce his or her motivation for speech communication. Attempts at speech communication do not appear to diminish. This conclusion is supported by a number of published and unpublished reports (see Table 2.2). There appears to be little (if any) reason, therefore, to be concerned about reducing a client's chances for improving speech by intervention with a nonspeech communication mode regardless of the mode used or the reason for speech being inadequate for communication.

TABLE 2.2. Impact of nonspeech communication modes on attempts at speech communication.

Reference	Number of Clients	Children or Adults	Diagnosis	Nonspeech Mode	Impact on Speech Attempts		
					INCREASED	DECREASED	NONE
Balick, Spiegel, & Greene (1976)	5	Children	Mental Retardation	Mime	5		
Brookner & Murphy (1975)	1	Child	Mental Retardation	Total Communication			1
Creedon (1975)	30	Children	Multiply-Handicapped	Total Communication	"Some"		
Duncan & Silverman (1977)	32	Children	Mental Retardation	Amerind Sign	15		17
Eagleson, Vaughn, & Knudson (1970)	31	Adults	Expressive Aphasia	Hand Signals	"Success with this nonspeech mode of communication increased the apparent motivation of patients to persevere in learning verbal modes of communication."		
Ellsworth & Kotkin (1975)	1	Child	Apraxia (?)	Manual Sign Language	1		
Fulwiler & Fouts (1976)	1	Child	Autism	Ameslan	1		
Gitlis (1975)	1	Child	Cerebral Palsy	Total Communication	1		
Goodwin & Goodwin (1969)	2	Children	Aphasia	Edison Responsive Environment	2		

Study							"Symbol use appeared to encourage vocalization and speech."
Kates & McNaughton (no date)	19	Children	Cerebral Palsy	Blissymbolics	2		2
Kimble (1975)	4	Adolescents	Mental Retardation	Signed English	1		2
Kladde (1974)	3	Children	Cerebral Palsy	Communication Board	2		3
Konstantareas et al (1975)	5	Children	Autism	Total Communication	2		
Lebeis & Lebeis (1975)	27	Children	Mental Retardation	Ameslan	6		21
Levett (1971)	12	Children	Cerebral Palsy	Mime	1		11
Linville (1977)	4	Adolescents	Mental Retardation	Ameslan	2		2
Miller & Miller (1973)	19	Children	Autism	Total Communication	2		17
Offir (1976)	30	Children	Autism	Ameslan	20		10
Ontario Crippled Children's Centre Symbol Communication Programme (1974)	141	Children	Physically Handicapped	Blissymbolics	45	2	94
Schaeffer et al (1976)	3	Children	Autism	Total Communication	3		
Schlanger (1976)	5	Adults	Aphasia	Pantomime	3		2
Schmidt, Carrier, & Parsons (1971)	10	Children	Mental Retardation	Plastic Symbols (Non-SLIP)	10		
Skelly et al (1974)	6	Adults	Verbal Apraxia	Amerind Sign Language	5		1
Wilson (1974)	26	Children	Mental Retardation	Ameslan	5		21

TABLE 2.3. Other impacts of nonspeech communication modes.

Reference	Number of Clients	Children or Adults	Diagnosis	Nonspeech mode	Impacts
Balick, Spiegel, & Greene (1976)	5	Children	Mental Retardation	Mime	Attention span increased; hyperactivity decreased
Brookner & Murphy (1975)	1	Child	Mental Retardation	Total Communication	Temper tantrums lessened
Bullock, Dalrymple, & Danca (1975)	1	Child	Cerebral Palsy	Auto-Com Communication Board	Child "... became more self-confident and independent;" She also became a "... more involved member of the class"
Duncan & Silverman (1977)	32	Children	Mental Retardation	Amerind Sign	13 of the children were reported to have had noticeable changes in behavior —i.e., reduction in frustration behavior such as temper tantrums and being more willing to participate in language activities
Fulwiler & Fouts (1976)	1	Child	Autism	Ameslan	Increased social interaction; increased attentiveness

Study	N	Age	Disability	Method	Results
Fouts (1973) (Cited in Fulwiler & Fouts, 1976)	1	Child	Autism	Ameslan	Increased ".. attentiveness of the child to the therapist."
Hagen, Porter, & Brink (1973)	4	Children	Cerebral Palsy	Morse Code Oscillator	3 became more relaxed physically
Harris-Vanderheiden (1976b)	7	Children	Cerebral Palsy	Auto-Com Communication Board	Facilitated educational progress; enhanced self-confidence; increased independence
Helfrich (1976)	1	Child	Oral Apraxia	Total Communication	Reduced frustration behavior
Kates & McNaughton (no date)	19	Children	Cerebral Palsy	Blissymbolics	Children showed evidence of greater self-assurance and self-confidence
Kimble (1975)	4	Adolescents	Mental Retardation	Signed English	Increased willingness to interact with others; increased attention span
Konstantareas et al (1975)	5	Children	Autism	Total Communication	Increased ".. awareness, interaction with other persons, and improvements in self-care skills."
Levett (1971)	12	Children	Cerebral Palsy	Mime	"All of the children were reported to be easier to handle both in and out of school."

TABLE 2.3. (*Continued*)

Reference	Number of Clients	Children or Adults	Diagnosis	Nonspeech mode	Impacts
Lucas & Dean (1976)	1	Child	Autism	Ameslan	"Disruptive behavior had dramatically decreased with increased appropriate attending and social behaviors."
Vanderheiden & Harris-Vanderheiden (1976)	9	Children & Adolescents	Cerebral Palsy	Auto-Com Communication Board	Observed "...a major beneficial effect upon the students' educational progress, their productive educational time, ... personal development, motivation, and independence."
Webster et al (1973)	1	Child	Autism	Ameslan	Reduction in "bizarre behaviors"

Can learning and using a nonspeech communication mode have any impact on verbal output? The answer to this question appears to be yes. The use of a nonspeech communication mode seems to facilitate speech (i.e., increase verbal output) in some children and adults (see Table 2.2). The proportion of users who are likely to be so affected judging by the data summarized in Table 2.2 is at least 40 percent. Thus, *intervention with nonspeech communication modes can be rationalized for the purpose of speech facilitation as well as improving message transmission.* This form of intervention, in fact, appears to be as likely as any to be successful for facilitating speech in "speechless" children and adults.

The rationalization of nonspeech communication modes as speech-facilitation techniques can be useful in gaining acceptance for them from clients and their families. Speech pathologists' recommendations to their clients that they learn to use nonspeech communication modes may be interpreted by them and their families to mean that no further attempts will be made to develop or improve speech. This, obviously, could result in resistance to the use of such a communication mode (or modes) by a client, his family, or both. If the nonspeech communication mode (or modes) were presented to the client and his family as a means of facilitating *both communication and speech,* such resistance probably could be minimized. (This topic is dealt with further in Chapter 8.)

Other Impacts on Users

A third question necessary to answer when assessing a therapy method is concerned with its impacts other than those directly related to a person's communication behavior. An intervention strategy that influences communication behavior can influence other aspects of a person's functioning as well. Such impacts can be classified as *physical* or *behavioral* (i.e., psychological) and as *desirable* or *undesirable.* An example of an undesirable physical impact would be a skin lesion at the point where a pointing or switching mechanism was attached to a client's body. (Interfacing pointing and switching mechanisms with people is dealt with in Chapter 5.) An example of an undesirable behavioral impact would be depression arising from having to rely on a device to communicate.

The noncommunication impacts of nonspeech communication modes on users that have been reported are *overwhelmingly desirable* (see Table 2.3). Whether the paucity of reports of undesirable impacts is due to there not being any, or to a failure by clinician-investigators to evaluate for them and report them, is uncertain. Whatever the reason, the reports summarized in Table 2.3 suggest that intervention with nonspeech communication modes can have several desirable impacts on users, including decreased temper tantrums, increased willingness to participate in group activities, increased attention span, decreased hyperactivity, increased self-confidence, increased independence, and improved performance in the classroom.

Acceptance by Users and Others

The fourth and fifth questions necessary to answer when assessing a therapy method are concerned with its acceptability to the client and to those with whom he or she interacts (e.g., parents or spouse). As indicated previously, if a method is unacceptable to a client and those with whom he or she interacts, its potential impact on the client will be reduced.

There appear to have been very few attempts to systematically determine the level of acceptability of nonspeech communication systems to users and others. Relevant data that have been reported (Duncan & Silverman, 1977) suggest that such systems are acceptable to most users and those with whom they interact if they understand the following:

1. Intervention with a nonspeech communication mode does not necessarily mean that the speech pathologist has given up on improving speech.
2. The nonspeech communication system is intended to *supplement* the speech the person has; the goal is *total communication*. (The concept of total communication is dealt with in Chapter 4.)
3. Learning and using a nonspeech communication system is highly unlikely to result in reduced attempts at speech.
4. Learning and using a nonspeech communication system appears to *facilitate* speech in some clients. *The use of such a system may be, in fact, one of the most successful speech facilitation techniques for "speechless" children and adults* (see Table 2.2).
5. It is important for the patient to have an alternative mode of message transmission to meet his immediate communication needs if speech is not adequate for the purpose.

Investment Required

The sixth question is concerned with the investment required of the client and clinician. This investment may be of several kinds, including money, time, and willingness to use a communication mode that initially would make one feel uncomfortable.

All nonspeech communication systems require some financial investment. If the system does not contain electronic components, the financial investment is likely to be nominal. If it does contain such components, the cost will be determined by their complexity or sophistication. The cost of components for some electronic scanning systems is less than $50.00 (see Appendix D). For electronic communication systems that contain components such as electric typewriters, teletypewriters, strip printers, or speech synthesizers, the investment can be hundreds or thousands of dollars (these components of electronic communication systems are described in Chapter 5). The nonspeech communication systems that tend to be the most expensive are those that provide some form of hard copy (i.e., typewritten).

A second kind of investment required is time. The clinician has to assemble the hardware and software components of the system and teach the client how to use the system. The amount of time it will take for a clinician to do this ranges from a few hours (e.g., to construct and teach an apraxic adult to use a simple communication board) to hundreds of hours (e.g., to teach the use of American Sign Language or Blissymbolics to mentally retarded children).

A third kind of investment that *may* be required to implement a nonspeech communication system is for the client to be willing to tolerate being uncomfortable when initially using the system. He may feel that using the mode will call undesirable attention to him. This is the same sort of concern that a person who is hard of hearing may have initially about using a hearing aid. After he has used it for a while, he probably will find that people are not reacting to him in the manner he had anticipated, and the problem will solve itself.

Long-Term Impact

The seventh and final question is concerned with the impact of the therapy method on the patient following termination of formal therapy. Does the impact on a patient of using a nonspeech communication mode tend to increase, decrease, or remain approximately the same? How likely are patients to continue using a nonspeech communication system once they are no longer seeing a clinician on a regular basis? Answers to these questions obviously are important for assessing the impact of any nonspeech communication system. There are a number of individual case studies which suggest that such communication systems continue to be used and continue to have an impact following termination of therapy; their generality (or representativeness), however, is uncertain. There is a need, therefore, for clinicians to collect systematic follow-up data from clients using all types of nonspeech communication systems. (For a discussion of the role of clinicians in therapy outcome research, see Chapter 2 in Silverman, 1977b.)

REFERENCES

BALICK, S., SPIEGEL, D., & GREENE, G. Mime in language therapy and clinician training. *Archives of Physical Medicine and Rehabilitation, 57,* 35-38 (1976).

BONVILLIAN, J.D., & NELSON, K.E. Sign language acquisition in a mute autistic boy. *Journal of Speech and Hearing Disorders, 41,* 339-347 (1976).

BROOKNER, S.P., & MURPHY, N.O. The use of a total communication approach with a nondeaf child: A case study. *Language, Speech, and Hearing Services in Schools, 6,* 131-137 (1975).

BULLOCK, A., DALRYMPLE, G.F., & DANCA, J.M. The Auto-Com at Kennedy Memorial Hospital: Rapid and accurate communication by a multihandicapped student. *American Journal of Occupational Therapy, 29,* 150-152 (1975).

CARLSON, F.L. *An adapted communication project for a nonspeaking child.* Paper presented at the 51st Annual Meeting of the American Speech and Hearing Association, Houston (1976).

CHARBONNEAU, J.R., COTE, C., & ROY, O.Z. *NRC'S "Comhandi" communication system technical description and application at the Ottawa Crippled Children's Treatment Center.* Paper presented at the seminar "Electronic Controls for the Severely Physically Handicapped," Vancouver, British Columbia (1974).

CHEN, L.Y. Manual communication by combined alphabet and gestures. *Archives of Physical Medicine and Rehabilitation, 52,* 381-384 (1971).

CLAPPE, C., GRANT, M., HAZARD, G., LANG, J., & TOMLINSON, R. *The Morse code visual translator—A means of communication for the anarthric patient.* Paper presented at the 48th Annual Convention of the American Speech and Hearing Association, Detroit (1973).

Computerized device speaks for handicapped youngsters. *Journal of the Acoustical Society of America, 59,* 1520-1521 (1976).

CREEDON, M.P. (Ed.) *Appropriate Behavior Through Communications: A New Program in Simultaneous Language.* Available from Dysfunctioning Child Center, 2915 Ellis, Chicago, Illinois (1975).

DUNCAN, J.L., & SILVERMAN, F.H. Impacts of learning American Indian Sign Language on mentally retarded children: A preliminary report. *Perceptual and Motor Skills, 44,* 1138 (1977).

EAGLESON, H.M., VAUGHN, G.R., & KNUDSON, A.B. Hand Signals for dysphasia. *Archives of Physical Medicine and Rehabilitation, 51,* 111-113 (1970).

EGAN, J.J., ANTHONY, G.M., & HONKE, L.E. *Joan: A case study of manual communication with a severe cerebral palsied dysarthric.* Paper presented at the Annual Meeting of the American Speech and Hearing Association, Houston (1976).

ELLSWORTH, S., & KOTKIN, R. If only Jimmy could speak. *Hearing & Speech Action, 43,* 6-10 (November/December, 1975).

FEALLOCK, B. Communication for the nonverbal individual. *American Journal of Occupational Therapy, 12,* 60-63, 83 (1958).

FENN, G., & ROWE, J.A. An experiment in manual communication. *British Journal of Disorders of Communication, 10,* 3-16 (1975).

FULWILER, R.L., & FOUTS, R.S. Acquisition of American Sign Language by a noncommunicating autistic child. *Journal of Autism and Childhood Schizophrenia, 6,* 43-51 (1976).

GERTENRICH, R.L. A simple mouth-held writing device for use with cerebral palsy patients. *Mental Retardation, 4,* 13-14 (August, 1966).

GITLIS, K.R. *Rationale and precedents for the use of simultaneous communication as an alternate system of communication for nonverbal children.* Paper presented at the 50th Annual Meeting of the American Speech and Hearing Association, Washington, D.C. (1975).

GLASS, A.V., GAZZANIGA, M.S., & PREMACK, D. Artificial language training in global aphasics. *Neuropsychologia, 11,* 95-103 (1973).

GOLDBERG, H.R., & FENTON, J. *Aphonic Communication for Those with Cerebral Palsy: Guide for the Development and Use of a Conversation Board.* New York: United Cerebral Palsy of New York State (1960).

GOLDSTEIN, H., & CAMERON, H. New method of communication for the aphasic patient. *Arizona Medicine, 8,* 17-21 (1952).

GOODWIN, M., & GOODWIN, T.C. In a dark mirror. *Mental Hygiene, 53,* 550-563 (1969).

HAGEN, C., PORTER, W., & BRINK, J. Nonverbal communication: An alternative mode of communication for the child with severe cerebral palsy. *Journal of Speech and Hearing Disorders, 38,* 448-455 (1973).

Handicapped youth "talks" with eyes. *News Journal* (Mansfield, Ohio) (October 22, 1974).

HARRIS-VANDERHEIDEN, D. Blissymbolics and the mentally retarded. In Gregg C. Vanderheiden and Kate Grilley (Eds.), *Non-vocal Communication Techniques and Aids for the Severely Physically Handicapped.* Baltimore: University Park Press, pp. 120-131 (1976a).

———— . Field evaluation of the Auto-Com. In Gregg C. Vanderheiden and Kate Grilley (Eds.), *Non-vocal Communication Techniques and Aids for the Severely Physically Handicapped.* Baltimore: University Park Press, pp. 144-151 (1976b).

HELFRICH, K.R. *Total communication with the oral apractic child.* Videotape presented at the 51st Annual Meeting of the American Speech and Hearing Association, Houston (1976).

HILL, S.D., CAMPAGNA, J., LONG, D., MUNCH, J., & NAECHER, S. An explanation of the use of two response keyboard as a means of communication for the severely handicapped child. *Perceptual and Motor Skills, 26,* 699-704 (1968).

HOFFMEISTER, R.J., & FARMER, A. The development of manual sign language in mentally retarded deaf individuals. *Journal of Rehabilitation of the Deaf, 6,* 19-26 (1972).

JACK H. EICHLER: Builds communication device. *Case Alumnus* (Publication of Case Institute of Technology Alumni Association, Cleveland, Ohio), 211 (June, 1973).

JENKINS, R. Possum, a new communication aid. *Special Education* (Great Britain), *56,* 9-11 (1967).

KATES, B., & MCNAUGHTON, S. *The first application of Blissymbolics as a communication medium for non-speaking children: History and development, 1971-1974.* Distributed by Blissymbolics Communication Foundation, 862 Eglinton Avenue East, Toronto, Ontario, Canada (no date).

KIMBLE, S.L. *A language teaching technique with totally nonverbal, severely mentally retarded adolescents.* Paper presented at the 50th Annual Meeting of the American Speech and Hearing Association, Washington, D.C. (1975).

KLADDE, A.G. Nonoral communication techniques: Project summary No. 1, August, 1967. In Beverly Vicker (Ed.), *Nonoral Communication System Project 1964/1973.* Iowa City: Campus Stores, The University of Iowa, pp. 57-104 (1974).

KONSTANTAREAS, M., OXMAN, J., WEBSTER, C., FISCHER, H., & MILLER, K. *A five week simultaneous communication programme for severely dysfunctional children: Outcome and implications for future research.* Distributed by Clarke Institute of Psychiatry, Toronto, Ontario (1975).

LEBEIS, S., & LEBEIS, R.F. The use of signed communication with the normal-hearing, nonverbal mentally retarded. *Bureau Memorandum* (Wisconsin Department of Public Instruction), *17* (1), 28-30 (1975).

LEVETT, L.M. A method of communication for nonspeaking severely subnormal children—Trial results. *British Journal of Disorders of Communication, 6,* 125-128 (1971).

LINVILLE, S.E. Signed English: A language teaching technique with totally nonverbal severely mentally retarded adolescents. *Language, Speech and Hearing Services in Schools, 8,* 170-175 (1977).

LUCAS, E.V., & DEAN, M.B. *An alternative approach to oral communication for an autistic child.* Videotape presented at the 51st Annual Meeting of the American Speech and Hearing Association, Houston (1976).

MCDONALD, E.T., & SCHULTZ, A.R. Communication boards for cerebral palsied children. *Journal of Speech and Hearing Disorders, 38,* 73-88 (1973).

MILLER, A., & MILLER, E.E. Cognitive-developmental training with elevated boards and sign language. *Journal of Autism and Childhood Schizophrenia, 3,* 65-85 (1973).

MYKLEBUST, H.R. *Auditory Disorders in Children.* New York: Grune & Stratton (1974).

NICOL, E. Breakthrough to communication. *Special Education, 61* (4), 25-28 (1972).

OFFIR, C.W. Visual speech: Their fingers do the talking. *Psychology Today, 10* (1), 72-78 (June, 1976).

Ontario Crippled Children's Centre Symbol Communication Programme Year End Report 1974. Distributed by the Ontario Crippled Children's Centre, 350 Rumsey Road, Toronto, Ontario (1974).

RATUSNIK, C.M., & RATUSNIK, D.L. A comprehensive communication approach for a ten-year-old nonverbal autistic child. *American Journal of Orthopsychiatry, 44,* 396-403 (1974).

RICE, O.M., & COMBS, R.G. Practical aids for non-verbal handicapped. *Proceedings of the 1972 Carnahan Conference on Electronic Prosthetics* (1972).

RICHARDSON, T. Sign language for the SMR and PMR. *Mental Retardation, 13,* (3), 17 (1975).

SCHAEFFER, B., MCDOWELL, P., MUSIL, A., & KOLLINZAS, G. Spontaneous verbal language for autistic children through signed speech. *Research Relating to Children* (ERIC Clearinghouse for Early Childhood Education), Bulletin *37,* 98-99 (1976).

SCHLANGER, P.H. *Training the adult aphasic to pantomime.* Paper presented at the 51st Annual Meeting of the American Speech and Hearing Association, Houston (1976).

SCHMIDT, M.J., CARRIER Jr., J.K., & PARSONS, S.D. *Use of a nonspeech mode in teaching language.* Paper presented at the 46th Annual Meeting of the American Speech and Hearing Association, Chicago (1971).

SILVERMAN, F.H. Criteria for assessing therapy outcome in speech pathology and audiology. *Journal of Speech and Hearing Research,* 20, 5-20 (1977a).

———. *Research Design in Speech Pathology and Audiology.* Englewood Cliffs: Prentice-Hall (1977b).

SKELLY, M., SCHINSKY, L., SMITH, R., DONALDSON, R., & GRIFFIN, J. American Indian Sign: A gestural communication system for the speechless. *Archives of Physical Medicine and Rehabilitation, 56,* 156-160 (1975).

SKELLY, M., SCHINSKY, L., SMITH, R.W. & FUST, R.S. American Indian Sign (AMERIND) as a facilitator of verbalization for the oral verbal apraxic. *Journal of Speech and Hearing Disorders, 39,* 445-456 (1974).

TOPPER, S.T. Gesture language for a non-verbal severely retarded male. *Mental Retardation, 13* (1) 30-31 (1975).

VANDERHEIDEN, D.H., BROWN, W.P., MACKENZIE, P., REINEN, S., & SCHEIBEL, C. Symbol communication for the mentally handicapped. *Mental Retardation, 13,* 34-37 (1975).

VANDERHEIDEN, G.C., & HARRIS-VANDERHEIDEN, D. Field evaluation of the
    Auto-Com, An auto-monitoring communication board. *Research
    Relating to Children,* Bulletin 37, 86-87 (1976b).
VICKER, B. *Nonoral Communication System Project 1964/1973.* Iowa City:
    Campus Stores, The University of Iowa (1974).
WEBSTER, C.D., MCPHERSON, H., SLOMAN, L., EVANS, M.A., & KUCHAR, E.
    Communicating with an autistic boy by gestures. *Journal of Autism and
    Childhood Schizophrenia, 3,* 337-346 (1973).
WENDT, E., SPRAGUE, M.J., & MARQUIS, J. Communication without speech.
    Teaching Exceptional Children, 38-42 (Fall, 1975).
WILSON, P.S. *Sign language as a means of communication for the mentally
    retarded.* Paper presented at the Eastern Psychological Association
    (April, 1974).

II

NONSPEECH COMMUNICATION MODES

Classification of Nonspeech Communication Modes

3

All nonspeech communication modes, or systems, that have been developed can be assigned to one of three categories: gestural, gestural-assisted, or neuro-assisted. The category to which a mode, or system, would be assigned would be a function of (1) whether any instrumentation were needed to encode or transmit messages and (2) if instrumentation were needed, whether it is controlled by muscle gestures (i.e., patterned movements of muscle groups) or bioelectrical signals (i.e., electrical signals generated by the nervous system such as muscle action potentials). The defining characteristics of these categories are summarized in Table 3.1.

Gestural Modes

The defining characteristic of a gestural mode is that it requires no instrumentation, only patterned muscle gestures, or movements. Messages are encoded into muscle gestures and transmitted visually. The muscle groups involved are primarily those of the upper extremities (one or both) and/or of

TABLE 3.1. Defining characteristics of gestural, gestural-assisted, and neuro-assisted communication systems.

	Type of Mode		
	GESTURAL	GESTURAL-ASSISTED	NEURO-ASSISTED
Instrumentation Necessary	No	Yes	Yes
Muscle Gesture Control of Instrumentation	No	Yes	No
Neuro-Activity Control of Instrumentation	No	No	Yes

the head and neck. Patterned movements of other muscle groups (e.g., those of the lower extremities) also could be used. The only requirement is that the gestural code be meaningful to the person using it and to those with whom he or she is communicating.

The gestural mode is *not an abnormal one* for encoding and transmitting messages. All persons use facial and body gesture to some extent for this purpose. We all, at times, indicate what we want by pointing. We answer questions by nodding or shaking our heads yes or no. We partially convey our messages through the facial and body gestures that accompany speech. (We all, therefore, use a form of Total Communication; see Chapter 4.) When we feel that we are not making ourselves understood (e.g., when we are attempting to communicate with someone who does not understand English well), we resort to pantomime. We shrug our shoulders when we want to indicate we don't know. We may use hand signals while driving a car. We raise our right arm when we want to signal someone to stop. We all use many types of gesture, alone or in combination with speech, for encoding and transmitting messages.

Persons who lack adequate speech for their communicative purposes are likely to use gesture to some extent to encode and transmit messages *without being taught* to use it. In fact, unless they are taught a formal nonspeech communication mode or are able to communicate by writing, this probably will be the way they communicate.

While almost all speechless persons exhibit some normal gestural communication, it should not be assumed that their ability to communicate gesturally is normal. Their gestural communication may be limited for several reasons. First, the musculature used to produce particular gestures may not function normally, due to a neuromuscular disorder or apraxia. Such a condition is particularly apt to limit gestural communication if it affects the musculature of the upper extremities and head and neck.

A second reason for gestural communication being limited is the presence of aphasia. Aphasics may have similar difficulties using gestures propositionally as they do using speech propositionally. They may not be able to reliably signal yes and no by shaking their heads or to communicate a message through pantomime. Such deficits have been observed in both aphasic children (Myklebust, 1954) and adults (Duffy, Duffy, & Pearson, 1973).

A third reason for gestural communication being limited is the presence of developmentally inappropriate cognitive ability. Persons with this condition do not function intellectually (i.e., do not solve problems and see relationships) as well as would be expected for someone their age. Included here would be children and adults who are congenitally mentally retarded as well as those who were developing normally but lost normal cognitive ability as a result of brain damage. Since the acquisition of the ability to communicate gesturally follows a predictable developmental sequence, such persons would be more limited in their use of some types of gestural communication than of others. The types that are most likely to be affected are those which develop last and are relatively abstract (e.g., pantomime).

Gestural communication systems are taught to speechless persons to *enhance* their abilities to transmit messages gesturally. They can supplement normal gestural communication in two ways. First, they can provide additional information for messages that can be transmitted by normal gestural communication, thereby increasing the *redundancy* and hence the intelligibility of such messages. And second, they can increase the number of messages that can be encoded and transmitted gesturally; that is, they can be used to encode and transmit messages that cannot be encoded and transmitted by normal gestural communication.

It should be noted that speech enhances normal gestural communication in the same manner as do gestural communication systems. First, it increases the redundancy and hence the intelligibility of messages that can be communicated by facial and body gestures. And second, it increases the number of messages that can be encoded and transmitted gesturally. Speech can be viewed as a gestural communication mode because messages are encoded and transmitted by gestures of the articulators. The gestural nature of speech, incidentally, is particularly evident while speechreading.

How might the use of a formal gestural system, such as fingerspelling, increase the redundancy of normal gestural communication? Suppose that a person was feeling depressed. He or she might communicate this by facial expression and overall body posture; he or she might "look depressed." If the person were to fingerspell the message "I feel depressed," this would increase its redundancy and thereby the probability that it would be understood. Fingerspelling, in this instance, would increase the probability that the message would be understood because the facial and bodily postural signs of depression may not be obvious to the person or persons to whom the message was being transmitted.

Gestural communication systems also supplement normal gestural communication by providing a gestural means for encoding and transmitting messages that could not be encoded and transmitted by facial and other bodily gestures. The gestures used for this purpose (as well as for the previous one) are of two types. Those of the first type stand for, or signify, *linguistic units* such as letters, phonemes, or morphemes. Messages (or message segments) that are encoded and transmitted by means of such gestures are *directly translatable* into a natural language such as English. Thus gestures of this first type can be used to encode and transmit a message or message segment by—

1. spelling the words in it letter by letter (e.g., through the use of the manual alphabet);
2. signaling the phonemes of the words in the message phoneme by phoneme (e.g., through the use of cued speech); or
3. signaling morphemic information contained in it, such as verb tense (e.g., through the use of Signed English).

Gestures of the *second* type stand for, or signify, *concepts* rather than linguistic units. Messages encoded by means of such gestures are not similar in structure to English or other Indo-European languages. They have a different linguistic structure. For example, they cannot be segmented into letters or phonemes. In addition, they may have a different syntactic structure (i.e., the ordering of signs for a message does not necessarily correspond to the ordering of the words used to express it). Finally, they may have a different semantic structure. There may not, for example, be a one-to-one correspondence between the number of words and number of gestures needed to encode and transmit a concept. For some concepts the number of gestures needed is less than the number of words, and for others the number needed is greater.

The gestures mentioned previously that signal morphemic information such as verb tense can be used with this type of gestural system. Their use for this purpose is discussed by Bornstein (1974).

The two basic types of gestures that have been described—those that signify linguistic units and those that signify concepts—are often used together for encoding and transmitting messages. When concept gestures exist, they are used. When they do not exist, the words necessary to communicate the concept are fingerspelled. Both types of gestures are combined in American Sign Language (Wilber, 1976), the gestural communication system used by the deaf in the United States.

Representative gestural communication modes are described in Chapter 4.

Gestural-Assisted Modes

The defining characteristic of a gestural-assisted communication scheme is that it contains a readout device (or display) that is activated directly or indirectly by muscle gestures, or movements. Users either *point to* or *cause to be reproduced* on the display the components of the message they wish to transmit. An example of a display that permits users to indicate message components by pointing is a communication, or conversation, board. (Several representative communication boards are reproduced in Chapter 5.) An example of a device that permits users to reproduce message components is an adapted electric typewriter. (Electric typewriters that have been adapted for persons who have neuromuscular disorders are described in Chapter 5.)

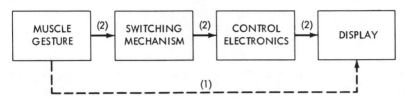

FIGURE 3.1. *Two approaches for indicating message components on a display with gestural-assisted modes. The first (1) is direct and the second (2) is indirect.*

Muscle gestures can be used to indicate message components *directly* or *indirectly*. Both approaches are diagrammed in Figure 3.1. With the first (number 1 in Figure 3.1) muscle gestures are used directly to indicate or reproduce message components on a display. The display is controlled directly by the person, not indirectly by an electronic switching mechanism. An example of a display that would use such an approach for indicating is a communication board. Muscle gestures that can be used to directly indicate message components include: movements of one or both upper extremities; movements of the head (in conjunction with a headpointer); and movements of the eyes. The first two also can be used to directly reproduce message components. (This approach is described in depth in Chapter 5.)

The second approach (number 2 in Figure 3.1) uses muscle gestures *indirectly* to indicate or reproduce message components on a display. The display is controlled by an *electronic switching mechanism* that is activated by one or more muscle gestures. Almost any movement resulting from the contraction of a muscle group can be used to activate a switching mechanism. Gestures that have been used for this purpose include finger movements, head movements, foot movements, and eyebrow movements. (A number of gestures that can be used to activate electronic switching mechanisms are described in Chapters 5 and 7.) The types of switches that can be activated by muscle gestures that have been used to control electronic displays include mechanical microswitches, magnetic proximity switches, and photoelectric switches. (The use of these and others is dealt with in Chapter 5.)

The *control electronics* (which are located in Figure 3.1 between the switching mechanism and display) make it possible for the switching mechanism to control the display. The functions performed by the control electronics are determined in part by the nature of the switching mechanism and display. In some instances (e.g., when eyeblink Morse code is used to control an electric typewriter) a component of the control electronics is a small computer. (The functions of control electronics are discussed further in Chapter 5.)

Electronic switching mechanisms (with appropriate control electronics) can be used to indicate or reproduce message components on several types of *displays* or readout devices. These are described in Chapter 5.

Gestural-assisted communication systems, to be maximally effective in meeting each client's communication needs, have to be individually designed. While commercial communication boards can meet most clients' communication needs temporarily and those of a few permanently, they are not as functional for most clients as would be individually designed boards. (Factors that should be considered when developing a communication board for a client are indicated in Chapter 5.) Also, standard combinations of switching mechanisms, control electronics, and displays are apt not to be maximally effective in meeting most clients' communication needs. (The design of electronic gestural-assisted communication systems is dealt with in Chapter 5.)

Representative gestural-assisted communication systems, or modes, that have been used with dysarthric, aphasic, apraxic, mentally retarded, and autistic children and adults are described in Chapter 5.

Neuro-Assisted Modes

The defining characteristic of a neuro-assisted communication system is that it contains a readout device or display that is activated by *bioelectrical* signals —electrical signals originating from within the body such as muscle action potentials (electrical signals transmitted by lower motor neurons to muscle fibers, which causes them to contract).

The only way in which neuro-assisted communication systems differ from electronic gestural-assisted ones (see Figure 3.1) is that they are activated by an electrical signal rather than gestural manipulation of a switching mechanism. The components of neuro-assisted communication systems can be diagrammed as in Figure 3.2. Note that the only difference between this system and that diagrammed in Figure 3.1 is that it interfaces with the user by means of an electrode-activated signal detection, amplification, and modification mechanism rather than by a gesture-activated switching mechanism. The same displays can be used with both types of systems. (The design of neuro-assisted communication systems is dealt with in Chapter 6.)

Neuro-assisted communication systems have not been refined to the same degree as have gestural and gestural-assisted ones. There appear to be several reasons for the relative lack of interest in this type of communication system. First, the communication needs of almost all speechless children and

FIGURE 3.2. *Components of neuro-assisted communication systems.*

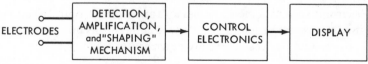

adults can be met by gestural and gestural-assisted communication systems. Second, neuro-assisted communication systems tend to be more sophisticated electronically, and hence more expensive than comparable gestural-assisted ones. And third, such systems (in part because they tend to be relatively complex electronically) are not as reliable as comparable gestural-assisted ones.

Neuro-assisted communication systems are dealt with in this book because there are a few children and adults who are so involved motorically that they cannot communicate adequately with a gestural or gestural-assisted communication scheme. A neuro-assisted system may facilitate communication for such a person. Representative systems of this type are described in Chapter 6.

REFERENCES

BORNSTEIN, H. Signed English: A manual approach to English language development. *Journal of Speech and Hearing Disorders, 39,* 330-343 (1974).

DUFFY, R.J., DUFFY, J.R., & PEARSON, K.L. *Impairment of gestural ability in aphasics.* Paper presented at the 48th annual meeting of the American Speech and Hearing Association, Detroit (1973).

MYKLEBUST, H. *Auditory Disorders in Children.* New York: Grune & Stratton (1954).

WILBER, R.B. The linguistics of manual language and manual systems. In Lyle L. Lloyd (Ed.), *Communication Assessment and Intervention Strategies.* Baltimore: University Park Press (1976).

$\boxed{4}$ Gestural Modes

The previous chapter presented the characteristics of three classes of non-speech communication systems, or modes: gestural, gestural-assisted, and neuro-assisted. This chapter describes *representative* communication modes of the gestural type. (Representative gestural-assisted modes are described in Chapter 5, and neuro-assisted in Chapter 6.) The descriptions will include information about the following:

1. neuromuscular functions that must be intact for the mode to be used;
2. its "intelligibility" to untrained observers;
3. its ability to convey messages concerning the "here and now";
4. its ability to convey messages *not* concerned with the "here and now";
5. its syntactic and semantic structure;
6. the similarity of its linguistic structure to English;
7. its ability to convey messages containing abstract concepts;
8. the time and "energy" investment required to learn to use it;
9. the time and "energy" investment required to learn to comprehend it;
10. the level of acceptability of the mode to users and interpreters;
11. the populations with which it has been used;
12. examples of gestures—photographs or drawings;
13. sources of dictionaries of gestures; and
14. sources of materials for teaching children and adults how to use the system.

Specific applications of the modes described are indicated at the end of the chapter.

American Sign Language (Ameslan)

American sign language, or Ameslan, is the manual gestural communication system used by the deaf in the United States. Each gestural sign in this system performs one of the following linguistic functions:

1.   It signals a *letter* of the alphabet. The set of twenty-six such signs is known as the American Manual Alphabet (see Figure 4.1).

2.   It signals a *word* or *phrase*. There are more than 5,000 such signs (Bornstein, 1974).

3.   It signals *morphological* or *syntactic* information (e.g., verb tense). The twelve sign markers in Signed English (Bornstein, 1974) have this function (see Figure 4.2).

4.   It signals a *phoneme*. The system known as Cued Speech (Lykos, 1971) contains such signs.

Signs having the first two functions are the most frequently occurring ones in messages transmitted by American Sign Language.

Communication with Ameslan usually involves the transmission of an *ordered* series of signs. When fingerspelling, signs are ordered to spell words. The ordering of the signs for a word corresponds to the ordering of the letters in it. Both words that are signed as units and those that are fingerspelled are ordered on the basis of syntactic rules, but *these rules are not necessarily those of spoken English.* (The Signed English system of Bornstein, 1974, is an

FIGURE 4.1. *American Manual Alphabet (from Bornstein, 1974).*

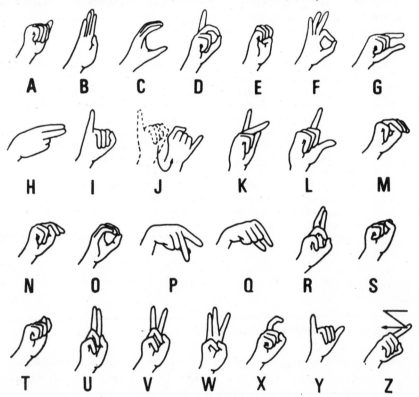

FIGURE 4.2. *Sign markers used in Signed English (from Bornstein, 1974).*

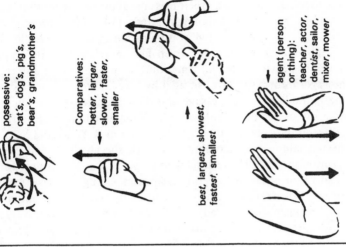

possessive:
cat's, dog's, pig's,
bear's, grandmother's

Comparatives:
better, larger,
slower, faster,
smaller

best, largest, slowest,
fastest, smallest

agent (person
or thing):
teacher, actor,
dentist, sailor,
mixer, mower

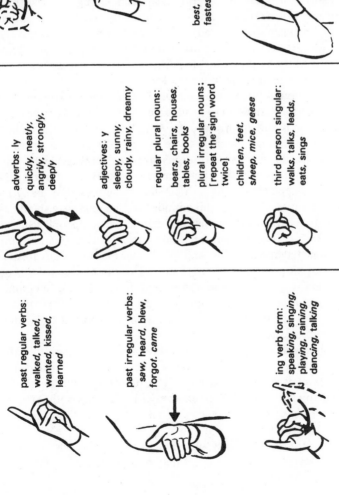

adverbs: ly
quickly, neatly,
angrily, strongly,
deeply

adjectives: y
sleepy, sunny,
cloudy, rainy, dreamy

regular plural nouns:
bears, chairs, houses,
tables, books

plural irregular nouns:
[repeat the sign word
twice]

children, feet,
sheep, mice, geese

third person singular:
walks, talks, leads,
eats, sings

past regular verbs:
walked, talked,
wanted, kissed,
learned

past irregular verbs:
saw, heard, blew,
forgot, came

ing verb form:
speaking, singing,
playing, raining,
dancing, talking

attempt to develop a manual sign system that has a syntax similar to spoken English.)

Some users of Ameslan say their message at the same time that they sign it. Simultaneous speaking and signing is referred to as *total communication.* Presumably, such a person could communicate more successfully in this manner than by speech or sign alone. Even if his speech were relatively poor, it probably would provide some information that would help to interpret his signed message. Information transmitted by speech, however limited, would add to the redundancy of a message and thereby increase its intelligibility. (For further discussion of the role of redundancy in communication, see the writings of such information theorists as Shannon & Weaver, 1963.)

Ameslan (alone or in combination with speech) has been used as a communication medium by persons whose speech was inadequate for their communicative purposes for several reasons, including deafness, mental retardation, childhood autism, and dysarthria. Its use as a communication medium for the mentally retarded, autistic, and dysarthric is relatively recent (see Appendix A). Its use by persons in these three groups, incidently, tends to be more limited than that by the deaf: they tend to use fewer signs and their signed utterances tend to be less complex syntactically.

The functioning of the musculature of *both* upper extremities must be reasonably good for Ameslan to be useable. It does not have to be normal. So long as a person is able to produce the Ameslan signs at a reasonable rate of speed accurately enough for them to be recognizable, he can use the system.

The majority of Ameslan signs are *not* intelligible to untrained observers. The amount of training necessary to learn to interpret a person's Ameslan signs depends on the number he or she uses. For many mentally retarded and autistic children this number will be relatively small (less than 200). When the number of signs used is relatively small, people usually can be taught to interpret them in a short period of time. Clinician instruction, videotaped (or filmed) demonstration, and worksheets on which signs are illustrated by drawings, photographs, or both (Lake, 1976) can be used for this purpose.

Ameslan is a very flexible sign system. It can be used to communicate any message concerning present, past, or future that could be communicated by English. It is one of the most flexible, if not the most flexible, of the nonspeech communication systems.

The time and energy investment necessary for a person to learn to use Ameslan is a function of several factors, including (1) his or her mental age and (2) the level of proficiency desired. The lower the mental age, the longer it would tend to take to attain a given level of proficiency with Ameslan. And the higher the level of proficiency desired, the greater the time and energy investment necessary to attain it.

The level of acceptability of Ameslan to persons who use it to communicate appears to be fairly good. Many persons who are mentally retarded or autistic have used Ameslan as a communication mode for a year or longer (see Table 2.1 for studies in which Ameslan was used).

The level of acceptability of Ameslan to interpreters may not be particularly good (see Olson, 1976). The problem is that many Ameslan signs cannot be understood by persons who have not been taught to interpret them. If a person used only a few such signs and interacted with only a few people (which would be the case, for example, for some institutionalized, mentally retarded persons), the training of interpreters probably would not be a serious problem. On the other hand, if a user had a relatively large Ameslan vocabulary, or had a need to communicate with persons who had not been trained to interpret the signs he or she used, or both of these, this could counterindicate the use of Ameslan. Of course, a person could be taught to use Ameslan only when communicating with those who understood it; when communicating with others, another nonspeech system, such as a communication board, could be used. This situation, incidently, is somewhat similar to that in which a person who spoke only English would find himself when visiting a country where English is not the national language. He would use English to communicate with those who understood it and something else (e.g., pantomime) to communicate with others.

A source from which Ameslan dictionaries and other materials for teaching Ameslan (including Signed English) can be obtained is the bookstore at Gallaudet College in Washington, D.C.; they publish a list of such materials that can be ordered by mail from them. This list contains materials appropriate for all age groups, preschool through adult. Some representative materials for teaching Ameslan are listed in Appendix B.

A comprehensive bibliography of papers dealing with the use of Ameslan with populations *other than the deaf* is included in Appendix A.

American Indian Sign Language (Amerind)

American Indian Sign Language, or Amerind, is a manual gestural communication system that was used by North American Indians for inter-tribal communication—for communication between tribes whose members did not speak a common language (Tomkins, 1969). They also used it to communicate with the early Spanish and English-speaking European settlers. It functioned as what linguists currently refer to as an auxilliary international language, or interlanguage (Pei, 1965). It is probably one of the most successful such languages ever developed since it was actually used for intercultural communication by large numbers of persons. It is interesting to note in this regard that

> the International Boy Scout movement . . . resolutely adopted the Indian sign language and proceeded to develop a science of pasimology, or gestures, which

serves the Jamborees in perfect fashion. Representatives of as many as thirty-seven nations have met at various times and carried on both general business and private conversations in pasimology. The use of Indian sign language for international purpose has repeatedly been advocated. Sir Richard Paget and the American Tourist Association, in recent times, have both advocated the possibility of "handage" to replace language (Pei, 1965, p. 17).

The gestural signs in Amerind are (kinetic) pictographic and ideographic rather than phonetic. They represent ideas and in many cases are kinetic pictorial representations of the ideas conveyed. Figure 4.3, the Amerind sign for cry, illustrates the pictographic and ideographic nature of the signs in this system.

The Amerind signs for some words, or concepts, consist of an ordered series of gestures rather than a single gesture. The meanings of the individual gestures indicate the meaning of the composite. This process (which is referred to as *agglutination*) greatly increases the number of words, or concepts, that can be communicated by Amerind. The items in Table 4.1 illustrate the agglutination process.

The syntactic structure of Amerind is less complex than that of English and other spoken languages. Its grammatical rules, according to Tomkins (1969), include the following:

1. Every question begins with, or is preceded by, a question sign (see Figure 4.4). Thus, "Where are you going?" in Amerind sign would be QUESTION YOU GOING? "The sign for 'question' covers the words WHAT, WHY,

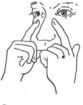

FIGURE 4.3a. *Amerind sign for cry. With both hands at eyes tears are indicated as flowing by tracing their course down the face (from Tomkins, 1969).*

Pleurer
Weinen   Cry

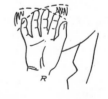

FIGURE 4.3b. *Amerind sign for question. Right hand is held palm outward at height of shoulders with fingers and thumb extended, separated, and pointed upwards. The hand is turned slightly by wrist action two or three times (from Tomkins, 1969).*

Question
Frage   Question

TABLE 4.1. Agglutinated Amerind sign sequences for 10 words, or concepts*.

Word or Concept	Amerind Sign Sequence
Aid	WORK, WITH
Bachelor	MAN, MARRY, NO
Boil	WATER, KETTLE, FIRE
City	HOUSE, MANY
Cook	MAKE, EAT
Generous	HEART, BIG
Hospital	HOUSE, SICK, MANY
Midnight	NIGHT, MIDDLE
Read	BOOK, LOOK
Store	HOUSE, TRADE

*From Tomkins, 1969

WHERE and WHEN. It is made to attract attention, to ask, to inquire, to examine" (pp7-8).
2. "*Present* time is expressed by adding the sign for NOW or for TODAY. Past tense is expressed by adding LONG TIME" (p. 8).
3. "What we understand to be the first person singular is indicated by pointing to one's-self. The plural WE is made by the signs ME and ALL. YOU, ALL, means YE; while HE, ALL means THEY" (p. 8).
4. "Gender is shown by adding the signs MAN or WOMAN" (p. 8).
5. "Such words or articles, as A, THE, AN, IT, etc., are not used" (p. 8).

The items in Table 4.2 illustrate several aspects of the syntactic structure of Amerind sign language. (For other examples of Amerind sign equivalents of English utterances, see Tomkins, 1969, pp. 97-100).

Many Amerind signs stand for more than one English word. The question sign (see Figure 4.3), for example, can be interpreted as WHAT, WHERE, WHY, or WHEN. The intended meaning of this type of Amerind sign is inferred from context.

Amerind was adapted for use with aphasics, oral apraxics, dysarthrics, dysphonics, and persons who have had glossectomies, by Dr. Madge Skelly and her associates at the St. Louis Veteran's Administration Hospital (Skelly, Schinsky, Smith, Donaldson, & Griffin, 1975; Skelly, Schinsky, Smith, & Fust, 1974). They eliminated signs not applicable to present day use and developed signs for contemporary activities (e.g., driving a car) and other concepts it would be important for a person to be able to communicate, particularly in a hospital setting. (The signs they developed, incidently, were shown to native American users of Amerind and judged by them to be compatable with the system.) In addition, they developed a one-hand version of Amerind for use by hemiplegics. (Both the one-hand and two-hand versions

TABLE 4.2.   Amerind sign equivalents of 10 English utterances*

English	Amerind Sign Equivalent
I want a drink of water.	I WANT WATER.
Do you understand Indian Sign Language?	QUESTION YOU KNOW INDIAN SIGN LANGUAGE?
Look, it is raining.	SEE RAIN.
When do we eat, at noon?	QUESTION FUTURE-TIME ME ALL EAT, SUN HIGH?
What is your name?	QUESTION YOU CALLED?
Don't wait for me, I'll come pretty soon.	WAIT ME NOT. I COME SHORT-TIME FUTURE.
Be quiet, listen to the speaker.	QUIET: LISTEN: MAN TALK.
We like to walk.	ME ALL FOND WALK.
The girl is running.	GIRL RUN.
I do not each much for breakfast.	I EAT NOT MUCH SUNRISE.

*From Tomkins, 1969

of Amerind as adapted by Madge Skelly and her associates are demonstrated in a series of eight videotapes available on interlibrary loan from the Learning Resources Center of the St. Louis Veteran's Administration Hospital; see Appendix A.) Their version of Amerind also has been used with nonvocal mentally retarded children (Duncan & Silverman, 1977).

To use Amerind a person must have essentially normal neuromuscular functioning of at least one upper extremity. While Amerind signs normally are formed using both hands, many can be encoded with one hand. (The one-hand version of Amerind is demonstrated in the fourth tape of the *Amerind Video Dictionary;* see Appendix A.) It also is desirable, *but not essential,* that the functioning of the musculature of the face and neck be essentially normal since "facial expression" appears to be a component of some Amerind signs (e.g., BAD ODOR).

Amerind can be used to convey messages about the "here and now" as well as the past and future. While it can be used to convey both abstract and concrete concepts, one probably would tend to be more successful using it to convey the latter than the former.

The time and energy investments required to learn to *use* Amerind do not seem to be excessive. Based on reports in the literature, most children and adults can acquire enough Amerind to have a significant impact on their ability to communicate in two months or less. Obviously, the speed at which a given person would achieve a particular level of proficiency with Amerind would be influenced by several factors including his or her intellectual level. The *Amerind Video Dictionary* (1975), which presents demonstrations of 193 two-hand Amerind signs and 42 one-hand Amerind signs, can be used both to reduce the time necessary for a client to learn Amerind (assuming that the dictionary is used for self-instruction) and to minimize the clinician's time investment.

The time and energy investment necessary for learning to *comprehend* Amerind is usually minimal for several reasons. First, it is more than 50 percent intelligible to most untrained observers (Skelly, Schinsky, Smith, Donaldson, & Griffin, 1975). Second, its syntactic structure is relatively simple. There are only a few rules governing the ordering of signs in utterances. And third, Amerind signs tend to be relatively easy to learn because almost all are concrete, or representational. (The representational nature of some Amerind signs may not be obvious before you are told what they mean. However, once you are told, you usually are able to perceive how they are suggestive, or representational, of their meanings. The same is true for agglutinated signs. After you learn what one means you usually can understand how the meanings of the individual signs that make it up concretely indicate its meaning.) The *Amerind Video Dictionary* (1975), incidently, can also be used for improving comprehension of Amerind signs. Some persons can learn the meanings of relatively large numbers of Amerind signs merely by viewing these videotapes several times (Bady & Silverman, 1978).

Amerind appears to be reasonably acceptable to most users and interpreters (Duncan & Silverman, 1977; Skelly, Schinsky, Smith, Donaldson, & Griffin, 1975; Skelly, Schinsky, Smith, & Fust, 1974). The majority of persons who are taught it appear to use it for communicating outside the therapy room. Duncan and Silverman (1977) have reported that it was sufficiently acceptable to the parents of a group of thirty-two mentally retarded children who were being taught it for them to request that their children continue receiving instruction in it after a ten-week experimental program in which they had been enrolled terminated. There may be some initial resistance to using it, however, because using it may at first make the person feel uncomfortable, or as one aphasic put it, feel "crazy" (Melvin Cohen, personal communication). Such resistance probably can be reduced or overcome by positive experiences with Amerind and by counseling. (Counseling users of nonspeech communication modes and their families is dealt with in Chapter 8.) Resistance from this source, incidentally, can occur with the introduction of any nonspeech communication system.

There are several dictionary-like compilations of Amerind signs. The most useful clinically is the *Amerind Video Dictionary* (1975) that was produced by Skelly and her associates. In it are demonstrated 193 two-hand and 42 one-hand Amerind signs. Another such compilation is the book by Skelly (1979) which illustrates by drawings and verbal descriptions the Amerind signs in the *Amerind Video Dictionary.*.

Information about materials for teaching Amerind can be obtained from the Learning Resources Center, Veteran's Administration Hospital,

St. Louis, Missouri. Available materials include two series of videotapes: *American Indian Sign Language: Gestural Communication for the Speechless* (1974) and *Amerind Video Dictionary* (1975).

Other Gestural Communication Modes

Pantomime (Mime)

Pantomime, or mime, can be defined as "the art or technique of portraying a character, mood, idea, or narration by gestures and bodily movements" (Stein, 1966, p. 911). It differs from manual sign systems, such as Ameslan and Amerind, in several ways. First, it uses the musculature of the entire body, not only that (or primarily that) of the upper extremities. Second, the gestures tend to be dynamic rather than static. Meaning is conveyed primarily by the sequential relationships between gestures, rather than by the configurations of individual gestures. Third, more gestures usually are needed to convey a message than with the manual systems. And fourth, the gestures are an analogue of the message—that is, they are a dramatization of the message. Their structure is similar (or isomorphic) to that of the message. Because a pantomime tends to be similar in structure to what is being pantomimed, its meaning will be conveyed to most observers *without training*.

All persons use pantomime. It is a medium for message transmission (an aspect of nonverbal communication) as well as a theatrical art form. It occurs in interpersonal communication both alone and simultaneously with speech.

Pantomime has been used with both children and adults who lack adequate speech for their needs to facilitate communication (Balick, Spiegel, & Greene, 1976; Levett, 1969, 1971; Schlanger, 1976; Schlanger, Geffner, & DiCarrado, 1974). The clinical populations with which it has been used include cerebralpalsied children, mentally retarded children, and aphasic adults. The purposes for which it has been used with persons in these populations include the following:

1. To provide a means for encoding and transmitting messages.
2. To facilitate speech. Users are encouraged to speak their message while they pantomime it. Some aphasics have reported that this activity helps them to formulate more complete sentences and minimize word-finding problems. Communicating by pantomime also seems to increase the verbal output of some persons.
3. To facilitate receptive and expressive manual communication. Pantomime is more concrete than either Ameslan or Amerind. It usually can provide a more complete (or representational) impression of an idea or concept than either of them. For this reason, it is easier to both understand and do than Ameslan or Amerind. It is not surprising that it has been used, therefore, as an initial gestural communication system. Using this strategy, a person is first taught to

mime a relatively small set of concepts (usually fewer than 100). Manual signs are then slowly introduced, the first ones being primarily for abstract concepts that are difficult to mime. With the passage of time, a smaller and smaller percentage of the person's gestural communication would consist of mime.

4. To increase spontaneity and attention span and improve auditory and visual memory (see Balick, Spiegel, & Greene, 1976).

The concepts it is possible to mime range from the relatively concrete to the relatively abstract. The concrete end of the continuum includes the following (from Levett, 1969): above, big, car, broken, down, good, hungry, knife, light, mother, nurse, plate, shut, small, tired, train, where, bad, boat, cup, father, heavy, house, letter, long, money, on, open, sleep, spoon, toilet, up, who, both, bus, book, doctor, fork, I, I don't know, in, love, no, pain, quick, quiet, stop, tomorrow, and wash. The following pantomime, which a person used to communicate that someone he knew had adopted a baby, is representative of the other end of the continuum:

> Mr. M. outlines a large store window. He looks into the window and watches what appears to be moving objects on display. He waves at them, smiles and emits a vocalization that sounds like "kitchy, kitchy koo." He then outlines a door which he opens. He goes into the room and summons someone out to show her something in the window. He gives the woman money from his wallet as he continues pointing at one thing in the window. He goes into the store, picks up the object from the window, cuddles it, uses his forefinger to stimulate a smile from the baby in his arm (Schlanger, 1976, pp. 3-4).

The musculature of the entire body is used in mime. However, muscle function does not have to be completely normal to use it. Some cerebral-palsied children have used mime successfully (Levett, 1969, 1971). Mime does not appear to require as high a level of functioning of the musculature of the upper extremities as do manual sign systems such as Ameslan and Amerind.

Mime, if done reasonably well, should be highly intelligible to untrained observers. Photographs and drawings of the mime used by a person can be made available to those with whom he interacts to improve their understanding of it.

Mime can convey messages concerning the past and future as well as the present. While it can convey messages containing either abstract or concrete concepts, it is more suited to the concrete, particularly when the user is relatively inexperienced.

Mime does not have a standard, nationally accepted semantic or syntactic structure. No dictionary-like compilations illustrating standardized mime-gesture sequences for specific concepts are available. Also, there are no formal, generally accepted sets of rules for ordering mime gesture sequences.

The time and energy investments usually required for learning to use and comprehend mime do not appear to be excessive (see Table 1 in Levett,

1971). The level of acceptability of mime to at least some users and interpreters seems to be quite high (Balick, Spiegel, & Greene, 1976; Levett, 1971; Schlanger, 1976).

There are a number of books about mime as an art form that may provide information useful for teaching it. Also, the services of a professional mime can be useful both for training clients to use the technique and for training clinicians to teach it (Balick, Spiegel, & Greene, 1976). The theater department at a local college or university may be able to help you locate such a person.

Left-Hand Manual Alphabet

Aphasia resulting from a stroke, or CVA, usually is accompanied by right hemiplegia (this is because the left half of the cerebral cortex is dominant for speech for almost everyone). Persons who have this condition who were right-handed prior to their stroke probably would not have adequate control of the musculature of their right hand to use the American Manual Alphabet (see Figure 4.1). Chen (1968, 1971) has devised a left-hand manual alphabet for use by such persons (see Figure 4.4). His manual alphabet is more concrete than the American Manual Alphabet because the finger gestures used in it more closely approximate printed letters. This should make it easier for many aphasics to learn.

The linguistic and other characteristics of Chen's system appear to be the same as for the American Manual Alphabet (see section on Ameslan).

Limited Manual Sign Systems for Hospitals and Nursing Homes

Several limited manual sign systems have been developed for use with aphasic, dysarthric, and dysphonic adults. These systems are limited in the sense that they are intended primarily for communicating basic needs in a hospital or nursing home setting. The systems of Chen (1968, 1971), Eagleson, Jr., Vaughn, and Knudson (1970), and Goldstein and Cameron (1952) are representative.

Manual Shorthand. Chen (1968, 1971) has devised a gestural system for basic needs, that he refers to as manual shorthand, by combining letters from his left-hand manual alphabet (Figure 4.4) with other gestures. All gestures in this system can be made with the left hand. Needs that cannot be communicated by the manual shorthand can be spelled out using the left-hand manual alphabet. Chen refers to the combination of the manual shorthand and left-hand manual alphabet as the "talking hand" system.

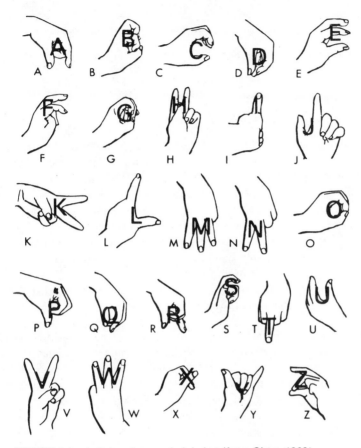

FIGURE 4.4. *Left-hand manual alphabet (from Chen, 1968).*

The following are included in Chen's manual shorthand system (Chen, 1971, pp. 381, 383):

O.K.—Make a sign of "O" and "K".
Water—Make a sign of "W" then point the finger to mouth.
Milk—Make a sign of "M" and then point the finger to mouth.
Tea—Make a sign of "T" and then point the finger to mouth.
Coffee—Make a sign of "C" and point the finger to mouth.
Juice—Make a sign of "J" and point the finger to mouth.
Open—Palm up and extend all fingers and then point to the object to be opened.

Close—Flex all fingers to make a fist and then point to the object to be closed.
Light on—Make a sign of "L" and then palm up with extend fingers.
Light off—Make a sign of "L" and then flex fingers to make a fist.
Too cold—Make a sign of "C" and put left hand at right shoulder and shrug the shoulders.
Too hot—Make a sign of "H" and then wipe the forehead with left hand.
Thirsty—Make a sign of "T" and "H" and then point the finger to mouth.
Pain—Make a sign of "P" and then point to the site of pain.
Urinal—Make a sign of "U." with
Bedpan—Make the sign of "B" and "P."
Bathroom—Make the sign of "B" and "R."

Chen used his "talking hand" system with aphasic, dysarthric, and dysphonic patients. Approximately 50 percent were "able to learn all the manual alphabet and to communicate using manual shorthand or to spell out any word that . . . [they] wanted" (Chen, 1971, p. 383). Results were poorest for aphasics, particularly sensory aphasics. While Chen does not report outcome data for the manual shorthand separately, it seems reasonable to assume that the success rate would be higher for it than for the entire system.

This system probably would be usable in at least some hospital and nursing home settings. Training patients to use it and staff to interpret it should not involve much of a time or energy investment in most cases (see Chen, 1968, 1971 for relevant data).

Manual Self-Care Signals. Eagleson, Jr., Vaughn, and Knudson (1970) devised twelve self-care signals for use as an interim communication system for expressive aphasics who have right hemiplegia (see Figure 4.5). All can be made with the left hand. They attempted to teach the signals to thirty-one expressive aphasics, and felt they were successful in all cases.

This system, like the previous one, probably would be usable in at least some hospital and nursing home settings. The training required to teach patients to use it and staff to interpret it should be minimal. An enlarged copy of Figure 4.5 could be attached to the patient's bed or wheelchair to facilitate his and the staff's use of the system.

Hand Talking Chart. Goldstein and Cameron (1952) have devised a set of 20 self-care hand signals. They are reproduced on a chart (see Figure 4.6) that also functions as a communication board. A copy of the chart is given to the patient. He uses it to learn the hand signals and to communicate by pointing to the letters of the words in his message with his left hand (assuming he has a right hemiplegia). The chart also is used by physicians, nurses, family members, and others to interpret his hand signals. All can be made with the left hand. The system is reported to have been used successfully with more than 200 aphasics (Goldstein & Cameron, 1952).

This system, like the previous two, should be usable in at least some hospital and nursing home settings. The training required to teach patients to

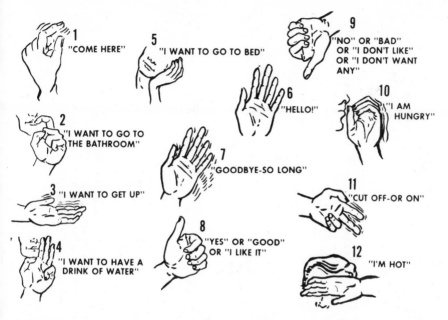

FIGURE 4.5. *Manual self-care signals (from Eagleson, Jr., Vaughn, & Knudson, 1970).*

use it and staff to interpret it should be minimal, in part because of the presence of the chart. Making the chart large (e.g., 1 ft. by 2 ft.) may facilitate its use by patients who have visual acuity problems.

Gestures for "Yes" and "No"

It is extremely important for any nonvocal patient, child or adult, to develop reliable gestural signals for yes and no as quickly as possible. Once these signals are developed the patient can communicate *by answering questions* (assuming his or her ability to understand speech is relatively intact). The strategy used frequently to facilitate such communication is similar to that of the game known as *twenty questions*. After a patient indicates he wants something, he is asked a series of questions beginning with the carrier phrase "Do you want _____?" The questioning continues until he signals yes. While this is obviously not a highly efficient communication strategy, it may be the only one that can be used with some patients who are severely involved motorically.

A second reason why it may be important for a patient to develop reliable yes and no signals is to make it possible for him to use a communication board with a scanning response mode. (The use of scanning response modes with communication boards is dealt with in Chapter 5.)

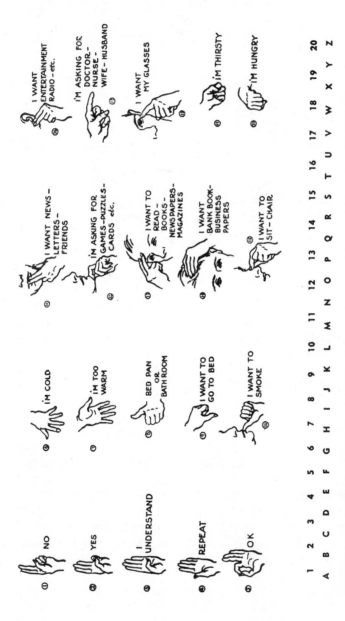

FIGURE 4.6. Hand talking chart (from Goldstein and Cameron, 1952). The sign language in the designs speaks for itself. The figures and letters across the bottom are independent of the designs. By pointing with pencil or finger to the letters or figures needed to further a conversation, communication between patient and friend can be amplified even to the "dictation" of a letter by the patient who otherwise would remain completely inarticulate.

NO ①

YES ②

I UNDERSTAND ③

REPEAT ④

OK ⑤

I'M COLD ⑥

I'M TOO WARM ⑦

BED PAN OR BATH ROOM ⑧

I WANT TO GO TO BED ⑨

I WANT TO SMOKE ⑩

I WANT NEWS — LETTERS — FRIENDS ⑪

I'M ASKING FOR GAMES — PUZZLES — CARDS etc. ⑫

I WANT TO READ — BOOKS — NEWSPAPERS — MAGAZINES ⑬

I WANT BANK BOOK — BUSINESS PAPERS ⑭

I WANT TO SIT — CHAIR ⑮

I WANT ENTERTAINMENT RADIO — etc. ⑯

I'M ASKING FOR DOCTOR — NURSE — WIFE — HUSBAND ⑰

I WANT MY GLASSES ⑱

I'M THIRSTY ⑲

I'M HUNGRY ⑳

1 2 3 4 5 6 7 8 9 10 11 12 13 14 15 16 17 18 19 20
A B C D E F G H I J K L M N O P Q R S T U V W X Y Z

The term "reliable" has two meanings when applied to gestural signals for yes or no. First, it refers to the patient's use of them. He must signal yes when he means yes and signal no when he means no. Some patients, particularly aphasics, may not signal yes and no reliably. And second, it refers to the observer's interpretation of them. They must be distinctive enough for an observer to reliably perceive their presence and different enough for him to reliably differentiate between them. Obviously, if an observer cannot detect when a patient is attempting to answer a question or determine whether his answer is yes or no, reliable communication is impossible.

How might a patient signal yes and no gesturally? Any two gestures are usable for this purpose so long as they can be produced and interpreted reliably. Those that have been used include:

> 1. moving head from side to side for a no and up and down for a yes (This set of signals, if usable, is the most satisfactory because its meaning is universally understood.);
> 2. turning head to the right for a yes and to the left for a no (Carlson, 1976);
> 3. directing gaze to the right for a yes and to the left for a no;
> 4. blinking right eye for a yes and left eye for a no;
> 5. blinking once for a no and twice for a yes; and
> 6. forming a fist with the thumb pointed up for a yes and pointed down for a no (see Figure 4.5).

An attention-getting sign describing the patient's yes and no signals should be attached to his bed, wheelchair, or both.

Eye Blink Encoding

A person may be able to communicate a few basic needs by means of an eye-blink encoding system (Adams, 1966). A specific number of eye blinks would signal a particular need. One such system (which was adapted from that illustrated in Figure 4.5) is the following:

Number of Eye Blinks	Meaning
1	No
2	Yes
3	I want to go to the bathroom.
4	I want a drink of water.
5	I am hungry.
6	I am uncomfortable.

Cards describing the system would be placed where they could be seen by the patient and the person with whom he is attempting to communicate. A phonatory grunting could be used in such a system instead of an eye blink (Adams, 1966).

Gestural Morse Code

The Morse code, which encodes letters and digits in dots and dashes (see Table 4.3), can be used as a gestural communication mode. Dots and dashes can be signaled gesturally in several ways, including:

> producing a single gesture at two durations (e.g., a brief eye blink for a dot and one approximately twice as long for a dash) and
> producing two gestures—one signaling a dot and the other a dash (e.g., a blink of the left eye signaling a dot, and one of the right eye a dash).

In addition to serving by itself as a gestural communication system, Morse code can be used with switching mechanisms to activate such displays as electric typewriters. (This application of Morse code is dealt with in Chapter 5.)

TABLE 4.3.   The international Morse code.

Symbol	Code	Symbol	Code
A	. -	V	. . . -
B	- . . .	W	. - -
C	- . - .	X	- . . -
D	- . .	Y	- . - -
E	.	Z	- - . .
F	. . - .	1	. - - - -
G	- - .	2	. . - - -
H	. . . .	3	. . . - -
I	. .	4	. . . . -
J	. - - -	5	. . . . .
K	- . -	6	- . . . .
L	. - . .	7	- - . . .
M	- -	8	- - - . .
N	- .	9	- - - - .
O	- - -	0	- - - - -
P	. - - .	Period	. - . - . -
Q	- - . -	Comma	- - . . - -
R	. - .	?	. . - - . .
S	. . .	Error	. . . .
T	-	Wait	. - . . .
U	. . -	End	. - . - .

For a person to use gestural Morse code it only is necessary that he be sufficiently intact neuromuscularly to produce a single muscle gesture at two rates or two muscle gestures at a single rate. Any gestures can be used so long as they can be made and interpreted reliably.

While Morse code can be used to convey any message to an observer who can interpret it, it is unintelligible to an untrained observer. The time and energy investment necessary for learning to use and interpret it should not be excessive, particularly if cards on which the code is reproduced are available to both users and interpreters while messages are being transmitted. The linguistic structure of a Morse code message, of course, is that of English.

The level of acceptability of Morse code communication to at least some potential users and interpreters probably would be fairly high since it only would be used with persons who are severely involved motorically and it would permit such persons to communicate.

Morse code would be a particularly viable communication medium for persons who had learned it prior to the onset of their condition. Patients who are FCC-licensed amateur radio operators, for example, should know the code because they would have had to learn it to be licensed.

Pointing

A person may be able to signal a need or desire by pointing to something related to it. This communication strategy tends to be used frequently by persons who do not have a formal communication system. Most point with either a hand or an eye (by directing gaze). While pointing, by itself, is a very limited communication system (since it only can be used to signal needs or desires that are related to something in the immediate environment), when it is combined with a communication board it can facilitate a relatively flexible communication system. (The use of pointing responses to indicate message components on communication boards is dealt with in Chapter 5.)

Which System to Use?

Salient features of more than ten gestural systems have been summarized in this chapter. These systems make different demands on users and interpreters, and vary in flexibility and efficiency. With whom would each be used, and when? The comments in this section are an attempt to partially answer this question. All circumstances under which each would be used of course are *not* indicated, and the uses indicated are not necessarily applicable to all persons in the populations mentioned. The names of the systems are printed in capital letters to facilitate locating comments about particular ones.

1. All functionally speechless persons should be taught GESTURES FOR

YES AND NO if they do not have them. This should be done regardless of the other communication systems they are going to be taught. One of the first goals of therapy for clients who do not have these gestures should be to teach them. Once a client can reliably signal yes and no, he or she can communicate by answering questions.

2. AMESLAN would be the most appropriate communication system for the client (child or adult) who needs a communication system that approaches speech in flexibility and efficiency providing that (1) he can learn the system and (2) at least some of the persons with whom he needs to communicate know it or will learn it.

3. For the client (child or adult) who needs a communication system that will allow him to communicate reasonably effectively with persons in his environment who have had little or no training in the system, AMERIND probably would be the most appropriate, providing he could learn it. While it is not as flexible a system as AMESLAN, AMERIND signs tend to be easier to learn because of their concreteness, and they are more intelligible than AMESLAN ones to untrained observers.

4. For the client, particularly the expressive aphasic with right hemiplegia, who needs an interim system for communicating basic needs while in a hospital or nursing home, the MANUAL SHORTHAND, MANUAL SELF-CARE SIGNALS, or HAND TALKING CHART should be usable.

5. The communication ability of almost any client who can spell, and who has at least one hand that is normal motorically, can be enhanced by teaching the AMERICAN MANUAL ALPHABET or the LEFT-HAND MANUAL ALPHABET. These manual alphabets can be used in combination with AMESLAN signs, AMERIND signs, or MIME.

6. MIME may be useful for *introducing* gestural communication to clients (particularly mentally retarded ones). It is more concrete than either AMESLAN or AMERIND, and is thus easier to learn. Once a client has developed a basic MIME vocabulary, AMESLAN or AMERIND signs can be introduced.

7. The *mild* quadriplegic whose use of his hands is not adequate for AMESLAN or AMERIND may find MIME to be a usable communication system.

8. The *moderate* or *severe* quadriplegic may find EYE BLINK ENCODING or GESTURAL MORSE CODE to be a usable communication system. The latter, of course, would be more flexible than the former.

9. It is desirable that a person who is going to use a communication board develop a POINTING gesture. This also is desirable if a person is going to use an electronic communication system. A POINTING gesture can be used to activate the switching mechanisms that control such systems. (Both uses of POINTING gestures are dealt with in Chapter 5.)

REFERENCES

ADAMS, M.R. Communication aids for patients with amyotrophic lateral sclerosis. *Journal of Speech and Hearing Disorders, 31,* 274-275 (1966).
American Indian Sign: Gestural Communication for the Speechless. A series of four videotapes (VC 1 PT. 1 - PT. 4) distributed by the Learning

Resources Center, Veterans Administration Hospital, St. Louis, Missouri (1974).

Amerind Video Dictionary. A series of four videotapes (VC 76 PT. 1 - PT. 4) distributed by the Learning Resources Center, Veterans Administration Hospital, St. Louis, Missouri (1975).

BADY, J.A., & SILVERMAN, F.H. A Videotape approach to teaching interpretation of Amerind Signs. *Perceptual and Motor Skills, 47,* 530 (1978).

BALICK, S., SPIEGEL, D., & GREENE, G. Mime in language therapy and clinician training. *Archives of Physical Medicine and Rehabilitation, 57,* 35-38 (1976).

BORNSTEIN, H. Signed English: A manual approach to English language development. *Journal of Speech and Hearing Disorders, 39,* 330-343 (1974).

CARLSON, F.L. *An adapted communication project for a nonspeaking child.* Paper presented at the 51st annual meeting of the American Speech and Hearing Association, Houston (1976).

CHEN, L.Y. Manual communication by combined alphabet and gestures. *Archives of Physical Medicine and Rehabilitation, 52,* 381-384 (1971).

––––––– . "Talking hands" for aphasic patients. *Geriatrics, 23,* 145-148 (1968).

DUNCAN, J.L., & SILVERMAN, F.H. Impacts of learning American Indian sign language on mentally retarded children: A preliminary report. *Perceptual and Motor Skills, 44,* 1138 (1977).

EAGLESON, H.M., JR., VAUGHN, G.R., & KNUDSON, A.B. Hand signals for dysphasia. *Archives of Physical Medicine and Rehabilitation, 51,* 111-113 (1970).

GOLDSTEIN, H., & CAMERON, H. New method of communication for the aphasic patient. *Arizona Medicine, 8,* 17-21 (1952).

LAKE, S.J. *The Hand-Book.* Tucson, Arizona: Communication Skill Builders (1976).

LEVETT, L.M. A method of communication for nonspeaking, severely subnormal children. *British Journal of Disorders of Communication, 4,* 64-66 (1969).

––––––– . A method of communication for nonspeaking severely subnormal children—Trial results. *British Journal of Disorders of Communication, 6,* 125-128 (1971).

LYKOS, C.M. *Cued Speech: Handbook for Teachers.* Washington, D.C.: Gallaudet College Cued Speech Program (1971).

OLSON, T. Return of the nonverbal. *Asha, 18,* 823 (1976).

PEI, M. *The Story of Language.* Philadelphia: J.B. Lippincott (1965).

SCHLANGER, P.H. *Training the adult aphasic to pantomime.* Paper presented at the 51st annual meeting of the American Speech and Hearing Association, Houston (1976).

SCHLANGER, P.H., GEFFNER, D.S., & DiCARRADO, C. *A comparison of ges-*

tural communication with aphasics: Pre- and post-therapy. Paper presented at the 49th annual meeting of the American Speech and Hearing Association, Las Vegas (1974).

SHANNON, C.E., & WEAVER, W. *The Mathematical Theory of Communication.* Urbana: University of Illinois Press (1963).

SKELLY, M. *Amer-Ind Gestural Code.* New York: Elsevier (1979).

SKELLY, M., SCHINSKY, L., SMITH, R., DONALDSON, R., & GRIFFIN, J. American Indian Sign: A gestural communication system for the speechless. *Archives of Physical Medicine and Rehabilitation, 56,* 156-160 (1975).

SKELLY, M., SCHINSKY, L., SMITH, R.W., & FUST, R.S. American Indian Sign (AMERIND) as a facilitator of verbalization for the oral verbal apraxic. *Journal of Speech and Hearing Disorders, 39,* 445-456 (1974).

STEIN, J. (Ed). *Random House Dictionary of the English Language.* New York: Random House (1966).

TOMKINS, W. *Indian Sign Language.* New York: Dover Publications (1969).

5 Gestural-assisted Modes

A number of representative nonspeech communication modes, or systems, that can be classified as gestural-assisted (see chapter 3 for definition) are described in this chapter. Those included were selected because they illustrate salient features of such systems. Information about other gestural-assisted communication systems can be obtained from the periodically updated *Master Chart of Communication Aids* published by the Trace Research and Development Center for Severely Communicatively Handicapped of the University of Wisconsin, Madison, and from the papers about gestural-assisted modes included in Appendix A of this book.

All gestural-assisted communications modes have three features:

1. a symbol system for encoding messages;
2. a display on which elements of the symbol system are reproduced (e.g., a television screen); and
3. a means of indicating (or reproducing) on the display in the appropriate sequence the elements of the symbol system that encode a message.

The displays used and the means of indicating symbols on a display tend to be different for electronic and nonelectronic systems. Those of each type are discussed separately for this reason. The symbol systems used for encoding messages with both types of systems are essentially the same. They are dealt with in the section that precedes the two describing the modes.

The description of each electronic and nonelectronic gestural-assisted mode includes the following information:

1. its components;
2. the manner in which its components are assembled;
3. its portability, cost, and commercial availability;
4. sources of plans and components;
5. neuromuscular functions that must be intact for it to be usable;

6. the time and energy investment required to learn to use it;
7. its level of acceptability to users and interpreters;
8. the speed at which messages can be communicated with it; and
9. the populations with which it has been used.

Specific applications of the symbol systems and communication modes that are described are indicated at the end of the chapter.

Symbol System

A symbol system is a set of sensory (visual, auditory, or tactile) images, or signs, that suggest, or stand for, something else by reason of relationship (association) or convention. Visual signs that singly or in combination can function as symbols include photographs, drawings, Blissymbolics, rebuses, Yerkes lexigrams, printed words, and tokens (e.g., plastic symbols used in the Non-SLIP program). Auditory signs that can serve this function include both phoneme sequences (e.g., synthesized speech) and noise sequences (e.g., patterned bursts of noise used for communication by Morse code). Tactile signs that can serve it include the raised-dot configurations of the Braille alphabet.

A sign can function as a symbol because of a *structural relationship* (isomorphism) between it and what it symbolizes, or by reason of *convention* (it being assigned a particular meaning or meanings). A sign bears a structural relationship to its referent (or is isomorphic to its referent) if it is somehow similar to it in appearance, or is somehow associated with (or suggestive of) it, or both of these. A drawing of a house can serve as a symbol for the concept *house* because it is similar in appearance to this referent. A photograph of a person who looks unhappy can serve as a symbol for the concept *pain* because it is suggestive of this meaning. And a drawing of a person drinking something can serve as a symbol for the concept *thirsty* because it is both similar in appearance to and suggestive of this referent.

Many signs function as symbols because of convention. Any sign can have any meaning that all (or an influential group) of those who use it wish it to have. Conventional signs usually are not related to their referents by appearance or association. Examples are words and some types of pictographs (e.g., Yerkes symbols).

The description of each symbol system includes information concerning the following:

1. its intelligibility to untrained observers;
2. its ability to convey messages concerning the "here and now";
3. its ability to convey messages not concerned with the "here and now";
4. its ability to convey abstract concepts;
5. its syntactic and semantic structure;

6. the similarity of its linguistic structure to English;
7. the time and energy investment required to learn to use and interpret it; and
8. the populations with which it has been used.

Photographs and Drawings

Photographs and drawings are used frequently with persons who cannot speak, write, or read English as a symbol system for communicating basic needs. Users include functionally speechless children and adults who (1) have not learned to read, (2) are dyslexic because of cortical damage, and (3) are able to read one or more languages, but not English. (A patient in a hospital or nursing home who is unable to speak or write English could use such a symbol system for communicating basic needs to the staff.)

Sets of pictures used as symbols in gestural-assisted communication schemes vary on several dimensions, including size, level of abstraction, degree of complexity, degree of ambiguity, and number of messages that can be encoded. Pictures used as symbols should be large enough to be seen by both users and interpreters, but no larger than necessary—so that the display on which they appear can be kept as small as possible. Picture size is a particularly important variable when users or interpreters have visual acuity or visual field disturbances or when the display is located at a distance from them.

The *level of abstraction* of a picture is a function of the amount of detail (or information) present in the object or event depicted that is included in the picture. The more detail (or information) omitted, the higher the level of abstraction. Suppose you wanted a picture for a communication board to which a patient could point to indicate that she is thirsty. The following pictures, which are ordered from relatively high level of abstraction to relatively low level of abstraction, might be used for this purpose:

a line drawing of a woman drinking from a glass;
a line drawing of a woman drinking from a glass that resembles the one the patient uses;
a black and white photograph of a woman drinking from a glass that resembles the one the patient uses;
a color photograph of a woman drinking from a glass that resembles the one the patient uses; and
a color photograph of the patient drinking from the glass she uses.

There are, of course, many more gradations possible here than the five described; these were selected solely to illustrate what is meant by the abstraction continuum.

Is the level of abstraction an important consideration when selecting picture symbols for gestural-assisted communication systems? It appears to be, particularly for patients who have cortical damage. Some patients who have such lesions tend to exhibit what has been referred to as abstract-con-

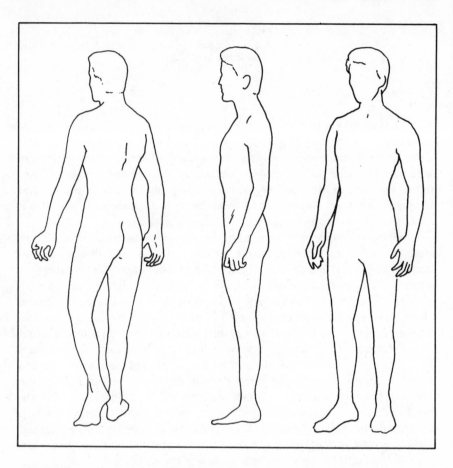

FIGURE 5.1. *Line drawings of back, side, and front of body on which sites of pain can be indicated by pointing.*
(Photo courtesy of Cleo Living Aids, Cleveland, Ohio)

crete imbalance (Wepman, 1951). They are more concrete than normal in their conceptual functioning. Consequently, they have more difficulty than usual in recognizing relatively abstract representations of objects and events. They might not, for example, recognize a line drawing of a glass. Persons with abstract-concrete imbalance also tend to have more difficulty than is usual with categorization. They may fail to perceive the abstract quality which results in objects and events that do not look alike being assigned to the same category. They do not abstract similarities and ignore differences as much as most people do. Consequently, they may not realize that by pointing to a photograph of a glass that does not look like the one they use they can communicate that they wish to drink from their glass.

The first pictures that are used as symbols with patients who have cortical damage should be as concrete as possible. For a picture symbol to which a patient who has this condition can point to indicate he is thirsty, you might use a Polaroid photograph of him drinking from his glass. Its use should place only a minimal demand on his abilities to recognize and categorize objects and events. It does place some demand on these abilities because he would have to recognize that a two-dimensional, static representation of a three-dimensional, dynamic event can portray, or symbolize, that event.

Following a period of therapy, spontaneous recovery, or both, it may be possible for a patient to utilize more abstract picture stimuli as symbols than those he was able to use initially. Increasing the abstraction level of picture stimuli, of course, should be done in relatively small steps.

The *degree of complexity* of a picture is partially a function of the extent to which its foreground stands out from its background. The foreground of a picture is the part that has symbol value—that is, the part that is necessary for

FIGURE 5.2. *Line drawings of back, side, and front of body superimposed on a matrix on which sites of pain can be indicated by linear scanning (see section on scanning in this chapter).*
(Body drawings courtesy of Cleo Living Aids, Cleveland, Ohio)

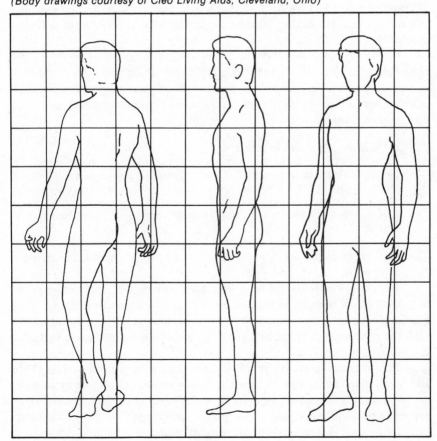

encoding the concept that the picture is intended to communicate. All other details or lines in a picture would constitute its background. The greater the separation between foreground and background, the lower the level of complexity. A photograph of a patient drinking from a glass (intended for encoding "thirsty") that was taken against a white background probably would be less complex than one of the same person drinking from the same glass with kitchen cupboards in the background. It is desirable to keep the level of complexity of picture symbols as low as is practical. (Backgrounds of photographs can be deemphasized by spraying them with a light coating of white watercolor paint using an airbrush. A frisket material can be used to cover foreground objects while the paint is being sprayed.)

The *degree of ambiguity* of a picture is a function of the number of concepts it could be used to encode. The more meanings that could reasonably be assigned to it, the greater its ambiguity. A picture of a person sitting at a kitchen table that has a glass of milk on it could be used to encode a number of concepts, including drink, milk, person, kitchen, sit, and table. It is, of course, desirable to select picture symbols that would have only the desired meaning to most persons. (Reducing complexity, incidentally, is one way of reducing ambiguity.)

The dimensions that have been discussed thus far are relevant to *individual* pictures. A dimension that applies to *sets* of pictures is the *number of messages* that can be encoded. Some sets can encode more messages than others. There are several factors that influence the number of messages a set of pictures can encode, including:

the number of pictures in the set;
the possibility of message expansion by agglutination (e.g., pointing to a picture of a glass and a picture of a carton of milk to encode a glass of milk); and
the possibility of combining concepts encoded by several pictures into an utterance (e.g., pointing to a picture of a person carrying something, a picture of a milk carton, and a picture of a glass to encode the message "Bring me a glass of milk").

The smallest set of pictures should be selected by which necessary messages can be encoded.

Picture symbols should be intelligible to untrained observers, particularly if an effort is made to minimize their complexity and ambiguity. Any question regarding their intelligibility can be eliminated by printing above each the concept it is intended to encode (assuming the observers can read English).

Pictures usually are better suited for encoding messages about the "here and now" than the past or future. The ability of a set of picture symbols to encode messages about the past and future can be enhanced by including in it a picture that would signal past time (e.g., a caveman) and one that would signal future time (e.g., a space colony on another planet.).

Pictures are better suited for encoding concrete than abstract concepts, but they can be used for encoding both. The more abstract a concept, the more ambiguous a picture depicting it tends to be. (Pictures suitable for encoding many relatively abstract concepts can be found in the *Peabody Picture Vocabulary* Test—Dunn, 1959—and other picture tests of receptive-language functioning.)

The linguistic structure of a message encoded in picture symbols usually differs from one encoded in English on morphological, syntactic, and semantic levels. Pictures depicting specific morphemic forms in English (e.g., singular vs. plural) usually are not used; appropriate English morphemic forms are inferred from context. Also, the ordering of picture symbols in a message does not necessarily correspond to that for English words. (A message encoded in picture symbols, though, may have a subject-predicate form—pictures that encode a noun and a verb may be used together.) In addition, picture symbols do not necessarily correspond to individual English words. A message encoded by a picture symbol may require two or more English words to encode. It may, in fact, be equivalent to an entire English utterance (e.g., pointing to a picture of someone drinking from a glass could be equivalent to, "I'm thirsty, I want a drink").

The time and energy investments required for learning to use and interpret picture symbols should be minimal, particularly if their levels of complexity and ambiguity are relatively low and the messages they are intended to encode are printed above them.

What picture symbols should be included in the set intended for a particular child or adult? While this would be partially determined by his environment (home, hospital, etc.) and specific communication needs, many of the following picture symbols probably should be included:

Picture	*Message Encoded*
Person eating	I am hungry.
Person drinking	I am thirsty.
Person sleeping	I am tired.
Person near fire	I am too warm.
Person sitting on ice	I am too cold.
Smiling face	I am happy.
Sad face	I am unhappy.
Bedpan, urinal, toilet	I want (bedpan, urinal, toilet).
Television set	I want the TV turned on (or off).
Nurse	I want a nurse.
Doctor	I want a doctor.
Photographs of family members	I want (family member).
Wheelchair	I want my wheelchair.
Eyeglasses, dental plates or hearing aid	I want my eyeglasses (dental plate, hearing aid).
Pills, hypodermic needle	I want my medication.
Book, magazine	I want to read.
Pencil, pen	I want to write.

Pictures of foods the person   I want_____to eat.
  might want to eat
Pictures of things the person   I want_____to drink.
  might want to drink, e.g.,
  water and coffee
Caveman   Past (time)
Spaceship   Future (time)
Line drawings of front, back,   My _____hurts.
  and side of body on which person
  can indicate where he hurts by
  pointing (see Figure 5.1) or
  scanning (see Figure 5.2)

English (or another language)

If the user of a gestural-assisted communication system and those with whom he intends to communicate can read English (or another language), this probably would be the most advantageous symbol system for them to use. It can encode as many messages as any of the other symbol systems mentioned in this section. In fact, it can be used to transmit any message if the sender can accurately spell the words used and the receiver can read them. In addition, if the sender can spell fairly well, it requires a smaller number of symbols for encoding a given number of messages (as long as this number exceeds 36) than any of the other symbol systems. An English symbol system usually would contain a minimum of thirty-six elements—twenty-six letters and ten digits. While the digits are not essential, they increase the efficiency of the system. One consequence of needing only a small number of symbols is that they can be displayed in a relatively small area. This increases both the portability of a display and its usefulness to persons who have a restricted range of movement.

While an English-language message can be encoded with a symbol set containing as few as thirty-six elements, the use of such a set would be relatively inefficient because every word would have to be spelled out. For this reason, English symbol sets intended for gestural-assisted communication systems usually contain some frequently used words and phrases in addition to letters and digits. The words and phrases on the communication board reproduced in Figure 5.3 are representative of those included in such sets.

An English symbol system can be used by itself or combined with other symbol systems. If it is combined with another system, the English symbols may be printed above those of the other system (e.g., pictures or Blissymbolics) to assist observers in interpreting them, or they may be used to encode messages that cannot be encoded with the other system. The first mode of combining English with those of another system (Blissymbolics) is illustrated by the communication board reproduced in Figure 5.4 and the second by that reproduced in Figure 5.5

Either capital or lower-case letters can be used in displays. The letters should be large enough to be readable by both users and interpreters and in a

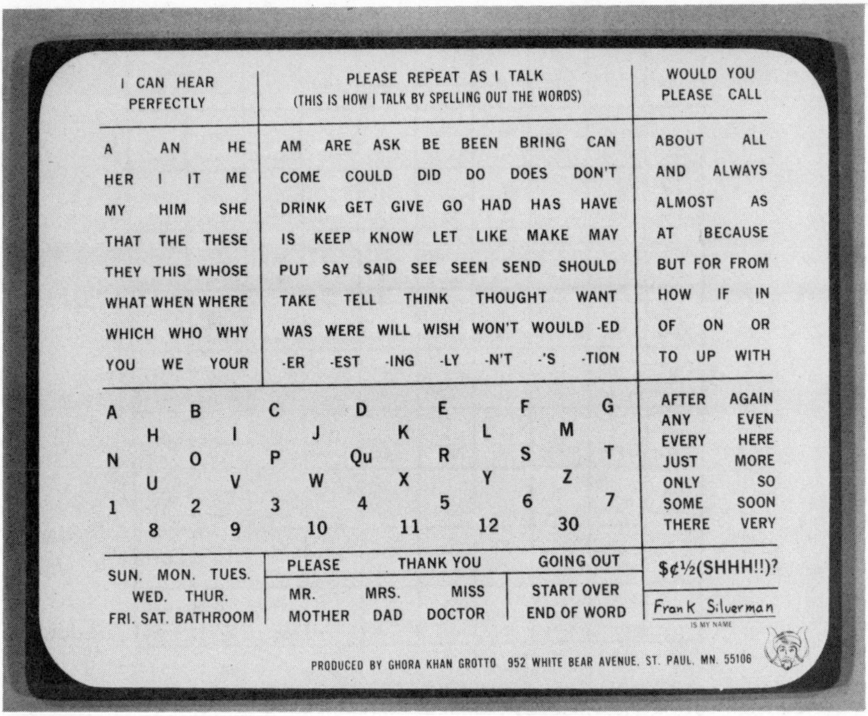

I CAN HEAR PERFECTLY	PLEASE REPEAT AS I TALK (THIS IS HOW I TALK BY SPELLING OUT THE WORDS)						WOULD YOU PLEASE CALL	
A AN HE	AM	ARE	ASK	BE	BEEN	BRING CAN	ABOUT	ALL
HER I IT ME	COME	COULD	DID	DO	DOES	DON'T	AND	ALWAYS
MY HIM SHE	DRINK	GET	GIVE	GO	HAD	HAS HAVE	ALMOST	AS
THAT THE THESE	IS	KEEP	KNOW	LET	LIKE	MAKE MAY	AT	BECAUSE
THEY THIS WHOSE	PUT	SAY	SAID	SEE	SEEN	SEND SHOULD	BUT FOR	FROM
WHAT WHEN WHERE	TAKE	TELL	THINK	THOUGHT		WANT	HOW IF	IN
WHICH WHO WHY	WAS	WERE	WILL	WISH	WON'T	WOULD -ED	OF ON	OR
YOU WE YOUR	-ER	-EST	-ING	-LY	-N'T	-'S -TION	TO UP	WITH

A	B	C	D	E	F	G	AFTER	AGAIN
H		I	J	K	L	M	ANY	EVEN
N		O	P	Qu	R	S	T	EVERY HERE
U		V	W	X	Y	Z	JUST	MORE
1		2	3	4	5	6	7	ONLY SO
8		9	10	11	12	30		SOME SOON
							THERE	VERY

SUN. MON. TUES. WED. THUR. FRI. SAT. BATHROOM	PLEASE THANK YOU GOING OUT MR. MRS. MISS START OVER MOTHER DAD DOCTOR END OF WORD	$¢½(SHHH!!)? Frank Silverman IS MY NAME

PRODUCED BY GHORA KHAN GROTTO. 952 WHITE BEAR AVENUE, ST. PAUL, MN. 55106

FIGURE 5.3. *Representative English language communication board. (Photo courtesy of the Ghora Kahn Grotto, St. Paul, Minnesota)*

relatively plain (unembellished) type style. The letters can be drawn with black ink, or black rub-on letters or vinyl letters can be used (both of which can be purchased at an art or stationery store).

English symbol systems can be used to convey any message. The only requirement is that users be able to spell the words they wish to encode and interpreters be able to read them.

Blissymbolics*

Blissymbolics (or Semantography) is a pictographic, ideographic writing system developed by Charles K. Bliss (Bliss, 1965) that can be read (decoded) in all languages. It was intended to function as an auxillary language system for written international communication. As such, it is one of a relatively large number of auxillary languages intended for international communication constructed during the past 500 years. None, with the possible exception of Esperanto, have been widely accepted even though few people seem to view learning such a language as undesirable. This may be partially because few people know they exist (see Silverman & Silverman,

*The Blissymbols illustrated herein are in accordance with B.C.I. approved symbols as of January, 1979. ©C.K. Bliss and exclusive worldwide licensee. Blissymbolics Communication Institute, Toronto, Canada.

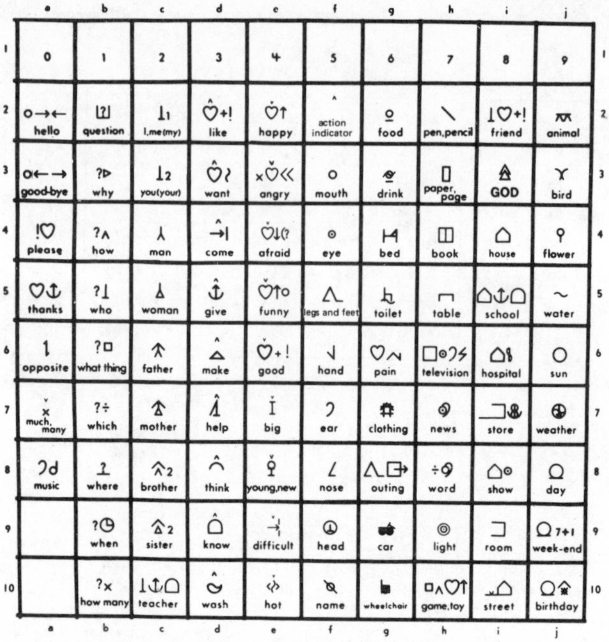

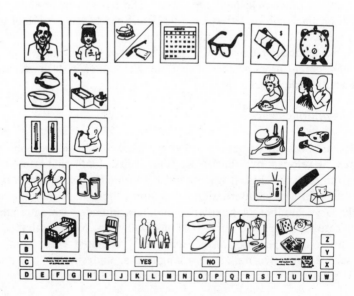

	a	b	c	d	e	f	g	h	i	j
1	0	1	2	3	4	5	6	7	8	9
2	hello	question	I,me(my)	like	happy	action indicator	food	pen,pencil	friend	animal
3	good-bye	why	you(your)	want	angry	mouth	drink	paper,page	GOD	bird
4	please	how	man	come	afraid	eye	bed	book	house	flower
5	thanks	who	woman	give	funny	legs and feet	toilet	table	school	water
6	opposite	what thing	father	make	good	hand	pain	television	hospital	sun
7	much, many	which	mother	help	big	ear	clothing	news	store	weather
8	music	where	brother	think	young,new	nose	outing	word	show	day
9		when	sister	know	difficult	head	car	light	room	week-end
10		how many	teacher	wash	hot	name	wheelchair	game,toy	street	birthday

FIGURE 5.4. *Representative Blissymbolics communication board.*
(Photo courtesy of Blissymbolics Communication Institute, Toronto, Ontario)

FIGURE 5.5. *Representative combined English-picture communication board.*
(Photo courtesy of Cleo Living Aids, Cleveland, Ohio)

1979). The Blissymbolics system has been adapted for use as a communication medium for prereading, nonvocal children (Kates & McNaughton, 1975; Archer, 1977; Silverman, McNaughton, and Kates, 1978).

The Blissymbol system consists of approximately 100 pictorial ideographic and arbitrary symbols that when used singly (see Figure 5.6 for the seventy most frequently used symbols according to C.K. Bliss) or when combined in various ways (see Figure 5.7) can encode almost any message. The structure of Blissymbols (see Figure 5.4) is comparable to that of printed ideographic Chinese characters. Bliss views his system as a *simplified* Chinese ideographic writing system. this ideographic system has been understood and used for thousands of years by persons living in China, who *do not speak a common language.*

Most Blissymbols encode information on a semantic, or meaning, level (a few encode grammatical information). Each symbol element represents a *general* ideal, or concept. This general idea, or concept, usually includes a *set* of related ideas, or concepts, that would be encoded in English (or another language) by more than one word. The symbol for *water* (see Figure 5.6) with the addition of other elements (see Figure 5.7) can mean rain, steam, snow, cloud, lake, ocean, freezing, thawing, hail, current, river, or cloudburst.

The *specific* concept, or idea, encoded by a Blissymbol is indicated by the manner in which it has been manipulated or modified. There are a number of ways that a symbol may be manipulated or modified to change its meaning, including those that follow (see Figure 5.7).

1. Agglutination (see Figure 5.7a). Symbols are combined by superimposing or sequencing elements to form compound symbols. The meaning of such a symbol can be inferred from the *meanings of its elements plus context.* If a cross out symbol, for example, is combined with the symbol for ear, the result would be a compound symbol that could encode the concept deaf. Likewise, if the symbols for person, mouth, and musical note are combined, the result would be a compound symbol that could encode the concept "singer."

Most symbols may have more than one interpretation. The meaning in a particular message usually can be inferred from context. Also, the English equivalent is almost certain to be printed with it. (Bliss insists that all reproductions of his symbols be accompanied by English or other language equivalents.)

2. Use of the Three Grammatical Class Indicators (see Figure 5.7b). A given Blissymbol can function as the English equivalent of a noun, verb, adverb, or adjective. Its grammatical class is specified by the indicator that appears above it. A *small square* (which indicates a "chemical THING") appearing above a symbol gives it a concrete *noun* meaning. A *small cone pointing upward* (which indicates a "physical ACTION") appearing above a symbol gives it a *verb* meaning. And a *small cone pointing downward* (which indicates a "human EVALUATION") appearing above a symbol gives it an *adjective* or

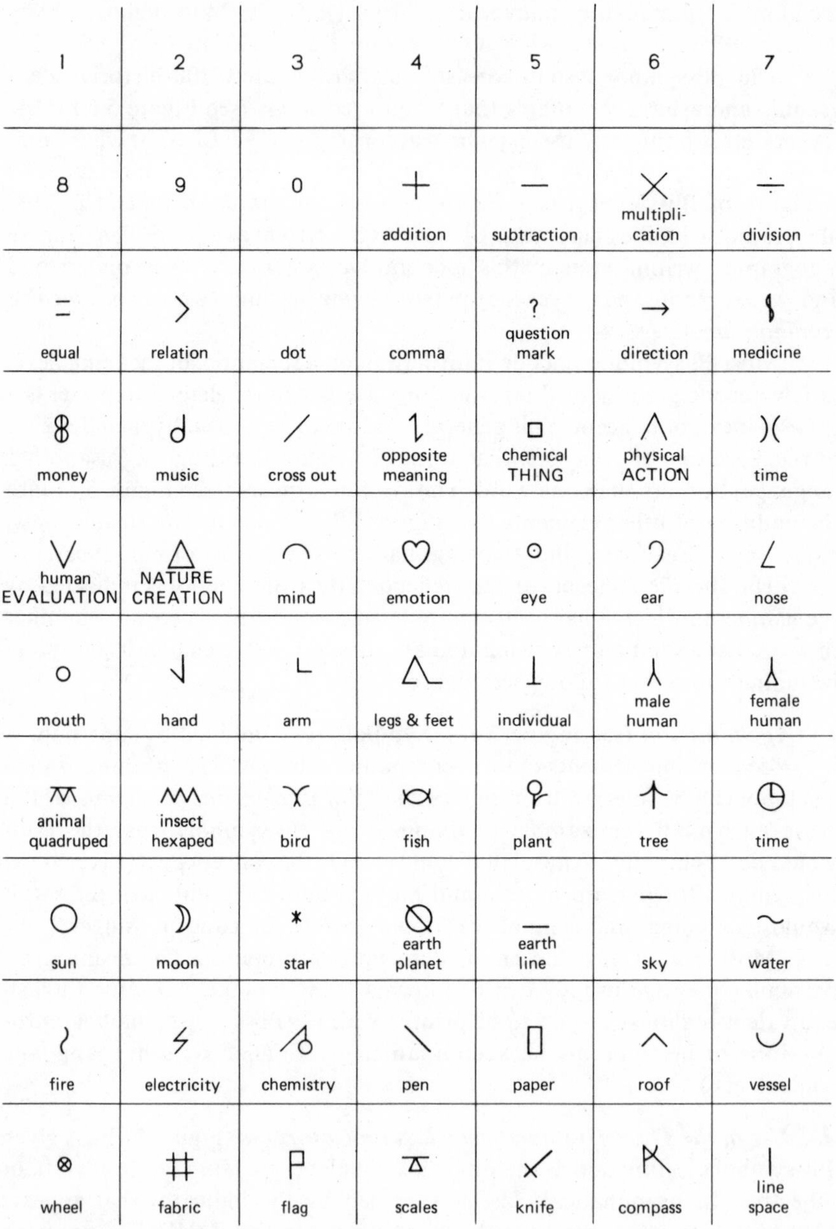

1	2	3	4	5	6	7
8	9	0	+ addition	— subtraction	✕ multipli- cation	÷ division
≝ equal	⟩ relation	dot	comma	? question mark	→ direction	∫ medicine
₿ money	♂ music	/ cross out	⌐ opposite meaning	□ chemical THING	∧ physical ACTION	)(time
∨ human EVALUATION	△ NATURE CREATION	⌒ mind	♡ emotion	⊙ eye	⌐ ear	∠ nose
○ mouth	√ hand	∟ arm	⌴ legs & feet	⊥ individual	⋋ male human	⋏ female human
ⱍ animal quadruped	Ɱ insect hexaped	⋎ bird	⋈ fish	⚲ plant	⋏ tree	◔ time
○ sun	☽ moon	* star	⊘ earth planet	— earth line	— sky	～ water
⟨ fire	⚡ electricity	⚗ chemistry	\ pen	▯ paper	∧ roof	∪ vessel
⊗ wheel	♯ fabric	⊓ flag	⟁ scales	✕ knife	⋉ compass	⎮ line space

FIGURE 5.6. *The main basic Blissymbol elements (from Bliss, 1965).*

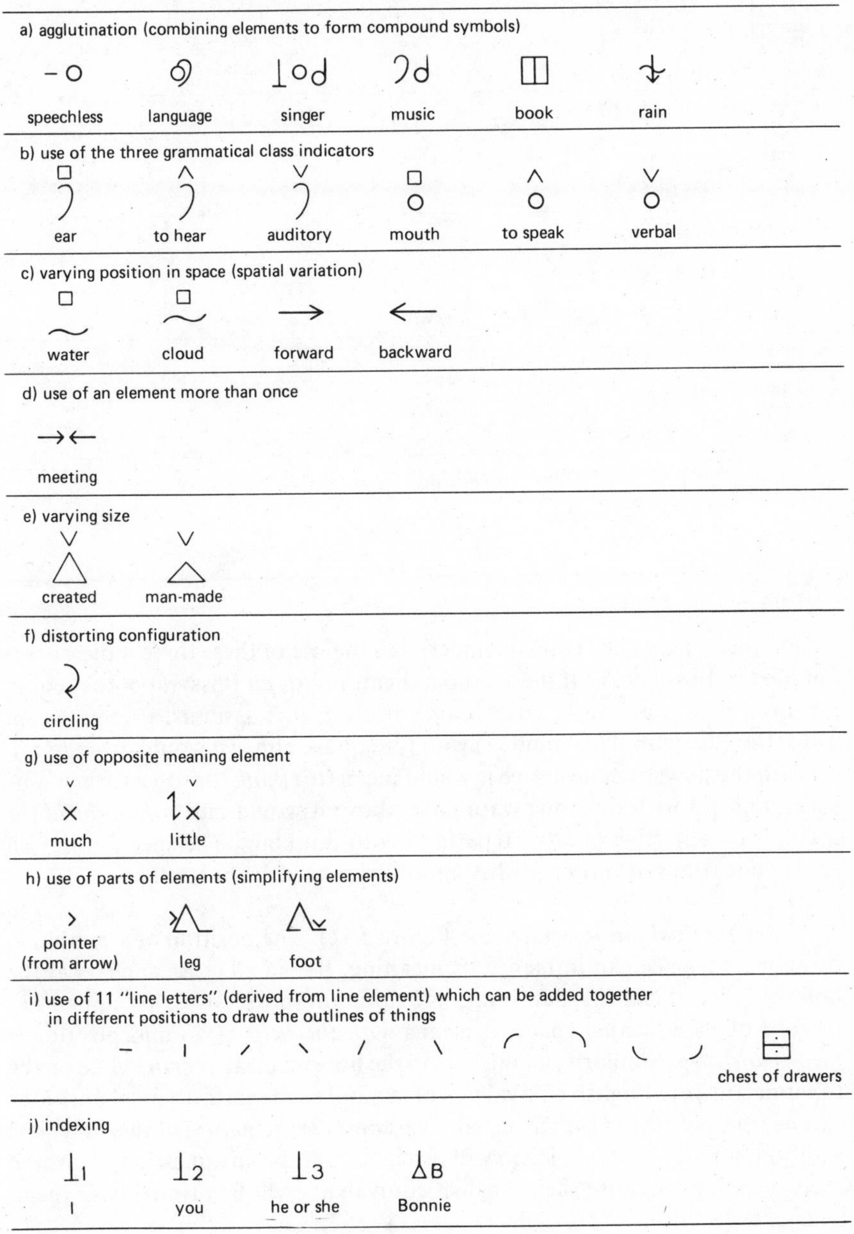

a) agglutination (combining elements to form compound symbols)

–o	⌒)	⊥od	)d	☐	⊥
speechless	language	singer	music	book	rain

b) use of the three grammatical class indicators

☐)	^)	˅)	☐○	^○	˅○
ear	to hear	auditory	mouth	to speak	verbal

c) varying position in space (spatial variation)

☐ ～	☐ ～	→	←
water	cloud	forward	backward

d) use of an element more than once

→←

meeting

e) varying size

˅ △	˅ △
created	man-made

f) distorting configuration

𝟤

circling

g) use of opposite meaning element

˅ ✕	˅ 𝟣✕
much	little

h) use of parts of elements (simplifying elements)

⟩	✕∧	∧～
pointer (from arrow)	leg	foot

i) use of 11 "line letters" (derived from line element) which can be added together in different positions to draw the outlines of things

— ∣ ╱ ╲ ╱ ╲ ⌐ ⌐ ∪ ⌣   ⊞

chest of drawers

j) indexing

⊥₁	⊥₂	⊥₃	∧B
I	you	he or she	Bonnie

FIGURE 5.7. *Strategies for vocabulary expansion by manipulation of Blissymbol elements.*

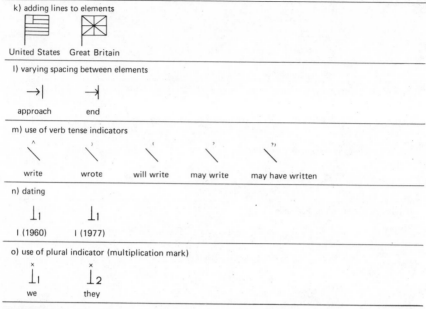

FIGURE 5.7. *(Cont.)*

adverb meaning. (The rationale underlying the use of these three indicators is outlined in Bliss, 1965.) If there is no indicator above a Blissymbol that could function as a noun, verb, adverb, or adjective, it is assumed to be a noun. Thus, the Blissymbol for mind (1) with the square above it would mean *brain*, (2) with the upward cone above it would mean (to) *think* (or some form of this verb), and (3) with the downward cone above it would mean *thoughtful* (or some other adjective or adverb pertaining to thinking). The specific English equivalent (translation) of a Blissymbol is inferred from context.

3. Varying Position in Space (see Figure 5.7c). The position of a symbol in its allocated space can influence its meaning. If a small cross appears at the *bottom* of its allocated space, it means *belongs to* (possessive); if it appears at the top of its allocated space, it means *with the help of;* in mid position it means *and also.* Similarly, a long line on the bottom means *earth*, while on the top it means *sky.* English equivalents of symbol elements in atypical positions can be inferred from (1) their usual meanings, (2) the nature of their atypical position, and (3) context. There will rarely, if ever, be any question regarding their meanings because their English equivalents will be printed with them.

4. Use of an Element More Than Once (see Figure 5.7d). The same element may appear in a compound symbol two or more times. It may appear each time in approximately the same position in its allocated space or in different positions in this space. The latter is illustrated in Figure 5.7d (the two arrows of *meeting* are pointing in opposite directions). The meaning of symbol elements that are used more than once in a compound symbol such as (to) *surprise* can be inferred from (1) their meaning when used alone, (2) the number used and their relationships to each other, and (3) context.

5. Varying Size (see Figure 5.7e). A given symbol may occur in more than one size, and the size in which it is drawn influences its meaning. A circle can be used to encode either *sun* or *mouth* depending on its size. The square can encode *enclosure* in full size, *thing* in a half size, and, in a quarter size, is used to designate a concrete noun. The meanings of symbol elements that are smaller or larger than normal can be inferred from (1) their meaning when a normal size, (2) how their size differs from normal, and (3) context.

6. Altering Configuration (see Figure 5.7f). The configuration of a symbol may be distorted in some manner (e.g., a straight line may be curved). Thus, curving the straight-line portion of the arrow (as in Figure 5.7f) changes its meaning from *down* to *turn*. The shape of *person* is visible in (to) *kneel*. The meanings of distorted symbol elements can be inferred from (1) their meanings when unaltered, (2) the nature and pictographic significance of the alteration, and (3) context.

7. Use of the Opposite Meaning Symbol (see Figure 5.7g). Placing the *opposite meaning* symbol (see Figure 5.6) before another symbol changes its meaning to the opposite of what it would be without it. Thus, placing an opposite meaning symbol before the symbol for (to) *love* changes its meaning to (to) *hate*; and the *opposite meaning* plus *much, many* becomes *few, little*.

8. Use of Parts of Symbols (see Figure 5.7h). A part of a symbol may appear in a compound symbol. The part will have either the same meaning as the entire symbol or a related meaning. The tip of the arrow (see Figure 5.7h) can be used as a *pointer* to indicate locations on other symbols. The location of the pointer determines the meaning of the *symbol*.

9. Use of Eleven "Line Letters" (see Figure 5.7i). There are eleven types of line segments (derived from the line element) that can be combined in different positions to draw the outlines of things. These segments are referred to as *line letters*. They can be used by themselves or combined with other symbol elements (e.g., the wheel element to outline a vehicle). Blissymbols formed from line letters are pictographic—their outlines indicate their meanings (see the *chest of drawers* in Figure 5.7i).

10. Indexing   (see Figure 5.7j). Digits can be used as subscripts with other symbols to indicate a specific subpopulation, or subset, of the objects or events referred to by them. (This strategy was adopted from General Semantics; see Korzybski, 1933.) The symbol for an individual (see Figure 5.6) with the subscript *1* means *I*, with the subscript *2* means *you*, and with the subscript *3* means *he* or *she*. Another type of indexing that is sometimes used is placing the *first letter* of the name of a person referred to after the symbol for man or woman.

11.   *Adding Lines to Elements* (see Figure 5.7k). Lines can be added to symbol elements to indicate pictographically a specific subpopulation, or subset, of the objects or events referred to by them (lines used in this manner perform the same function as indexing). Thus, *eye* plus the symbol for *cross out* means *blind*; the symbol for *air* plus the *forward* symbol (arrow) means *wind*.

12.   *Varying Spacing between Elements* (see Figure 5.7l). The amount of spacing between the elements in a compound symbol can influence its meaning. The combination of an arrow and a vertical line means *approach* if there is a space between the tip of the arrow and the line and *end* if there is no space between them.

13.   *Use of Verb Tense, Mood and Voice Indicators* (see Figure 5.7m). The tense of a Blissymbol (functioning as a verb) can be designated by placing the appropriate tense, mood or voice indicator above it. Verb indicators are small *time action* and *question mark* symbols (see Figure 5.6), used singly or in combination. The use of seven of them is illustrated in Figure 5.7m.

14.   *Use of the Plural Indicator* (see Figure 5.7o). The placement of a small multiplication sign above a Blissymbol functioning as a noun changes it from singular to plural. Thus, placing a multiplication sign above the Blissymbol for *I* changes its meaning to *we*, and *you* (singular) changes its meaning to *you* plural.

For further information about Blissymbols as a symbol system, see Bliss (1965, 1975), the film "Mr. Symbol Man" (Film Board of Canada), and for its application publications of the Blissymbolics Communication Institute, Toronto.*

Blissymbolics have been used since the early 1970s, originally as a symbol system for prereading children who were non-speaking due to physical handicaps. It is now being used by all ages with its use being explored for the mentally retarded, dysarthric (or both) and stroke victims (Vanderheiden, Brown, MacKenzie, Reinen, & Scheibel, 1975; McNaughton, 1976a, 1976b; Harris-Vanderheiden, 1976; *Ontario Crippled Children's Centre Symbol*

---

*In 1975, the Blissymbols Communication Institute was established to further the use and development of Blissymbols as a means of communication for individuals lacking fundamental speech.

Communication Programme, 1974; Olson, 1976; McNaughton & Kates, 1974; Kates & McNaughton, no date; Carlson, 1976). Their use with handicapped children originated at the Ontario Crippled Children's Centre. They have been used on communication boards (see Figure 5.4) and on the displays of electronic communication systems (these are described later in this chapter). They also have been used for writing stories and other narrative materials.

While Blissymbols by themselves would not be highly intelligible to many untrained observers, when they are used on communication boards and electronic displays they are highly intelligible to almost all such observers, because the English or other language equivalent of each Blissymbol is printed with it. Thus, to understand Blissymbols it is only necessary that the observer be able to read English or the other language.

Blissymbolics can be used to convey messages about the "here and now" as well as the past and the future. It can encode both abstract and concrete concepts. In fact, it can be used to encode such sophisticated material as poetry and the Bible.

The linguistic structure of Blissymbolics can be made compatible with that of English. The order of the Blissymbols in a sentence or utterance can correspond to that for English words. While the morphological structure of Blissymbolics differs from that of English, morphological variations in Blissymbolics have English equivalents. There are Blissymbols for most, if not all, English words that should be in the vocabulary of a prereading child.

A substantial time and energy investment appears necessary for a child to learn to use Blissymbolics as a communication medium. However, this investment appears to be *less* than would be required to achieve any given level of proficiency with written English. Children seem to be able to learn to comprehend pictographic, ideographic symbol systems such as Blissymbolics more easily than phonetically based ones such as written English.

The use of Blissymbolics appears to facilitate learning to read English. Children often acquire a sight vocabulary just through frequent exposure to the English words that are printed with the Blissymbols they use.

There are several dictionary-like compilations of Blissymbols. The most comprehensive is in Bliss's book *Semantography* (1965). The Blissymbolics Communication Institute (Toronto) has published a compilation of Blissymbols, *Blissymbols for Use,* that have been used with handicapped children.

Materials for teaching the Blissymbol system are distributed by the Blissymbolics Communication Institute, Toronto. Available materials include a *Handbook of Blissymbolics for Instructors, Users, Parents and Administrators,* the book *Symbol Secrets* (McNaughton, 1975), the film "Symbol Boy" (Film Board of Canada), "Say It with Symbols" (a series of teaching slides), and 100 Blissymbol stamps from which displays may be created to fit the needs of individual users. Displays can be used, with either electronic or nonelectronic indicating systems. These systems are described later in this chapter.

Rebuses

Rebuses are predominantly pictographic symbols (i.e., line drawings) that represent whole words or parts of words (see Figure 5.8). The object or event depicted in a rebus may indicate its *meaning* or how all or a part of the equivalent English word "sounds" (i.e., the phoneme sequence of the entire word or one or more of its syllables). The rebuses in Figure 5.8 for *boat* and *breakfast* are representative of the first type, and those for *bottleneck* and *boxer* of the second type. The part of a word represented by a drawing can be a morpheme. Thus, rebuses can have phonological, morphological, or semantic significance.

A rebus may consist of (1) a single drawing, (2) several drawings, or (3) a combination of letters of the alphabet and drawings. The rebuses in Figure 5.8 for *boot, bowl,* and *breakfast* are representative of the first type; those for *bookshelf, boyfriend,* and *breadboard* of the second type; and those for *boxer, brain,* and *breaker* of the third type.

Variants of root words (morphemic variations) usually are indicated by adding an appropriate English suffix to a rebus (see Figure 5.9). Those used include the following (paraphrased from Clark, Davies, & Woodcock, 1974, pp. 8-9):

1. adding an *s* to a rebus to indicate more than one (see Figure 5.9a);
2. adding an *'s* to a rebus to indicate the possessive case (see Figure 5.9b);
3. adding *s, ed,* or *ing* to a rebus for a verb to indicate its tense (see Figure 5.9c);
3. adding *er* or *est* to a rebus to indicate a comparative form (see Figure 5.9d); and
5. adding *y* or *ly* to a rebus to denote an adjective or adverb (see Figure 5.9e).

Special rebuses are used for irregular verbs and nouns that do not form the plural by adding *s*.

Rebuses are easier to learn and remember than spelled words (Clark, Davies, & Woodcock, 1974). Consequently, they have been used as an initial symbol system for teaching reading to both normal preschool children and mentally retarded children (Woodcock, 1958, 1965, 1968; Woodcock, Clark, & Davies, 1968, 1969). Also, they have been used with Ameslan (see Chapter 4) vocabulary in the MELDS (Minnesota Early Language Development Sequence) Program to facilitate the development of language skills in children who use Ameslan (Clark, Moore, & Woodcock, 1973). In addition, because they are easier to decode than spelled words, they have been used as a symbol system on communication boards intended for persons who are aphasic or have a neuromuscular disorder and are unable to read adequately (Clark, Davies, & Woodcock, 1974).

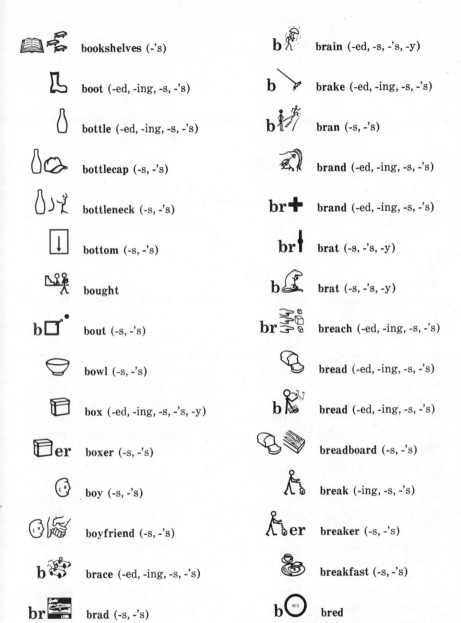

bookshelves (-'s)

boot (-ed, -ing, -s, -'s)

bottle (-ed, -ing, -s, -'s)

bottlecap (-s, -'s)

bottleneck (-s, -'s)

bottom (-s, -'s)

bought

bout (-s, -'s)

bowl (-s, -'s)

box (-ed, -ing, -s, -'s, -y)

boxer (-s, -'s)

boy (-s, -'s)

boyfriend (-s, -'s)

brace (-ed, -ing, -s, -'s)

brad (-s, -'s)

brain (-ed, -s, -'s, -y)

brake (-ed, -ing, -s, -'s)

bran (-s, -'s)

brand (-ed, -ing, -s, -'s)

brand (-ed, -ing, -s, -'s)

brat (-s, -'s, -y)

brat (-s, -'s, -y)

breach (-ed, -ing, -s, -'s)

bread (-ed, -ing, -s, -'s)

bread (-ed, -ing, -s, -'s)

breadboard (-s, -'s)

break (-ing, -s, -'s)

breaker (-s, -'s)

breakfast (-s, -'s)

bred

FIGURE 5.8. *Representative rebuses (from Clark, Davies, and Woodcock, 1974). (Drawing courtesy of American Guidance Service, Inc., Circle Pine, Minnesota)*

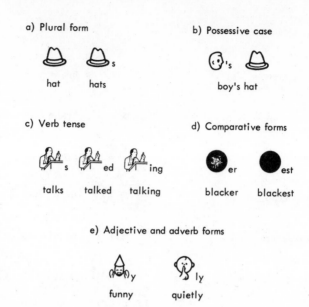

a) Plural form

hat   hats

b) Possessive case

boy's hat

c) Verb tense

talks   talked   talking

d) Comparative forms

blacker   blackest

e) Adjective and adverb forms

funny   quietly

FIGURE 5.9. *Representative morphemic variations of rebuses (from Clark, Davies, and Woodcock, 1974, pp. 8-9). (Drawing courtesy of American Guidance Service, Inc., Circle Pine, Minnesota.)*

Rebuses can be used in several ways with gestural-assisted communication systems. First, they can be used alone (not combined with symbols of another system). Second, they can be combined with English word equivalents. (The English word equivalent of a rebus could be printed below it, as is done with Blissymbols.) And third, they can be combined with English words that are not equivalents of the rebuses used. Rebuses would be substituted for English words that the person using the system could not read. (Presumably, the rebuses would be replaced by English word equivalents once he or she could read them.)

Most rebuses should be intelligible to untrained observers even without English word equivalents printed below them. Of course, if they are printed below them, messages encoded in rebuses would be intelligible to any observer who could read English.

Rebuses can be used to encode messages concerning the "here and now" as well as the past and future. Also, they can be used to encode both abstract and concrete concepts.

The morphological, syntactic, and semantic structures of messages encoded in rebuses can be made to correspond to those encoded in English. Messages can, in fact, be encoded with a combination of rebuses and English words.

The time and energy investments ordinarily required to learn to decode rebuses appears to be minimal. In one study (Woodcock, 1958) the subjects (children) took only thirty to forty-five minutes to learn the meanings of seventy-two rebuses.

A dictionary-like compilation of rebuses is available (Clark, Davies, & Woodcock, 1974). In it are rebuses for more than 2,000 alphabetically listed words, including those for almost all the objects and events one may wish to symbolize on a communication board. There are no restrictions on the right to reproduce and use the rebuses in this publication other than making appropriate acknowledgment of their source, since they are not copyrighted. (The rebuses in this compilation are available in rub-on form from American Guidance Service, Circle Pines, Minnesota. Being available in this form can facilitate their use on communication boards and other displays.)

Yerkish Language (LANA Lexigrams)

The Yerkish lexigram language was developed by Ernst von Glaserfeld (1977) for the LANA Project (LANA is an acronym for Language Analogue Project as well as being the name of a young chimpanzee) of the Yerkes Regional Research Center (see Rumbaugh, 1977, for a detailed description of the Project). The purpose of the project was to develop a computer-based language-training system for investigating the ability of chimpanzees to acquire language. The LANA technology, including Yerkish lexigrams (with different meanings than those for chimpanzees), has been used as a communication medium for persons who are severely or profoundly retarded and have no functional speech (Parkel, White, & Warner, 1977). A portable electronic conversation board has been developed that utilizes LANA lexigrams for encoding messages (Warner, Bell, & Brown, 1977).

The Yerkish language consists of nine design elements (see Figure 5.10) that when used singly and in combinations of two, three, and four yield 255 different lexigrams (von Glaserfeld, 1977). See Figure 5.10 for representative lexigrams. The design elements used were selected because they were readily discernable from each other, could be superimposed on one another, and once superimposed, would yield combinations that were still discernable (von Glaserfeld, 1977). Lexigrams are reproduced with one of seven background colors; the color-coding categorizes the lexigrams on the basis of meaning (e.g., a green background designates lexigrams that can encode a part of the body).

Each Yerkish lexigram has only one meaning, and this meaning almost always corresponds to that of an English word (the English equivalents of a few lexigrams are phrases. The meaning assigned to a Yerkish lexigram usually is not associated with its configuration in any way. Thus, Yerkish lexigrams differ from Blissymbols and rebuses in not being pictographic. They are similar to them, though, in being ideographic.

Yerkish lexigrams can be combined to form utterances. Most Yerkish utterances are between three and seven lexigrams in length. The ordering of lexigrams in an utterance corresponds generally to that for English words.

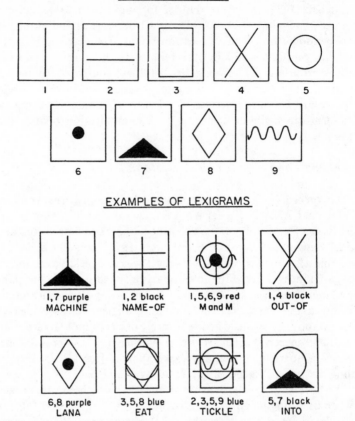

DESIGN ELEMENTS

1	2	3	4	5

6	7	8	9

EXAMPLES OF LEXIGRAMS

1,7 purple MACHINE	1,2 black NAME-OF	1,5,6,9 red M and M	1,4 black OUT-OF

6,8 purple LANA	3,5,8 blue EAT	2,3,5,9 blue TICKLE	5,7 black INTO

FIGURE 5.10. *Yerkish (LANA) design elements and representative lexigrams (from Von Glaserfeld. 1977, Table 2).*
(Drawing courtesy of Academic Press, Inc.)

The following are English equivalents of four representative Yerkish utterances (from von Glaserfeld, 1977):

> Please Tim make window open.
> ? Tim make machine give coke.
> This piece of apple black.
> Lana want apple.

For an in-depth description of Yerkish syntax, see von Glasersfeld's 1977 paper.

Since Yerkish lexigrams are conventional symbols (i.e., have assigned meanings), they are not intelligible to untrained observers. They were designed for conveying a relatively small number of relatively concrete messages concerning the "here and now." The time and energy investments required for adults to learn to decode messages encoded in Yerkish should not be very great, but the investments required to teach it to severely and profoundly retarded children could be considerable.

When this chapter was written, insufficient data were available to assess the potential of Yerkish as a symbol system for gestural-assisted communication modes. While it is reasonable to inquire whether the fact that it can be mastered by a chimpanzee indicates it is within the ability range of a mentally retarded child, it is not necessarily safe to assume that the language potential of a brain-damaged child is similar to that of a neurologically intact chimpanzee (Mayberry, 1976).

Premack-Type Plastic Word Symbols

David Premack, to investigate the ability of the chimpanzee to learn several aspects of human language ("reading and writing"), designed a symbol system consisting of pieces of plastic, each representing a specific word (Premack, 1970, 1971; Premack & Premack, 1972, 1974). The plastic symbols varied in color, shape, and size. Each was backed with metal so that it would adhere to a magnetic board. Sentences were "written" by arranging symbols vertically on the magnetic board in the proper sequence from top to bottom.

Premack's symbols are ideographic, but not pictographic. Each stands for a specific word or concept, but its configuration is not related to (or suggestive of) the word or concept it represents. (These symbols, therefore, are conventional symbols because their meanings are assigned.) The syntactic rules for sequencing these symbols were adopted from English. (For illustrations of some of these symbols and of the manner in which they are sequenced, see Premack & Premack, 1972.)

Premack taught a young chimpanzee named Sarah to "read" and "write" using his plastic symbols. She developed a receptive-expressive vocabulary of more than 130 "words." She was able to both encode (write) messages using the symbols and decode (read) messages that had been encoded with them. Premack described the program used to teach her to read and write in considerable detail (Premack, 1970, 1971; Premack & Premack, 1972, 1974). This program can be adapted for teaching the system to humans.

Adaptations of Premack's plastic language and the program developed for teaching it have been used with several populations of speechless persons including global aphasics (Glass, Gazzaniga, & Premack, 1973), autistic children (Premack & Premack, 1974), and mentally retarded children (Premack & Premack, 1974; Carrier, 1974a, 1974b, 1976; Carrier & Peak, 1975). They have *not* been taught in most instances to provide a symbol system for *communication,* but to provide an *introduction* to the *strategies* involved in using symbol systems, or languages. The assumption is made that learning this symbol system will facilitate the acquisition of other symbol systems, such as speech or manual communication. This assumption is reflected in the name that Carrier (1974a, 1974b, 1976) has given to his adaptation of Premack's symbol system—the "Non-Speech Language Initiation Program" (Non-SLIP)—and in the following statement: "Non-SLIP is not intended to be a comprehensive communication training program. Rather, it is a very carefully structured, finely graded, set of procedures for starting children through the process of learning communication skills." (Carrier & Peak, 1975, p. 10). The symbol system that these adaptations of Premack's plastic language are intended to facilitate is in almost cases speech.

Because Premack-type plastic symbols have not been used much as a communication medium does not necessarily mean that they are unusable for this purpose. They have several features that tend to make them desirable for use with certain clients, including the following:

1.   They can be identified either by sight or by touch—their configurations can be both seen and felt. This would tend to make them more usable with patients who have visual problems than the other symbol systems described in this section, with the exception of Braille.
2.   They place minimal demands on a patient's memory. He does not have to remember the portion of a message that has already been encoded, because it is visible on a display.
3.   It may be easier to learn and remember these symbols than strictly visual ones because they are recorded in both tactile and visual memory.

Premack-type plastic symbols can be fabricated quite easily from 1/8" sheet Plexiglass. (The protective paper covering should not be removed from the Plexiglass until after the pieces have been cut out and their edges sanded.) Some shapes that can be used for symbols are illustrated in Figure 5.11. The size of the symbols is dependent on several factors including the potential user's ability to grasp and his or her visual functioning. (A height of 3 inches would suffice for most persons.) The symbols can all be made the same color or be color-coded based on their grammatical function (e.g., red for all symbols functioning as nouns, blue for those functioning as verbs, etc.). The English word equivalent of each should be printed on it. The symbols can be backed with small magnets so that they can be displayed on a magnetic board or they can be displayed (without being backed) horizontally on a table top or vertically on a board with a ledge at the bottom (like a blackboard).

Premack-type plastic symbols would only be intelligible to untrained observers if English word equivalents were printed on them. They could be used to encode messages about the "here and now" as well as the past and the future if appropriate verb tense indicators were available. And they could be used to encode both abstract and concrete concepts. (Of course, the physical

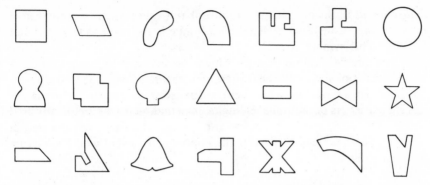

FIGURE 5.11. *Representative Premack-type word symbols (from Carrier, 1974; Premack & Premack, 1972).*

size of the symbols imposes a limit on the maximum number a person can use and, hence, the maximum number of messages that can be encoded with any set of such symbols.)

The time and energy investments required for learning to use Premack-type symbol systems is a function of several variables including the user's level of conceptual functioning and the complexity of the program being taught. If the English translation of each symbol is printed on it, no training should be necessary to learn to interpret them (unless the person to whom messages are being sent cannot read English).

There is a program commercially available that utilizes Premack-type symbols—the Non-SLIP, or *Non-Speech Language Initiation Program* (Carrier & Peak, 1975). This Program is intended for *introducing children to strategies for learning and using symbol systems* rather than for providing a symbol system for encoding messages in their environments. Because of the objective of the Program, the vocabulary used was not selected for encoding basic needs. While this Program does not develop a usable symbol system for communicating in one's environment, it may provide a vehicle for introducing children (particularly severely and profoundly retarded children) to such symbol systems.

Braille

A patient is occasionally encountered who lacks adequate speech for his or her communicative purposes and whose vision is inadequate for using any of the symbol systems described in this section (with the possible exception of Premack-type plastic symbols). The patient may be completely blind, or have a visual-field problem, a visual-acuity problem, or a visual agnosia. The visual problem may have antedated the condition responsible for the communicative disorder or it may have resulted from this condition or one that followed it. Such a patient would probably find a *tactile* symbol system more advantageous than a visual one. Braille is the most widely used and flexible tactile symbol system.

The Braille Symbol System, which was invented by Louis Braille in 1824, consists of sixty-three characters, each made up of a one to six raised-dot pattern in a six-position (i.e., cell) matrix (see Figure 5.12). These characters encode letters of the alphabet, digits, punctuation marks, frequently used words (e.g., *and*), and letter combinations (e.g., *ed*). They are embossed in lines on paper and read by passing the fingers lightly over them. Their structure is as follows:

> To aid in identifying the 63 dot patterns, or characters, that are possible within the six-dot cell, Braille numbered the dot positions 1-2-3 downward on the left and 4-5-6 downward on the right. The illustration [see Figure 5.12] shows the formation of each cell and its simplest designated meaning. The first ten letters of the alphabet are formed with dots 1, 2, 4, and 5. When preceded by the numeric indicator diagrammed in line 6, these signs have number values. The letters *k* through *t* are formed by adding dot 3 to the signs in line 1. Five of the remaining letters of the alphabet and five very common words are formed by adding dots 3 and 6 to the signs in line 1. When dot 6 is added to the first ten letters, the letter *w* and nine common letter combinations are formed (see line 4). Punctuation marks and two additional common letter combinations are made by placing the signs in line 1 in dot positions 2, 3, 5, and 6 (line 5). Three final letter combinations, the numeric indicator, and two more punctuation marks are formed with dots 3, 4, 5, and 6 as shown in line 6. The last seven dot patterns indicated in line 7 are formed by dots 4, 5, and 6 and have no true equivalents in ordinary written language (*Encyclopedia Britannica,* 15th Edition, Volume 3, 1974, p. 110)

Braille can be embossed ("written") on a sheet of paper by hand through the use of a device called a slate or by means of a typewriter-like machine.

Since Braille is a system for writing English, the linguistic structure of messages encoded in Braille is that of English. Any message that can be encoded in English can be encoded in Braille.

Braille is not intelligible to untrained observers. However, if the English equivalents of Braille characters are printed above them, messages encoded in Braille can be decoded by anyone able to read English. A communication board could be constructed on which each message component appears in both Braille and printed English. The user would locate message components by scanning the board with his fingers. When he located a component he wanted to transmit, he would point to it. The person to whom he was transmitting the message would note the English letter, letter combination, digit, word, or punctuation mark printed above it. The user would then locate the next message component and the process indicated would continue until the entire message had been transmitted.

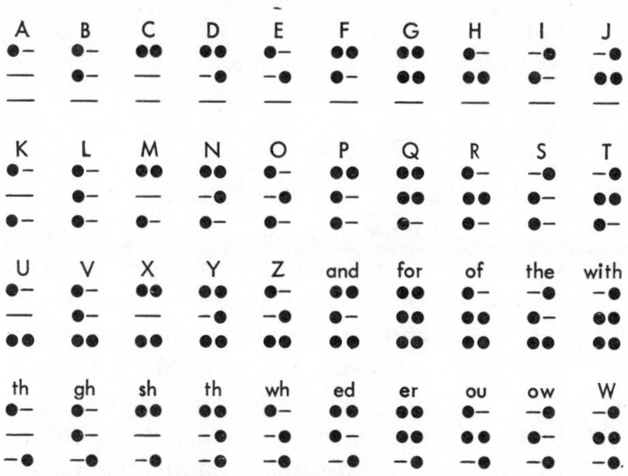

A B C D E F G H I J

K L M N O P Q R S T

U V X Y Z and for of the with

th gh sh th wh ed er ou ow W

FIGURE 5.12. *The Braille characters.*
(Drawing courtesy of the Encyclopaedia Britannica)

The time and energy investments necessary to learn to decode Braille well enough to identify a finite number of message components encoded in it on a communication board should not be too great. Learning it well enough to be able to read and write it fluently would, of course, take a great deal of training.

Machine-Generated Speech

Machine-generated (recorded or synthesized) spoken English has been used with electronic gestural-assisted communication systems for encoding messages (e.g., Ehrlich, 1974; Rahimi & Eylenburg, 1973; Reuter, 1974; Record-player "voice" for mutes, 1977; Microprocessor based voice synthesizer puts speech at its user's fingertips, 1977). Some such systems contain speech synthesizers that generate messages by stringing together phonemes. Others generate messages from recorded, pre-stored words and phrases (and possibly letters, prefixes, and suffixes). The speech elements are sequenced to create utterances that structurally are equivalent to those of spoken English.

Machine generated speech can be particularly useful to verbal apraxics, dysarthrics, and persons who have had glossectomies, for conversing on the telephone. One device designed for this purpose by Sidney Hamilton (Record-player "voice" for mutes, 1977) will generate the following words: yes, no, ok, hello, goodbye, maybe, correct, wrong, right, true, untrue, definitely, fine, too bad, why, when, what, how, where, who, good, and bad. It also will generate up to eight prerecorded phrases such as: please repeat; how are you; I'm fine, thanks; my name is ___; my address ___; I feel ill; please come as soon as possible; and I am using a device to speak because I have a voice problem. (Speech-generating devices are described later in this chapter.)

Morse Code

The International Morse Code (see Table 4.3) has been used as an *encoding* symbol system for indicating and generating message components in gestural-assisted communication systems. Messages are encoded in Morse Code, but translated into and displayed in another symbol system, such as written Engish. There are gestural-assisted communication systems, for example, that will translate messages encoded in Morse Code (by activation of a switching mechanism) into English and will either display them on a TV screen or print them with an electric typewriter. (Devices for translating Morse Code into English are described later in this chapter.)

When and with Whom Might Each Symbol System Be Used Advantageously?

Nine symbol systems are described in this section. When and with whom might it be advantageous to use each of them? The recommendations made here are intended to provide a tentative, partial answer to this question. The answer is tentative because data from clinical research may require some of the recommendations to be modified; it is partial because all possible applications of these symbol systems obviously are not mentioned and the uses indicated are not necessarily applicable to all persons in the populations specified. The names of symbol systems are printed in capital letters to facilitate locating comments about particular ones.

1. The *most flexible* and *efficient* symbol system for gestural-assisted communication modes is printed ENGLISH or another language. It can transmit any message that the user can spell and that those with whom he is communicating can read.

2. The *most concrete* symbol system and probably the *easiest* for most people to learn to use would consist of PHOTOGRAPHS, DRAWINGS, or a combination of the two. These can be used and understood by almost anyone who is sufficiently intact visually to identify the objects and events depicted. This type of symbol system is particularly useful for communicating *basic needs* in hospital and nursing home settings and as an *initial symbol system* for children's communication boards.

3. BLISSYMBOLICS is the most flexible symbol system for persons who are *unable* to *read* or *spell* ENGLISH words well enough to encode the messages they wish to transmit. It can encode almost any message that can be encoded in ENGLISH and is easier for most persons to learn to "read" than ENGLISH. Also, it tends to facilitate learning to read ENGLISH because the ENGLISH equivalent of each BLISSYMBOL is printed with it.

4. PHOTOGRAPHS and DRAWINGS, BLISSYMBOLICS, and printed ENGLISH can be used sequentially. A person could begin with PHOTO-

GRAPHS, DRAWINGS, or a combination of the two. BLISSYMBOLS could be gradually introduced and used along with PHOTOGRAPHS and DRAWINGS to increase the number of messages the person could encode. As his or her knowledge of BLISSYMBOLICS increased, BLISSYMBOLS could be substituted for PHOTOGRAPHS and DRAWINGS and BLISSYMBOLS for other concepts could be added to the symbol set. BLISSYMBOLS, in turn, could be replaced by ENGLISH words as the person's ability to read ENGLISH improved.

5.   REBUSES can supplement symbol systems consisting of PHOTOGRAPHS and DRAWINGS or ENGLISH words. They can be particularly useful with adults who have normal, or near normal, abilities to understand spoken ENGLISH and are dyslexic. REBUSES can be useful to such persons by helping them to remember the *auditory* symbol (spoken word) for the concepts or ideas that they are used to encode.

6.   PREMACK-TYPE PLASTIC SYMBOLS or BRAILLE can be used with persons who lack adequate vision to identify and discriminate between symbols visually. The latter, of course, can encode more messages than the former.

7.   MACHINE-GENERATED SPEECH can be used by almost any speechless person to facilitate *telephone* communication.

8.   The Non-SLIP adaptation of the PREMACK symbol system can be used to *introduce* children (particularly, severely or profoundly mentally retarded children) to the nature of symbol systems and the strategies involved in using them. A program combining LANA LEXIGRAMS with a computer system also can be used for this purpose.

9.   MORSE CODE can be used by *quadriplegics* to indicate message components on displays of electronic gestural-assisted communication systems.

Nonelectronic Gestural-Assisted Communication Systems

There are three types of nonelectronic gestural-assisted communication systems:

1.   systems in which the symbols are reproduced on a display known as a *communication board* (or *conversation board*), and in which messages are transmitted by the user indicating in the appropriate sequence the symbols on the board that encode them;

2.   systems in which the symbols are *manipulable*, and messages are transmitted by the user arranging the symbols that encode them in the appropriate sequence on a magnetic board, table top, or other surface; and

3.   systems in which the symbols are *drawn* or *written*, and messages are transmitted by the user writing or drawing the symbols that encode them in the appropriate sequence on a piece of paper or other material.

Representative systems of these three types are described in this section.

Communication (Conversation) Boards

Communication, or conversation, boards consist of one or more sheets of some type of material on which the elements of a symbol system are reproduced. Materials from which they can be made include paper, cardboard, cloth, plastic, Masonite, and plywood. The symbol elements may be reproduced on a single sheet of material or on several sheets (e.g., in booklet form). Each sheet may contain a single symbol element (see Figure 5.13) or a number of symbol elements (see Figures 5.3, 5.4, and 5.5). The symbol elements may be reproduced directly on the board or on pieces of material (usually paper or cardboard) that are attached to it. The symbol systems described in the first section of this chapter, except for Premack-type plastic symbols and Morse code, can be used on communication boards.

Aside from the symbol system to be used, there are a number of factors to consider when designing a communication board for a client, including those below.

1. Construction Material. Communication boards can be fabricated from a number of materials. That chosen for a particular client would be determined by several factors including:

a. the size of the board (the larger the board, the more sturdy the material needed);
b. the length of time it is intended to be used (the longer a board is intended to be used, the more durable the material needed);
c. how portable it has to be (the more portable it has to be, the lighter the weight of the material from which it would tend to be fabricated);
d. how it is to be mounted (a board that is intended to be used horizontally on a surface such as a table top does not have to be fabricated from as sturdy a material as one that is intended to be mounted at an angle and not rest on a surface);

FIGURE 5.13. *Communication bracelet.*
(Courtesy of Ideas, Tempe, Arizona)

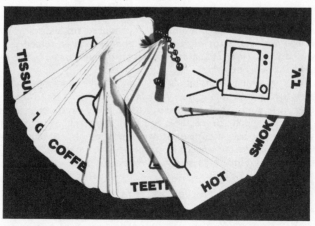

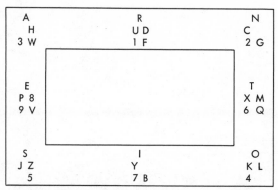

FIGURE 5.14. *ETRAN communication device.*
(Jack Eichler, drawing courtesy of Trace Center)

e.   how easy it has to be to clean (if a patient is likely to drool on or otherwise soil the board, it has to have a washable surface such as that afforded by clear plastic contact paper); and
f.   whether it has to be transparent (this is sometimes necessary if an eyepointing response mode is to be used as with the ETRAN and ETRAN-N boards—see Figures 5.14 and 5.15).

2.   *Size.* Rectangular sheets of material used for fabricating communication boards can range in size from a few inches on the longest side (e.g., see Figure 5.13) to more than 18 inches on the longest side (e.g., see Figure 5.5). The optimum size for a particular client would be determined by several factors including:

a.   the number of symbol elements in the set being used (the greater this number, the larger the board would have to be);
b.   the sizes of the symbol elements in the set being used (the larger they are, the larger the board would have to be);
c.   the method to be used for indicating symbol elements (e.g., if symbol elements were to be indicated by a directed gaze—i.e., eyepointing—rather than by pointing with a finger, there would have to be greater separation between elements and, hence, a larger board would be needed for a given number of elements);
d.   how the board is to be mounted (e.g., if a communication board is to be used as a tray on a wheelchair, this places some restrictions on its minimum and maximum size);
e.   the degree of portability desired (if a communication board has to be portable, it can not be too large to carry around); and
f.   the maximum number of sheets of material that can be used (the greater this number, the smaller each can be).

3.   *Method of Reproducing Symbol Elements on the Board.* Symbol elements can be reproduced on the board itself or on pieces of a material (usually

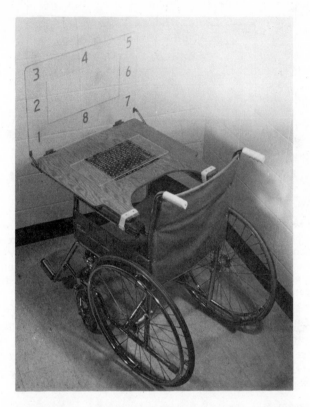

FIGURE 5.15. *ETRAN-N communication device attached to a wheelchair.*
(Photo courtesy of Trace Center)

paper or card stock) that can be attached to it. The latter frequently is done when symbol elements are introduced a few at a time or when the symbol elements on the board are to be updated periodically to meet the user's changing communication abilities and needs. (When this type of board is designed to be attached to a wheelchair as a laptray, the pieces of paper or card stock on which the symbols are reproduced can be sandwiched between the plywood base of the tray and the transparent Plexiglass sheet that covers it; see Vanderheiden, 1977, and Schurman, 1974.)

Symbol elements can be printed and drawn with felt-tip markers or lettering pens. Black ink can be used for all, or different color inks can be used to indicate a category to which each belongs (e.g., nouns, red; verbs, blue; etc.). If the symbol set includes letters of the alphabet (singly or in combination), they can reproduced with a primary typewriter. Rub-on letters also could be used.

Photographs can be attached to a board with rubber cement. Braille message components can be embossed on pieces of paper and attached to a board in this same manner.

4. *Method of Mounting the Board.* A communication board, to be usable, must be *positioned* so that message components that are indicated by the user are visible to the person (or persons) with whom he is communicating. It is necessary that the *full* board be both visible to the user and compatible with his or her motoric ability to indicate message components on it. For many persons and for most types of boards, a horizontal placement, such as on a table top or laptray, is satisfactory. About the only type of board for which horizontal positioning would never be satisfactory is a transparent plastic one, such as the ETRAN (Figure 5.14) and ETRAN-N (Figure 5.15), on which message components are indicated by eyepointing (this type of board usually is mounted vertically).

If a board can not be used when positioned horizontally, some type of stand (or support mechanism) will be needed to position it at an angle at which it can be used. One type of device that may be usable for positioning a communication board at an angle is the overbed table. The angle of the table surface is adjustable on some of them. A communication board could be attached temporarily or permanently to the table top. (If it were attached permanently, it could be sandwiched between the table top and a sheet of transparent Plexiglass the same size and shape. The communication board would then be available whenever the table was in place.)

A camera tripod tilthead attached (by a bolt with a ¼-20 thread) to some sort of supporting mechanism (e.g., a table top) also could be used to position a communication board at a desired angle. A piece of plywood that was slightly larger than the communication board could be attached to the tilt-head (by a piece of metal drilled and tapped with a ¼-20 thread attached to the center of the plywood), and the communication board could be mounted on the plywood.

5. *Board Surface (Covering).* The surface of a communication board may be covered to protect it. The two materials that are used most frequently for this purpose are transparent plastic contact paper and transparent sheet Plexiglass. The first, of course, only would be usable on communication boards that were not designed to be modified. The second would be usable also on those that were not so designed; when used on a board designed to be modified, it could be hinged to the board by means of a wide piece of tape (such as furnace duct tape) on one edge; the Plexiglass sheet then could be raised whenever necessary to modify the symbol set on the board.

For further information on constructing communication boards see

Vicker (1974), Vanderheiden and Grilley (1976), Vanderheiden (1977), McDonald and Schultz (1973), Sayre (1963), Feallock (1958), and Goldberg and Fenton (no date).

There are three types of strategies that can be used for indicating message components on a communication board: *scanning, encoding,* and *direct selection* (Vanderheiden, 1976). These, also, are used with electronic gestural-assisted communication systems for the same purpose. The *simplest* of the three for a patient to use is *scanning*. It demands less from him motorically than the other two. Scanning strategies include "any technique (or aid) in which the selections are offered to the user by a person or display, and where the user selects the characters by responding to the person or display. Depending upon the aid, the user may respond by simply signalling when he sees the correct choice presented" (Vanderheiden & Grilley, 1976, p. 21).

A communication board that would be usable with a scanning response mode is illustrated in Figure 5.16. Its format is that of a rectangular, row-column matrix. Each of the forty-two cells contains a message component—a letter of the alphabet, a digit, a mark of punctuation, or one or two words. (Of course, any of the other types of graphic symbol elements that were described in the first section of this chapter or a different size row-column matrix could have been used instead.) The scanning would be done by a person with whom the user wished to communicate. He or she would point to a *segment* of the board consisting of one or more cells and would ask the user whether it contains the message component he wishes to transmit. If the answer were *yes* and the segment contained more than one cell, he or she would point, in turn, to each of the cells in the segment and ask whether it contained the message component. This process would continue until there was a *yes* response. The message segment in the cell for which there was a *yes* response would be noted; and if the message consisted of more than one message segment, the process outlined would be repeated. The board would be scanned once for each symbol element in the message. Thus, the number of scans for a message would be equal to the number of cells whose contents are needed to encode it.

The simplest type of scanning strategy would be to point to the individual cells in a matrix one after the other and ask for each whether it contains the message component the person wishes to transmit, continuing until he or she gives a *yes* response. While any message can be transmitted by this strategy it is relatively time consuming. A slightly more complex type of scanning strategy (which can be referred to as *two-step scanning*) tends to be more efficient. With this strategy the board is divided into segments, each containing a number of cells (usually the same number of cells). A segment, for example, may be a row of cells. A person being communicated to would point to each of the segments (e.g., rows) one after the other and ask for each "Is it in this segment?" When the person doing the communicating gives a *yes*

	1	2	3	4	5	6	7
1	NEW WORD	A	E	I	O	U	NO
2	YES	.	?	B	C	D	F
3	G	H	J	K	L	M	N
4	P	Q	R	S	T	V	W
5	X	Y	Z	1	2	3	4
6	5	6	7	8	9	0	END

FIGURE 5.16. *Representative communication board for scanning or encoding.*

response for a segment, the person being communicated to points to the cells in that segment one after the other and asks for each "Is it in this cell?" This process continues until a second *yes* response is received. The two-step process outlined is repeated for each symbol element in (or segment of) a message. (For further information on scanning strategies, see Vanderheiden, 1976.)

For a person to use a communication board with a scanning response mode it is only necessary motorically that he or she be able to signal yes or no. There are a number of ways in which these can be signaled (see Chapter 4). He or she also must be sufficiently intact (1) *visually*, to identify the message components on the board, (2) *conceptually,* to understand their meanings, and (3) *auditorily,* (or visually if the person can speechread) to understand the questions asked.

Though almost anyone can use a communication board with a scanning response mode, it is *relatively slow*. It can require for most symbol elements in a message a yes-no response for almost every cell on the communication board used. The other two response modes—encoding and direct selection— allow messages to be transmitted at a faster rate (the latter more so than the former).

An *encoding* response mode consists of "a technique . . . in which the desired choice is indicated by a pattern or code of input signals, where the pattern or code must be memorized or referred to on a chart" (Vanderheiden, 1976, p. 22). The simplest type of encoding scheme would consist of (1) a large chart on which is printed a series of messages a person might want to transmit (e.g., "I am hungry") that are numbered consecutively and (2) a communication board of the type illustrated in Figure 5.16, with each cell containing one of the numbers that appears on the chart (the number of cells being equal to the number of messages on the chart). A one-step or two-step *scanning* mode could be used with the communication board to signal the number of the message on the chart the person wished to transmit. With this strategy only a *single scan* of a communication board is necessary to transmit a message. Of course, it has the limitation that only a relatively small number of predetermined messages could be transmitted using it. This limitation could be partially overcome by including a message on the chart similar to the following: "The message I want to communicate is not on the chart. Please use my other communication board." A communication board of the type illustrated in Figure 5.16 could be used with a one-step or two-step scanning-response mode to transmit the message. This type of system could be particularly useful for communication of basic needs in a hospital or nursing home.

Another encoding system that is only slightly more complex than the first will transmit the message component in any cell on a communication board similar in format to that depicted in Figure 5.16 by means of *two digits*. The first would indicate the row number of the cell containing the component, and the second the number of the column in which it appears. If there are sixty-four or fewer cells on the communication board (a maximum of eight rows and eight columns), the encoding device only has to display the digits from 1 to 8. Four devices that could be used to transmit a row-column, two-digit code are illustrated in Figure 5.17. The first (see Figure 5.17a), which is a two-row communication board, can be used with a one- or two-stage scanning response mode or a direct-selection response mode (i.e., the user points to the digits in some manner). The second (see Figure 5.17b), which is a single-row communication board, can be used with either a scanning or direct selection response mode. It is particularly advantageous for the person who is able to move his hand laterally, but not forward and backward well enough to reliably indicate (point to) message components arranged in rows. The third (see Figures 5.17c and 5.15) is a transparent Plexiglass communication board known as the ETRAN-N (Vanderheiden, 1976), intended for use with an eyepointing response mode. The fourth (see Figure 5.17d) is an electronic rotary pointer scanning device that can be stopped at any digit by a switching mechanism activated by the user (see Appendix D for a description of such a device). These, of course, are not the only types of devices that could be used to transmit a two-digit code.

The two encoding strategies that have been described are *indirect* in the sense that they indicate messages (or message components) to be transmitted on a chart rather than transmitting them directly. There is a type of encoding strategy that will transmit a message directly. It is used with the ETRAN Eye Signaling System (see Figure 5.14) for spelling out messages, developed by

a) Scanning or direct-selection communication board

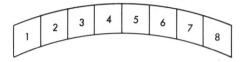

b) Direct-selection communication board

c) Eyepointing chart (ETRAN-N)

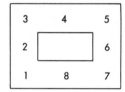

d) Electronic rotary pointer scanning device (see Appendix D)

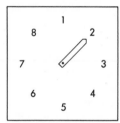

FIGURE 5.17. *Representative devices for encoding message components using two digits.*

Jack Eichler. (Construction details for the device used in this system are included in Appendix D.)

The ETRAN System functions as follows (Eichler, 1973):

General Arrangement

The sender and receiver sit facing each other 4 or 5 feet apart as in normal conversation. The chart stands upright midway between the two people permitting them to view each other through the large aperture at its center. The elevation of the chart should be adjusted so that the eyes of the sender appear to be at the center of the aperture as viewed by the receiver . . . . The chart faces the receiver. The sender reads backwards through it.

Method

The sender spells out words, one letter at a time by glancing at one of the eight distinct areas on the chart. It is easy for the receiver to see which area has been selected by watching the sender's eyes. Some letters require a redirection of the sender's eyes from the selected area to one of the four corners of the chart. [This is explained in the paragraph below on code.]

The sender's and receiver's eyes meet after each letter. The receiver should speak the letter while still watching the sender's eyes. This will permit any confirmation or correction that may be necessary. The receiver should then write the letter on his message paper and return his gaze to the sender which indicates he is ready for the next letter. Speeds of transmission usually improve up to a letter per second as a receiver gains experience.

The Code

Each of the eight distinct areas on the chart has one letter elevated above the remainder of the group. Taken all together, the elevated letters are the eight most frequently used letters in the English language. They have been incorporated into the code in such a way as to require only one glance by the sender. He directs his eyes to one of the chart areas and shifts immediately back to the receiver in order to specify the elevated letter in that area.

The selection of all letters and digits other than the elevated ones requires the sender to move his eyes to one of the four corners of the chart *after* selecting an area group and *before* returning his gaze to the receiver. A glance at the *upper right hand* corner of the chart indicates the *upper right hand* symbol has been selected, and so on, matching the corner of the chart to the position of the symbol among the three or four symbols in the original area selected. The fact that there has been a second glance rules out the elevated letter in the original areas.

The Sender

A patient starting out with the chart will be unfamiliar with the locations of the letters and will send false signals as he searches for the desired letter. If a patient wants to memorize the chart first, this can be done. However, the best way for him to become familiar with the chart is to begin using it. He will quickly learn all symbol locations, and the chart, from his standpoint, will become merely something on which to focus his eyes as he indicates the letters for the receiver.

The Receiver

Any adult, or child who can read, will "catch on" to the eye signaling system in three or four minutes of total instruction and practice. Inexperienced receivers should always write the message as it is being transmitted and should always use the chart as described above. Members of the patient's family and any attendants who use the system daily will develop their own shortcuts and will probably communicate without the chart at times. As in copying any code, receivers must not be too quick in chopping off a multi-syllable word merely because its first letters constitute a word. Request confirmation from the sender in such cases or request he punctuate words as well as sentences.

Punctuation

The dot in the chart's lower, center group represents all punctuation marks. If the receiver's imagination does not meet the degree of exactness needed in certain messages, he and the sender should assign numbers to any special symbols required.

A user and receiver who are thoroughly familiar with the chart can dispense with it; the receiver can "read" the user's eye movements (Handicapped youth 'talks' with eyes, 1974).

A *third type of response mode* used for indicating symbol elements on communication boards can be referred to as *direct selection*. This type of response mode, which is the most efficient of the three, includes "any technique in which the desired choice is directly indicated by the user" (Vanderheiden & Grilley, 1976, p. 26). He or she indicates the components of a message by *pointing* to them in the appropriate sequence. Since each gestural response indicates a message component, this mode requires fewer movements (but better controlled movements) to encode a message than do encoding or scanning. Thus, it transmits messages *faster* and with *less fatigue* than either of these response modes.

A number of different gestures (or patterned movements) of the musculature of the extremities, head and neck, and face can be used for indicating message components on a communication board. The three types that are used most frequently are (1) *hand* (or finger) gestures, (2) *eye* gestures (directed gaze), and (3) *head* gestures (used in conjunction with a *headstick*). The first is pointing with a finger or another part of the hand. This is the type used most often for indicating message components on communication boards. The hand used does not have to be completely normal neuromuscularly. A person who lacks adequate finger control for pointing may be able to do so with his knuckle or another part of his hand.

A person who is unable to point with a part of his hand may be able to do so by directing his gaze, or eyepointing. Even severe quadriplegics may have sufficient control of the musculature of the eyes to indicate message components in this manner. An eyepointing response mode can be used with a transparent, vertically mounted board such as the ETRAN or ETRAN-N (Figures 5.14 and 5.15) or with a standard communication board. For it to be usable with the latter, the message components on the board have to be fairly widely separated from each other.

Another response mode that can be used with someone unable to point with his hand is pointing with a headstick (see Figure 5.18). Many quadriplegics have sufficient head control to use such a device. An occupational therapist who has worked with persons who have neuromuscular disorders should be able to fabricate one and teach the person how to use. it.

For further information on scanning, encoding, and direct-selection response modes, see Vanderheiden (1976).

Another consideration when fabricating a communication board for a person is preparing *instructions* for its use. These instructions should be

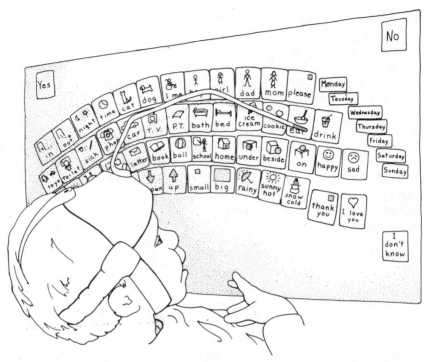

FIGURE 5.18. *Use of a headstick with a communication board (from McDonald, 1976, p. 115).*
(Drawing courtesy of Trace Center)

attached to the board, since persons who need to communicate with a patient may not know how to use the board. If the instructions are only a few sentences in length, they usually can be attached to the front of the communication board. Otherwise, they can be attached to the back of it (with a note on the front indicating so).

What kinds of information should be included in these instructions? The answer to this question would partially depend on the type of response mode the person used. A direct-selection response mode, for example, ordinarily would require fewer instructions than a scanning or encoding one. The following set of instructions that was prepared for use with the board illustrated in Figure 5.16 with a scanning response mode is representative:

This letter-number board is used by _____ to communicate. He (she) spells out the words in the message. Because _____ is unable to point to the letters and numbers on the board, the person with whom he (she) is communicating must do it for him (her). To communicate with _____ , you should point to the squares in the order diagrammed on the next page:

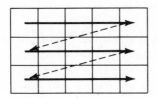

As you point to each square ask "THIS ONE?" and wait for a yes or no signal. _____signals yes and no as follows: _____

_____

As he (she) signals letters and numbers, print them with the attached pencil across the top of the board. _____ will indicate he (she) is finished by signaling the square in the lower right hand corner marked END.

The board for which these instructions were prepared was mounted with a blank space 3 inches high at the top, covered by transparent plastic contact paper. The message components signaled were printed in this space with a grease pencil.

Communication boards have been used with all populations of functionally speechless children and adults. Judging by the frequency with which they have been used, they would appear to be relatively acceptable to persons in at least a segment of these populations. The speed at which messages can be transmitted with a communication board is determined in large part by the response mode and symbol system used. The only neuromuscular requirement for using a communication board is somehow being able to signal yes and no. (Of course, a board can be used more efficiently if the user is sufficiently intact neuromuscularly to point to message components.) It should ordinarily take only a few minutes to teach the *mechanics* of using a communication board so long as a method of indicating is selected that will not overtax the user's neuromusuclar, sensory, and cognitive abilities. However, if he or she has to be taught to signal yes and no or to understand the symbol system used on the board, the time and energy investments required could be considerable; those necessary to teach a person to interpret messages transmitted by a communication board ordinarily would be nominal.

There are some communication boards available commercially. Those illustrated in Figures 5.3, 5.4, and 5.5 are representative. Most commercial communication boards are listed in the periodically updated *Master Chart of Communication Aids* published by the Trace Research and Development Center for the Severely Communicatively Handicapped of the University of Wisconsin Madison. Also, information regarding several of these boards is included in Appendix C.

Manipulatable Symbols

A second type of nonelectronic gestural-assisted communication system consists of sets of manipulatable symbols that can be arranged by the user on a magnetic board, table top, or other surface in appropriate sequences for encoding and transmitting messages. Premack plastic-symbol systems, such as Non-SLIP, are of this type. Any of the other symbol systems described in the first section of this chapter (with the exception of Morse Code) also could be used with such a system by having the symbol elements, or message components, reproduced on individual pieces of a material such as cardboard, cloth, wood, Masonite, or Plexiglass. With such systems, users select message components from those available to them and arrange them in appropriate sequences for encoding and transmitting their messages.

The main advantage of this type of system over that afforded by a communication board is that it makes fewer demands on a user's memory. He does not have to remember the portion of a message he has already encoded, because he can see it. These systems do, however, have several limitations when compared to those utilizing communication boards. First, they require better hand function. It is easier motorically to point to a message component than to pick up a small piece of a material on which it is reproduced and place it in the appropriate place on a display. And second, the number of manipulable symbols that it would be practical for a person to have within his reach probably could not exceed 75. If a larger set were used, it would be difficult to arrange them so that the user could easily locate and reach for the ones he needed. A communication board, on the other hand, can have as many as 400 symbols reproduced on it (as does one of the communications boards distributed by the Blissymbolics Communication Foundation).

Manipulatable symbols have been used with several populations of children and adults including aphasics (Gardner, Zurif, Berry, & Baker, 1976; Glass, Gazzaniga, & Premack, 1973), autistic children (Premack & Premack, 1974), mentally retarded children (Premack & Premack, 1974; Carrier, 1974a, 1974b, 1976; Carrier & Peak, 1975), and cerebral palsied children (material on Slip-n-Slide communication board in Vanderheiden, 1976). For further information about manipulatable symbol systems, see the section on Premack-type plastic word symbols in this chapter.

Drawn or Written Symbols

A third class of nonelectronic gestural-assisted communication systems includes those in which symbols are drawn or written. Messages are transmitted in such systems by writing or drawing the symbols that encode them in the appropriate sequence on a piece of paper or other material (e.g., a "magic slate").

The symbol system that is used most often in this manner is English or some other language. *If a person is able to print or write English or another language, this will afford him a more flexible and efficient communication system than any of the others described in this section.* It is desirable to develop as much as possible the ability of all speechless persons to communicate through writing.

There are two other symbol systems that can be used in this manner. These are Blissymbolics and Braille.

Is it possible for a person who has a neuromuscular disorder to learn to write or draw symbols that can be identified? The answer is yes, in some cases. A person who is hemiplegic on his dominant side can often be taught to write or draw with his nondominant hand. A person who has both hands affected (a quadriplegic or diplegic) may be able to use a mouth-held writing device (Gertenrich, 1966); or, through muscle training, positioning, or stabilization (or some combination of the three) it may be possible for him or her to improve the functioning of one hand sufficiently for it to be used for writing or drawing. An occupational therapist who is experienced in the area of neuromuscular disorders can often be helpful in teaching the use of a hand-held or mouth-held writing device.

Electronic Gestural-Assisted Communication Systems

All electronic gestural-assisted communication systems are fabricated from three types of components: switching mechanisms, control electronics, and displays (see Figure 3.1). There are a number of switching mechanisms and displays that can be used in such systems. Also, there are several features that can be incorporated into their control electronics. Representative switching mechanisms and displays that can be used in these systems are described in this section. The *electronics* that make it possible for specific switching mechanisms to *control* specific displays also are described. The intent of this discussion is to provide the reader with a good enough understanding of the functioning of switching mechanisms, displays, and control electronics so that he or she would be able to design a system for a particular person and describe it to the person responsible for fabricating it.

Switching Mechanisms

The switching mechanism interfaces the client with the communication system. The client's *gestural* manipulation of a switching mechanism *indicates or reproduces* on a display the components of messages he or she wishes to transmit.

All switching mechanisms perform two functions: (1) they connect directly or by means of a metallic substance the ends of two wires, thereby permitting an electrical current to flow from one to the other and (2) they separate the ends of the two wires or cause the metallic substance to separate from one or both ends of them, thereby interrupting the flow of electrical current between them. *Almost all switching mechanisms have such a metallic substance in them.* This substance functions in a manner similar to a drawbridge that connects the two shores of a river. When the drawbridge is down, the two shores are connected and traffic can flow from one to the other. When it is up, the two shores are not connected and traffic cannot flow between them.

The bridge function of switching mechanisms is illustrated in Figure 5.19. The circuit diagramed consists of a battery connected to a light bulb by means of two wires, one of which has been cut into two pieces. The piece of metal that could bridge the ends of these two pieces of wire in Figure 5.19a does not connect them; and the bulb, therefore, would not be lit. In Figure 5.19b, the piece of metal does bridge, or connect, the ends of these two wires, thereby permitting an electrical current to flow from one to the other causing the bulb to light.

The bridge function of a switching mechanism is illustrated further in Figure 5.20. The tilt switch in this figure consists of a small globule of mercury and the ends of two pieces of wire sealed in a glass bulb, or envelope. The glass bulb in the illustration is tilted in a manner that the globule of mercury does not bridge the ends of the two wires. The situation is thus comparable to that illustrated in Figure 5.19a. If the glass bulb had been tilted upward so that the tip was pointed at twelve o'clock (rather than between seven o'clock and eight o'clock as in the figure), the mercury globule would have bridged the two wire ends and the situation would have been comparable to that illustrated in Figure 5.19b.

Switching mechanisms that contain a bridge also contain a device for *raising and lowering* the bridge, which insulates the user from the electrical current that flows when the bridge is lowered. There are a number of types of devices that can perform this function. Switches are categorized primarily on the basis of the type of device that is used for this purpose. Some of these are described in this section. The scheme used for classifying switches was adapted from Holt and Vanderheiden (1974) and Holt, Buelow, and Vanderheiden (1976).

Push Switches. *Physical pressure* applied *directly* by a patterned movement (gesture) of a body part (e.g., finger) or *indirectly* by an implement controlled by a body movement (e.g., headstick) is used to either "lower the bridge" (turn on the switch) or "raise the bridge" (turn off the switch). The position of the bridge usually is maintained for as long as a physical pressure is applied. With such switches, the bridge is lowered the first time they are pushed and raised the second time.

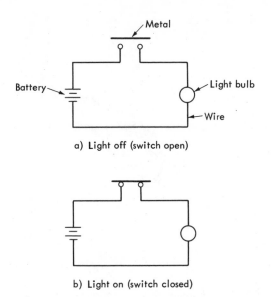

a) Light off (switch open)

b) Light on (switch closed)

FIGURE 5.19. *Open and closed switching mechanism.*

Push-switching mechanisms usually have three basic components: (1) a switch that can be activated by physical pressure, (2) a surface that will activate the switch when physical pressure is applied to it, and (3) some sort of housing for the switch and pressure surface. (In some such mechanisms the switch is activated by applying pressure to it directly.)

One type of switch that can be used in such mechanisms is known as a lever microswitch (see Figure 5.21). These switches are relatively inexpensive (less than $1.50 in 1979) and can be purchased at almost any store that sells electronic components. They are activated by applying pressure to the lever and can be wired so that pressure applied to it will either "lower the bridge" or "raise the bridge." Because they can be mounted at any angle in space, they can be activated by downward pressure, upward pressure, lateral pressure, or pressure applied from any other angle.

The surfaces to which pressure can be applied to activate switches in push-switching mechanisms are varied. *Push-buttons* can be made in almost any shape and size. (Most are round or rectangular.) They can be flush with the surface on which they are mounted, protrude outward from it, or be recessed (see Figure 5.22). The latter helps to prevent accidental activation. (The keys on an electric typewriter are push button switches. A guard made from a sheet of plastic with a hole at the location of each key can be mounted above the keyboard of an electric typewriter. This guard recesses the keys and helps to prevent them from being activated accidently. A keyguard mounted on an IBM electric typewriter is illustrated in Figure 5.23.)

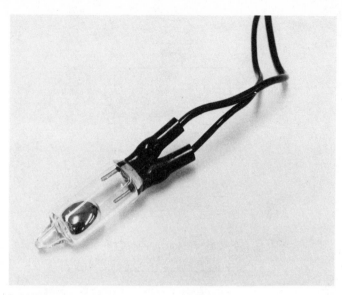

FIGURE 5.20. *Tilt switch (in open position).*

Push plates are similar to push buttons except they are larger. Downward pressure applied anywhere on the plate will activate a switch. They do not require as good a level of motor functioning as push buttons to use because they are larger. If they are pivoted at the center, they can be used in see-saw fashion to control two different switches (see Figure 5.24). (This see-saw arrangement, incidently, can be used to signal Morse code—activating

FIGURE 5.21. *Lever microswitch.*

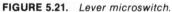

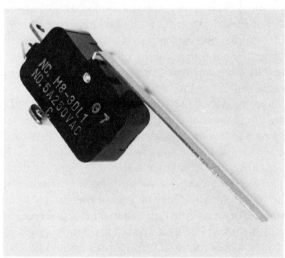

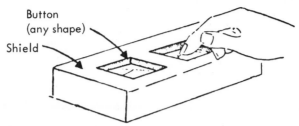

FIGURE 5.22. *Recessed ("shielded") push buttons for activating two microswitches. (Drawing courtesy of Trace Center)*

one switch would signal a *dot,* and the other a *dash.* Morse code signaled in this manner could be used to control the keys of an electric typewriter.)

Paddles have a pivoted arm that when pushed (see Figure 5.25) or blown (see Figure 5.26) up, down, to the side, or forward activates a switch. A paddle also can be used to activate two switches—pushing it to the right can activate one and pushing it to the left can activate the other (see Figure 5.25). They can be of any size and shape a user can manipulate. A spring mechanism can be used to return them to a neutral position after they have activated a switch.

Movement of a *sliding handle* (see Figure 5.27) or *foot trolley* (see Figure 5.28) along a slide, groove, or track may be used to activate a switch. These switches usually have two positions, one at each end of the slide, groove, or track. They can be fabricated so that sliding a handle or foot trolley

FIGURE 5.23. *IBM typewriter with Keyguard, Armrest, and Paper Roll. (Photo courtesy of IBM, Franklin Lakes, N.J.)*

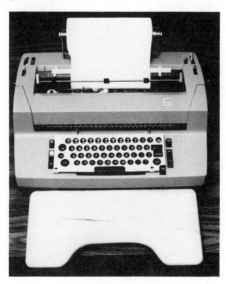

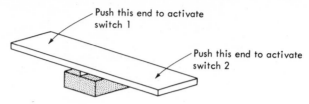

FIGURE 5.24. *See-saw rocking lever for activating two microswitches.*
(Drawing courtesy of Trace Center)

to one end turns on a device, and sliding it to the other turns the device off. Or they can be built so that sliding a handle or foot trolley to each end activates a different switch.

Wobblesticks are vertical sticks (see Figure 5.29) that when pushed off center in *any* direction activate a single switch. One variation consists of a rubber ball that can be suspended from an electrical cord (see Figure 5.30). Pushing the ball off center activates a single switch. *Joysticks* are vertical sticks which when pushed off center in a *specific* direction activate a particular switch (see Figure 5.31). Joysticks usually are designed to activate two to eight switches. (The one illustrated in Figure 5.31 can activate up to four switches.) Some use a gating scheme; this helps to guide the vertical stick to the desired switch when the stick is pushed.

With *pillows, pads,* and *squeeze bulbs,* pushing (or squeezing) a foam-padded or air-filled pillow, fabric or rubber pad, or air-filled bulb activates a single switch. These can be made in almost any size and shape. Several pressure sensitive switches have also been designed that can be activated by movements of specific body parts. These include: (a) an air-filled bulb or a push button that is squeezed between the chin and the chest and (b) a pressure-sensitive element molded into an artificial palate, which is activated by tongue pressure.

FIGURE 5.25. *Hand paddle for activating two microswitches.*
(Drawing courtesy of Ontario Crippled Children's Centre)

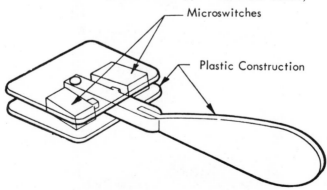

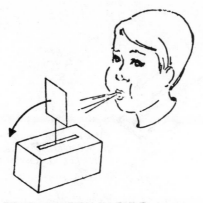

FIGURE 5.26. *Air paddle for activating one switch. (Drawing courtesy of the Trace Center)*

The switch and the surface to which pressure is applied should be mounted together in a suitable housing. The housing should permit this surface to be placed at a position in space where the user can apply pressure to it, and it should have some mechanism for keeping it from being accidently displaced from this point (e.g., suction cups).

Position Switches. A change of position (orientation) in space of the switch mechanism by a patterned movement (or gesture) of a body part such as an arm is used to either "lower the bridge" (turn on the switch) or "raise the bridge" (turn off the switch). The position of the "bridge" is maintained for as long as the body part remains at the same position in space.

Position switches (also known as tip or tilt switches) usually consist of a small globule of mercury and two wire ends in a glass envelope (see Figure 5.20). They can be attached to an arm or another body part that can be moved enough in space to change the position of the mercury globule. Particular

FIGURE 5.27. *Slide mechanism for activating two microswitches. (Drawing courtesy of Ontario Crippled Children's Centre)*

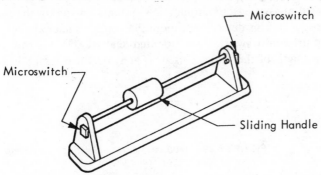

Microswitch

Microswitch

Sliding Handle

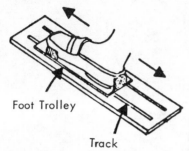

Foot Trolley

Track

FIGURE 5.28. *Foot-trolley for activating one or two microswitches. (Drawing courtesy of the Trace Center)*

patterned movements of this body part (see Figure 5.32) are used to position the mercury in the glass envelope to bridge the two wire ends.

Mercury position switches also can be activated by wobblesticks (see Figures 5.29 and 5.30). Pushing the stick off center would cause the mercury to bridge the two wire ends. It may be necessary to use three or four mercury switches in such a device. (They would be mounted so that pushing the stick off center in any direction would cause the mercury to bridge the wire ends in at least one of them.)

Proximity Switches. Bringing a body part (e.g., an arm) or a special object (e.g., a magnet) within a certain range of the "bridge" mechanism causes it to be "raised" or "lowered." The position of the bridge is maintained for as long as the body part or special object remains within this range.

One of the most frequently used types of proximity switches is the *magnetic reed* switch. This consists of two wire-like pieces of metal (reeds), each of which is attached to a wire end, that are mounted one directly over the other with a small air space separating them. The one on the bottom has on it a piece of metal (e.g., iron) that can be attracted by a magnet. If a magnet is placed over (on top of) the two reeds, the one on the bottom will be drawn upward and come into contact with the top one, thereby "bridging" the two wires and activating the switch. Reed proximity switches have been used in several gestural-assisted communication systems, including the Auto-Com (see Figure 5.33). This device used more than eighty such switches. (When a number of proximity switches are mounted relatively close to each other, the size and strength of the magnet used to activate them is important. If the

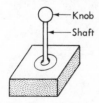

Knob

Shaft

FIGURE 5.29. *Wobblestick for activating one switch. (Drawing courtesy of Trace Center)*

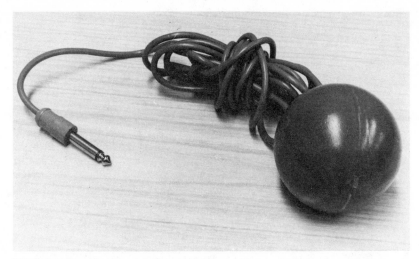

FIGURE 5.30. *Wobblestick switch (MED Call Ball).*

magnet used is either too large or too strong, it may activate more than one switch at a time.) The reed switches are covered by a sheet of Formica plastic on which a symbol is reproduced above each switch. (The magnet need not be in direct contact with a switch to activate it.)

Pneumatic Switches. Blowing into or sucking on the end of a tube changes the air pressure in it, thereby activating a pressure-sensitive device (transducer) that either "lowers the bridge" (turns on a switch) or "raises the bridge" (turns off a switch). These sometimes are referred to as *sip and puff* or *suck and blow* switches. Only very small pressure changes are needed to activate the pressure transducers in them. Their use is illustrated in Figure 5.34.

Pneumatic switches also can be activated in another way. A squeeze bulb or air-filled pillow can be attached to one by means of a piece of rubber tubing. Squeezing or pressing the bulb or pillow with some part of the body activates the transducer, which causes the position of the "bridge." The air paddle (see Figure 5.26) also can be classified as a pneumatic switch because it is activated by blowing.

Touch Switches. Touching a metal surface (contact) on a glove to a metal contact plate (see Figure 5.35) "lowers the bridge," turning on the switch. The person is the mechanism used for raising and lowering the bridge. Touching the metal contact plate with the metal contact surface on the glove is equivalent to bringing the two wire ends (see Figure 5.19) together. An electrical current would pass through the person when contact was made if it were not for the insulating property of the glove. This could, of course, be dangerous.

Touch switches can be activated by a part of the body other than a hand.

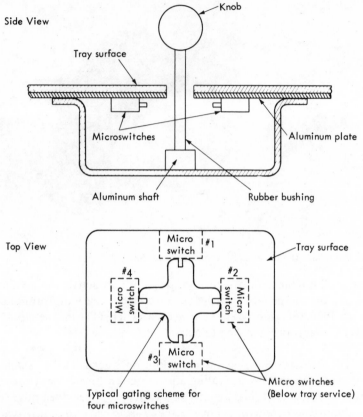

FIGURE 5.31. *Joystick with gating for four microswitches. (Drawing courtesy of Ontario Crippled Children's Centre)*

FIGURE 5.32. *Tip (or tilt) switch strapped to the arm. (Drawing courtesy of Trace Center)*

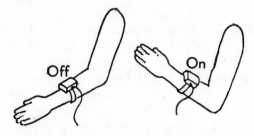

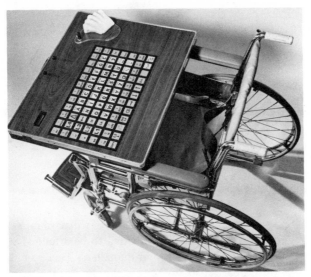

FIGURE 5.33. *Multiple proximity switch control for display. (Photo courtesy of the Trace Center, Auto-Com)*

A metal contact could, for example, be mounted on a sock (which adequately insulated the person from an electric shock) and touching the foot with the sock to a contact plate would "lower the bridge" (turn on the switch).

Sound-Controlled Switches. These switches are activated by sound energy that is transduced, or converted, into electrical energy by a microphone. The sound may be generated by a *device* (whistle, tone generator) or by the *vocal tract* (cough, hum, prolonged vowel). It may be audible or ultrasonic. If the sound is generated by the vocal tract, the microphone can be placed near the

FIGURE 5.34. *Pneumatic ("suck and puff") device for activating one switch. (Drawing courtesy of Trace Center)*

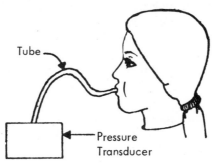

Tube

Pressure
Transducer

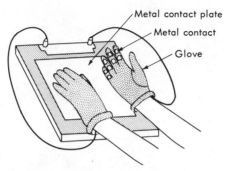

FIGURE 5.35. *Touch switch with contacts on a glove.*
(Cybernetics Research Institute, drawing courtesy of Trace Center)

user's mouth or attached to the throat by means of a disk of tape that is sticky on both sides. (Microphones that are intended to be attached to the throat usually are about the size of a nickle in diameter.) These switches can be designed so that only a particular sound (e.g., humming) at a particular intensity will activate them.

If a throat microphone is not used, there will be *no physical contact* between the user and the communication system. This eliminates the possibility of his receiving an electrical shock if the system malfunctions. It may also simplify mounting the components of his communication system (e.g., no part of the system would be mounted directly on his bed).

Detailed instructions for fabricating a voice-operated switch are included in Appendix D.

Light-Controlled Switches. These switches are activated by *directing* a beam of light at a photoelectric cell (transducer) or by *interrupting* a light beam that is directed at such a device. With the first of these, the beam from a light source that is attached to the user's head (or some other body part) is directed to a *spot* on a panel in front of him or her. The user can see the light spot on the panel and maneuvers it to the desired location. A large number of switches can be activated by such a device. (See Collins, 1974, for a description of the use of this type of switching mechanism with an electric typewriter.)

With the second approach, a beam of light that is directed at (shining on) a photoelectric cell is interrupted by an object or a part of the body (e.g., a hand) *passing between* the light source and the photoelectric cell. This type of switching mechanism is used in some alarm systems and on some automatic elevator doors.

With both of these approaches, there is *no physical connection* between the user and the communication system.

For further information on the switching mechanisms described in this section and others, see Holt, Buelow, and Vanderheiden, 1976.

What Factors Should be Considered when Selecting a Switching Mechanism for a Person?

A number of switching mechanisms are described in this section. What factors should be considered when deciding which to use with a particular person? The five indicated here are intended to provide a partial answer to this question.

1.   The *least sophisticated* (least complex) switching mechanism that will meet his or her communication needs should be selected, other things being equal. The more complex a switching mechanism, the more likely it is to malfunction. If both a push-button switch and a voice-operated switching mechanism would equally meet a person's needs, the push-button switch probably should be selected.

2.   A switching mechanism that requires a *gesture that does not have to be learned* (developed) would be preferable to one requiring a gesture that does have to be learned, other things being equal. Obviously, if he or she can do the gesture required to activate the switching mechanism for a communication system, he or she can begin to use it immediately.

3.   The *least energy consuming* switching mechanism that will meet his or her communication needs should be selected, other things being equal. Some switching mechanisms require more effort than others to activate. A person is apt to limit his use of a switching mechanism (and, hence, a communication system) if using it fatigues him.

4.   The switching mechanism selected for a person should be one that does *not interfere much* with his or her ongoing activities, other things being equal. One that requires something to be attached to the body (e.g., a head-mounted light source) is more likely to interfere with them than one that does not.

5.   The manner in which a switching mechanism is to be used may be an important consideration in its selection. Some switching mechanisms (e.g., push buttons) are easier to activate in a *sustained manner*—for more than a few seconds—than are others (e.g., suck or puff switches). Rotary scanning displays sometimes require a switch to be activated in this manner. Also, some switching mechanisms are more suited for signaling Morse code than are others.

Displays

All electronic gestural-assisted communication systems have at least one display. The elements of the symbol system (message components) used may be

all reproduced on the display, with those needed to encode a message somehow indicated in the appropriate sequence;

printed by the display on a piece of paper, on the surface of a cathode ray tube (i.e., television monitor), or on an illuminated alphanumeric display panel (e.g., the talking broach);

signaled by means of a noise, light, or vibration code (e.g., Morse code) generated by the display; or

transmitted as speech by the display.

These, of course, are not all usable with every symbol system.

Some representative types of displays that are usable in gestural-assisted communication systems are described below. For further information about these and other types of displays that have been used in such systems, see the periodically updated *Annotated Bibliography of Communication Aids* published by the Trace Research and Development Center for the Severely Communicatively Handicapped, of the University of Wisconsin, Madison.

Noise, Light, or Vibration Generators. These devices produce a noise, light, or vibration pattern when a switch is activated in a particular manner. The bursts of noise, light, or vibration emitted by them transmit messages in a code, such as Morse code (see Figure 4.3). They can be activated by any of the switching mechanisms described in this section.

The device of this type that probably has been used most frequently in gestural-assisted communication systems is a battery-operated, transistor, code audio-oscillator, which in 1979 could be purchased from almost any electronics store for less than $15.00 (see Figure 5.36). These emit a clear, crisp tone through a built-in loud speaker for as long as the switch is turned on. The switching mechanism is attached to the device by two wires. It is housed in a small plastic case (approximately 3" x 6"), that could be attached to a vertical surface, such as the side of a wheelchair, by four suction cups. These can be purchased at most hardware stores and are easily mounted on the bottom of the oscillator housing.

Almost any child or adult who uses a communication board could benefit from having this type of audio-oscillator and a switching mechanism attached to his or her wheelchair, bed, or both. Such persons can get the attention of others in the room with them or in an adjacent room when they want something, by activating the switch. Once they have someone's attention, they can use their communication board to indicate what they want. If a communication board user doesn't have such a system, he may have no *reliable* means of alerting people in his environment when he wants to use his board to communicate.

Coded messages also can be transmitted by a device that produces a vibration and light pattern when activated. One such device, the Code-Com, is distributed by the Bell Telephone Laboratories. It transmits, by telephone, messages coded as bursts of vibration and light.

Rotary Scanning Displays. These displays have a pointer (similar in appearance to a clock hand) that is attached to the shaft of an electric motor. The pointer and motor are mounted at the center of a sheet of material such as Plexiglass. Symbol elements (message components) are attached to this sheet around its perimeter. The motor (and thus the pointer) can be started and

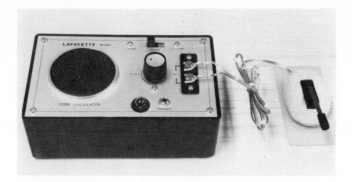

FIGURE 5.36. *Code oscillator alerting device with lever microswitch attached.*

stopped with almost any type of switching mechanism. With some displays of this type, the pointer will revolve in only one direction; with others it can be made to revolve both clockwise and counterclockwise. The speed of rotation of the pointer can be fixed (e.g., four revolutions per minute) or it can be variable. If the speed is variable, it may be fixed by an internal adjustment or it may be under the control of the user (e.g., the greater the pressure he applies to a push plate, the faster the speed of rotation). The sheet of material on which the motor and pointer are mounted can be of almost any size; the larger the sheet, the greater the number of symbols that can be mounted on it. The power source for the motor may be batteries or the unit may have to be plugged into an electrical outlet. Photographs of a representative display of this type and instructions for fabricating it are included in Appendix D.

The main limitation of the rotary scanning display is that only a limited number of symbol elements (message components) can be mounted on it if it is to be kept relatively small, because they can only be mounted at the edges. The type that is described next can utilize the entire board for displaying symbols.

Rectangular Matrix Displays. These consist of rectangular sheets of a material such as Plexiglass that are divided (or partitioned) into rows and columns (see Figure 5.37). The maximum number of symbol elements (message components) that can be displayed is equal to the number of cells in the resulting matrix, or the product of the number of rows *times* the number of columns. (If a matrix had three rows and five columns, this number would be 15.)

Only one symbol element (message component) would appear in each matrix cell. It could be printed or drawn directly on the display, or it could be attached to it. Any of the symbol systems mentioned in the first section of this chapter except for Braille, Morse code, and Premack-type plastic symbols can be used with this type of display.

a) Linear scanning

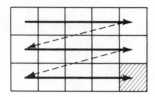

b) Row-column scanning

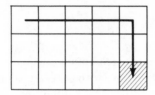

c) Directed scanning

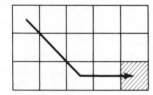

FIGURE 5.37. *Representative scanning approaches for indicating message components with an electronic rectangular matrix display.*

Displays of this type contain an electrical mechanism that makes it possible for a single cell selected by the user to *stand out* from the others for *longer than* a predetermined period of time. Two ways in which this is done are:

1. by placing a miniature bulb *in a corner of* each cell on the display board and lighting the bulb in the cell containing the message component to be transmitted for longer than a predetermined period of time; and
2. by placing a miniature light bulb *behind* each cell on the display board (the display board being either transparent or translucent plastic) and lighting the bulb behind the cell containing the message component to be transmitted for longer than a predetermined period of time.

A user can light a bulb in a cell that contains a message component that he wishes to transmit for longer than a predetermined period of time by manipulating a switching mechanism when the bulb is lit in that cell.

Most rectangular matrix displays use a *scanning* response mode for indicating (transmitting) message components. Bulbs are lit in a pattern that may be partially controllable by the user, each for the same predetermined period of time. The user activates a switch when the bulb is lit in the cell containing the message component he wishes to transmit. This causes the bulb to remain lit for longer than it would if the scanning process were continuing. After a certain period of time, or after the user activates the switching mechanism in a particular way, the scanning process begins again, permitting another message component to be transmitted. The user repeats this process until all the components of his message have been transmitted.

There are several scanning strategies that can be used with this type of display for indicating (transmitting) message components. Three of these are illustrated in Figure 5.37. The message component the user wishes to transmit in these illustrations is in the cell at the lower right hand corner of the display.

With a *linear scanning approach* (see Figure 5.37a) the bulbs in the top row of cells are lit one after the other. If the message component the user wishes to transmit is not in the top row, the bulb in the first cell of the second row would light after that in the last cell of the first row went off. This process continues until the user activates a switch, causing the light in the cell that was on to remain lit. The light in the illustration would go on and off *fourteen times* before going on in the cell containing the message component the user wished to transmit. A display that uses this type of scanning mode can be controlled by almost any kind of switching mechanism.

With a *row-column approach* (see Figure 5.37b), the bulbs in the top row of cells are lit one after the other until the one in the *column* containing the message component is lit. The scanning then *proceeds downward* until the bulb in the cell containing the message component is lit. The user then activates a switch causing the light in this cell to remain lit. The light in the illustration would go on and off *six times* before going on in the cell containing the message component the user wished to transmit. This type of scanning display can be controlled by three switches (one to begin the top row scan; one to stop the row scan and begin the column scan; and one to stop the column scan when the bulb is lit in the cell containing the message component). It also can be controlled by three activations of a single switch, if an appropriate switching mechanism is used.

With a *directed scanning approach* (see Figure 5.37c) the bulbs in the cells are lit one after the other that lie in the shortest path to the one containing the message component the user wishes to transmit. The path can be vertical, horizontal, angular, or combinations of the three. The light in the illustration would go on and off *four times* before going on in the cell containing the message component the user wished to transmit. Displays using this type of scanning mode usually are controlled by joystick switching mechanisms (see Figure 5.31).

Rectangular matrix displays can be fabricated that have a relatively large number of cells. Such devices containing more than 300 cells have been

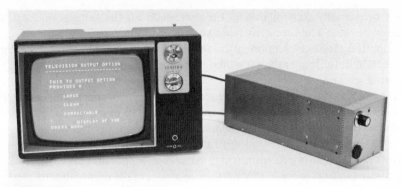

FIGURE 5.38. *Television display.*
(Photo courtesy of Trace Center)

built. Photographs and construction details for a representative display of this type are included in Appendix D.

CRT (Cathode-Ray Tube) Displays. These displays (which are modified television sets) print messages on a television screen—which is a cathode-ray tube (see Figure 5.38). Though they usually print messages character (letter or digit) by character, they can print them in larger units (words, phrases, or sentences). These devices usually have an editing capability which makes it possible for the user to insert or delete characters and move lines up and down. This capability can be used both to correct errors arising from such sources as accidentally activating the switching mechanism and for editing messages or responses which would be necessary if the communication system were used for schoolwork. They can be used alone or in conjunction with a printing device such as a strip printer, electric typewriter, or teletypewriter (these devices are described later in this section). When they are used in the second way, messages are formulated and edited on the CRT display and transferred to the printing device by activation of a switching mechanism. The advantage of formulating messages on a CRT display rather than directly on paper is that it is easier to correct errors and do other types of editing on a cathode-ray tube than on a piece of paper. Since almost any size television set can be modified to serve as a CRT display, it can be made relatively small or relatively large. CRT displays when in use are positioned so that they can be seen by both the user and those with whom he or she is communicating.

CRT displays have the following four components: (1) an input device such as a keyboard, (2) a character generator, (3) a CRT terminal, and (4) a display refreshing mechanism (Ralston & Meek, 1976). These are diagramed in Figure 5.39. Activation of the *input device* (which contains a switching mechanism such as a keyboard) causes letters, digits, or larger language units to be generated by the *character generator* and displayed on the *CRT terminal.*

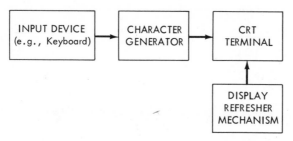

FIGURE 5.39. *Components of a CRT (cathode-ray tube) display.*

To keep the message on the CRT terminal from fading out, there is a mechanism that continuously refreshes the characters on it. The *editing function* of a CRT display is controlled by the input device.

There are input devices for CRT displays that can be activated by a computer. (In fact, CRT displays, referred to as alphascopes, are used as read-out devices in computer systems.) Small computers have been used in gestural-assisted communication systems to encode messages on CRT displays. One such application involves systems in which a Morse code input is used. A user of this type of system would signal the characters he or she wished to appear on the CRT in Morse code, using a switching mechanism that would be appropriate for the purpose. The Morse code signals for the characters would be entered into the computer. The computer would recognize the characters being signaled and would activate the character generator in a manner that would cause them to be generated and displayed on the CRT. Spacing and editing functions also would be controlled by Morse-code type signals. (Further information on the use of computers in gestural-assisted communication systems is presented later in this chapter in the section dealing with *control electronics.)*

LED (Light-Emitting Diode) Displays. These displays print out the words in a message character by character (or in larger units) on a panel. The characters are *outlined in light* by miniature transistors, known as light-emitting diodes (LEDs), that are arranged in rows and columns on the panel. This type of display is used in many electronic calculators. A representative arrangement of LEDs on such a panel is illustrated in Figure 5.40. This display panel has on it 231 LEDs, arranged in 7 rows and 33 columns. (A panel of this size, incidentally, is used in a gestural-assisted communication system that is referred to by Newell and Brumfitt, 1974, as the "Talking Broach," because it is pinned to the user's clothing.) Any letter or digit can be outlined by causing certain of the diodes to emit light. These panels usually display a single row of characters and can be fabricated in almost any length. While they can be controlled most efficiently by a keyboard, other types of switching mech-

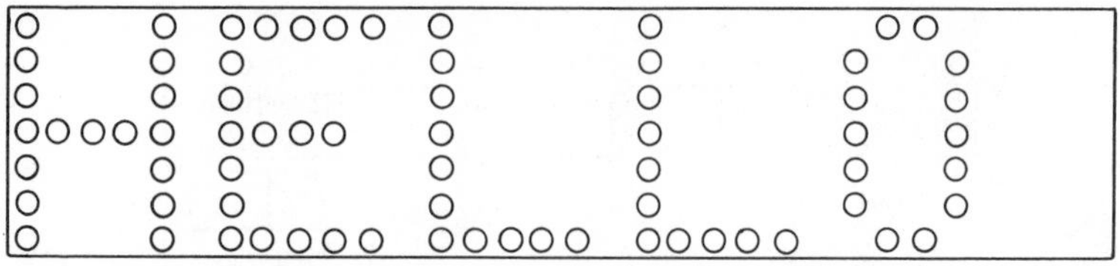

FIGURE 5.40. *A representative LED display, consisting of 231 light-emitting diodes arranged in a 7 x 33 matrix (adapted from Newell & Brumfitt, 1974).*

anisms can be used to activate the character generator that causes the diodes on the panel that outline the characters in the message to emit light.

Messages can be printed out in two ways on LED displays. First, a display can be filled with words, erased, filled again (if a message was not completed), erased, and so on, until a message is transmitted completely. Second, the characters in a message can be made to move across the display relatively smoothly from right to left in a manner similar to the "newscasts" on some buildings (e.g., the former Times building in New York City). This second approach is used with the LED display of the "Talking Broach" communication aid (Newell & Brumfitt, 1974). Only five characters are visible on this display at any one time. The manner in which each new character *gradually* moves from the right-hand end of the display, displacing those already present, is illustrated in Figure 5.41. The characters cease moving when all of them in a message have been displayed.

There is a type of display, known as a *Liquid-Crystal Display (LCD),* that provides the same type of readout as an LED and can be used in place of it. The characters usually are formed from combinations of short vertical and horizontal lines as illustrated below:

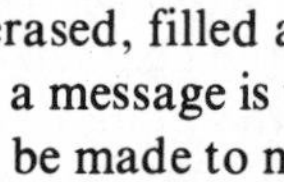

LCDs use less current than LED displays, so batteries last longer. Also, their use may make it possible to significantly reduce the size and weight of a portable communication system because they can be made thinner than LED displays. (LCDs have been used, incidentally, on digital watches and electronic calculators.)

Strip (Line) Printer Displays. These devices print messages made up of letters, digits, and punctuation marks on narrow strips of paper (usually heat sensitive) that are only wide enough to reproduce a single line of characters (see Figure 5.42). The paper, which is approximately the same width as telegraph ticker tape, is fed into the device in rolls. (The rolls may be in cassettes, which facilitates loading them into the printer.) The length of a paper strip on which a message is printed is a function of the number of

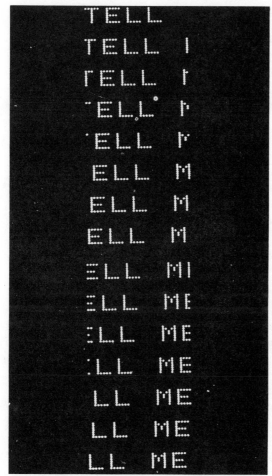

FIGURE 5.41. *Illustration of the floating display of the Talking Brooch.*
(Photo courtesy of Grune and Stratton)

characters in it. The strip can be any length that does not exceed that of the roll of paper in the device. If it is desired to save a message, the strip on which it is printed can be cut into sections and glued to a sheet of paper (as is done with telegrams). While strip printers can be controlled by almost any type of switching mechanism, keyboards are the most efficient for the purpose.

Strip printers are frequently used as displays in *portable* gestural-assisted communication systems intended for producing typewritten messages because they are smaller and less expensive than electric typewriters and teletypewriters and can be battery operated. The device in Figure 5.42 is representative of such portable systems.

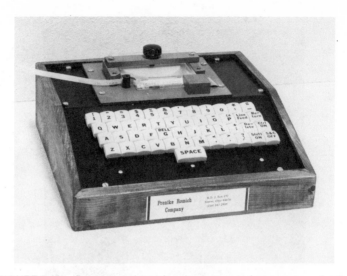

FIGURE 5.42. *Representative strip printer mounted on a communication device with a keyboard switching mechanism. (Photo courtesy of Prentke Romich Company)*

Messages can be typewritten directly with a strip printer or they can be composed on a CRT display with editing capability and transferred from this display to a strip printer after they have been edited. (For further information about the second approach, see the section on CRT displays.)

Electric Typewriters. Adapted electric typewriters (particularly those manufactured by IBM) have been used as display devices in a number of gestural-assisted communication systems (see Copeland, 1974, for a representative sample of systems utilizing electric typewriters for this purpose.) There are several ways in which such typewriters can be modified to make them usable by persons who have a neuromuscular disorder.

A device can be added that makes it possible to insert paper in *rolls* instead of sheets (see Figure 5.23). It is unnecessary with such a device for the user to have adequate control of the upper extremities to insert sheets of paper into the machines, though he or she would of course require assistance when a new roll of paper was needed. A *keyguard* can be mounted over the keys to help prevent them from being accidentally activated (see Figure 5.23). To activate a particular key, the user inserts a finger or a device (such as a mouth stick) into the hole in the keyguard that is over that key. The keyguard reduces errors resulting from the wrong key being activated. In addition, it eliminates a second source of errors. With a keyguard in place, the user's fingers rest on it instead of on the keys. Thus, keys can not be activated accidentally by the

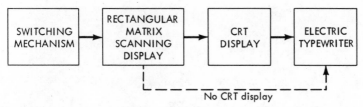

FIGURE 5.43. *Gestural-assisted communication system for controlling an electric typewriter with a scanning response mode. The CRT display is optional.*

weight and extraneous movements of fingers resting on them.

A device can be fabricated that the user can manipulate with some part of his or her body to push the typewriter keys. Such devices include head sticks and mouth sticks. An *armrest* can be installed to stabilize the user's arms (see Figure 5.23). Such a device would be advantageous if stabilizing the user's arms improved his or her ability to make the finger movements required to accurately activate the keys or reduced fatigue.

The keyboard can be modified so that the keys can be *individually electrically controlled,* such as through the use of *solenoids.* (Solenoids are electromagnets; when a solenoid mounted below a particular key is activated, that key is drawn downward by a magnetic force.) Almost any type of switching mechanism can be used to control a typewriter that has been modified in this manner. Several that have been used for the purpose are described in Copeland's (1974) book.

Messages can be typewritten directly or they can be composed on a CRT display with editing capability and transferred from this display to the typewriter after being edited. The transfer from CRT display to typewriter can be done by activation of a single switch. (See the section on CRT displays for further information about this approach.)

A rectangular matrix display that will function in a scanning mode can be used to control an electric typewriter. The symbols on the typewriter keys would be reproduced in the cells of the matrix, one key per cell. To activate a particular key, a scanning strategy (see Figure 5.37) would be used to light the bulb on the cell in which that key is reproduced (i.e., to stop the scan). The user could then activate a switch that would cause the corresponding key on the typewriter to be activated (pressed). A CRT display could be added to the system between the rectangular matrix display and the typewriter (see Figure 5.43). With the system modified in this manner, activating a switch after the bulb on the cell in which the key is reproduced is lit would cause that character or function (e.g., spacing) to appear or occur on the CRT display. After the message had been composed and edited, it could be transferred to the typewriter in the manner described elsewhere in this section.

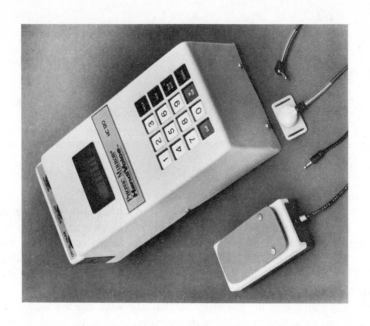

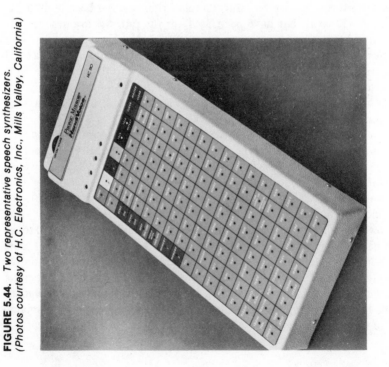

FIGURE 5.44. Two representative speech synthesizers. (Photos courtesy of H.C. Electronics, Inc., Mills Valley, California)

Teletypewriters. These devices which are similar in function to electric type-writers differ from them in two ways: (1) they print messages on a contin-uous roll of paper, usually 8½ inches wide, and (2) characters are printed in response to a *coded electrical signal* that can be generated by a *second teletypewriter* over a telegraph (or adapted telephone) line or by a *computer.*

They have been used instead of electric typewriters in gestural-assisted communication systems, particularly those in which the switching mechanism is not a keyboard *and* is being used to signal Morse code. One component of the control electronics of such systems is a small computer. (See the section on control electronics for further information about the use of small com-puters in these systems.) Since teletypewriters are designed to be used as dis-plays in computer systems, they are easier to interface with computers than are electric typewriters.

Teletypewriters also can be used by speechless persons in a second way—to communicate over telephone lines, particularly in an emergency. A teletypewriter is installed in the user's home or office. He or she can transmit a message that will be printed by another teletypewriter by dialing a telephone number at which one has been installed on the telephone line (e.g., the police department in some cities). The person called can respond by typing a message on his teletypewriter, which will be printed by the user's teletypewriter. Most teletypewriters will both send and receive messages.

Speech Generators (Synthesizers). These devices generate speech by either playing recorded speech segments (e.g., Record-player "voice" for mutes, 1977) or by synthesizing speech segments (e.g., Microprocessor based voice synthesizer puts speech at user's fingertips, 1977). Two representative devices of the synthesizer type are illustrated in Figure 5.44. Both are portable and will play a synthesized speech message through a built-in speaker. The unit on the left, which has a keyboard-type switching mechanism, is prepro-grammed with 373 words, 45 phonemes, 26 letters, 13 morphemes (word prefixes/suffixes), and 16 short phrases (e.g., "My name is . . . ."). To use this device requires essentially normal functioning of one hand (for activating the switching mechanism).

The unit on the right in Figure 5.44 can be controlled by a built-in key-board or by almost any of the switching mechanisms mentioned in this chapter. It can function in either a direct-selection or scanning *encoding response mode.* A maximum of 999 words, phonemes, letters, morphemes, or short phrases can be stored in its memory, each having a three-digit code. To generate one of these 999 speech segments, its three-digit code is inputed into the unit by means of the built-in keyboard (direct-selection) or an exter-nal switching mechanism (scanning). When used in a scanning mode, the three-digit numerals are displayed consecutively on an LED display located on the front of the device. The user activates a switch when the three-digit code of the speech segment he wishes to generate appears on this display. The segments of a relatively short message can be stored in its memory and played as a unit.

Speech-generator displays should be particularly useful for completely speechless persons who have normal hearing to communicate by telephone. Such persons should find them more flexible than the other two types that can be used for phone communication—code generators (e.g., Com-Code) and teletypewriters—because they do not require the person being communicated with to (1) learn Morse code or (2) have a special device installed on his telephone line.

What Factors Should be Considered when Selecting a Display (or Displays) for a Communication System?

A number of displays are described in this section. What factors should be considered when deciding which to use for a particular system? The six suggested here provide a partial answer to this question.

Need for Portability. If a communication system has to be portable, there will be limits on its maximum permissible size and weight. Rotary scanning displays, rectangular matrix displays, LED displays, strip printers, speech generators, and code oscillators tend to be more practical for portable systems than other types because they can be made both relatively small and relatively light in weight.

Need for Editing Capability. If it is important for the user to be able to edit the messages he or she has formulated, a CRT display with editing capability alone or in conjunction with a strip printer, typewriter, or teletypewriter probably would be the best choice.

Need for a Record of Messages Transmitted. If a communication system is not intended to be used only for conversation (e.g., if it is to be used for school work or business communication as well), it is desirable that it be capable of producing typed copies of messages. A strip printer, electric typewriter, or teletypewriter can provide this capability.

Need for Telephone Communication Capability. If the user of the system needs to be able to communicate by telephone, a code generator (e.g. Com-Code), a teletypewriter, or a speech generator can be used. The teletypewriter is the most flexible of the three because it can be used to communicate on any telephone with anyone who understands English.

The symbol system used. Rotary scanning displays and rectangular matrix displays tend to be more practical than other types for visual symbol systems not consisting of letters and digits (e.g., photographs, drawings, and Blissymbols).

Motivation of the user and those he communicates with to learn Morse Code. An audio code oscillator (with an appropriate switching mechanism) can provide an *inexpensive, flexible, portable* communication system if the user and those with whom he communicates are willing to learn Morse code. It can be used to communicate by telephone. A permanent record can be made of messages transmitted, by tape recording the audio code signals. For school work or business communication, the signals can be recorded on a dictating machine and transcribed by someone who either knows Morse code or is willing to consult a code chart.

It should be evident from the discussion in this section that gestural-assisted communication systems are likely to require *more than one* type of display to adequately meet users' communication needs. When designing these systems, it probably is safest to assume that more than one display is necessary unless there is evidence to the contrary.

Control Electronics

The control electronics *interface* the switching mechanism with the display (or displays). They make it possible to *reliably* indicate or generate message components on a display by activating a switching mechanism in a particular way. Reliability in this context pertains primarily to preventing a switching mechanism from being activated accidentally.

The control electronics of a gestural-assisted communication system perform two or more of the following functions:

1. connecting the switching mechanism to the display (or displays),
2. supplying electrical power to the display (or displays) and to other components requiring it,
3. transforming a user's activations of the switching mechanism into a form that will control the display (or displays),
4. "remembering" the components of a message until a user wishes to display them, and
5. preventing the switching mechanism from being activated accidentally.

The control electronics of *all* such systems perform the first two functions. The third and fourth functions, when needed, are performed by a small computer. The fifth can either be performed by a computer (if there is one in the system to perform the third and fourth functions) or by a separate delay circuit. Some components that are used to perform these functions are described briefly in the following paragraphs.

Connecting the Switching Mechanism to the Display (or Displays). This usually is done with electrical cable. The cable contains a number of insulated electrical wires. The number of wires in the cable is positively related to the number of switches in the switching mechanism. If it contains only one switch, the cable is likely to contain only two wires. If it contains a great many switches (as would a keyboard), the cable would contain at least two wires for each switch. The wires in a cable are color-coded to facilitate identifying them.

The cable may be attached permanently to the switching mechanism, the display, or both. (If it is only permanently attached to one of them, it usually is the switching mechanism.) An end that is not attached permanently to a component of the system has a male or female connector mounted on it. If the switching mechanism used contains a single switch, the connector is likely to be a male phone jack. (A more elaborate connector may be used instead to prevent the cable from accidentally being pulled-out of, or disconnected from, the display or switching mechanism.) It is not desirable for cables to be permanently attached to components because this makes them more difficult to replace. (The cables in a system tend to be among the components that are most likely to become defective.)

Systems with a computer or delay circuit in the control electronics, or with more than one display, usually have more than one connecting cable. One cable, for example, may connect the switching mechanism to the input of the computer while a second connects the output of the computer to the display.

The cables used to connect the components of a communication system should be adequately shielded from electrical radiation sources in the environment, such as fluorescent lamps and CB radios (the shielding is built into the cable). If shielding in inadequate, these extraneous, environmental energy sources may interfere with the functioning of the system. Such interference is particularly apt to occur when inadequately shielded cables are used that are relatively long.

When it is necessary (or desirable) for a display to be located at a distance from the user and it would be dangerous (or undesirable) to use an electrical cable to connect the switching mechanism to the display, there is another approach that may be usable. An example of such a situation would be a classroom in which a large CRT display was located where it could be seen by the teacher and the members of the class and in which the user was seated at a desk or in a wheelchair on which was mounted a keyboard-type switching mechanism such as an Auto-Com. The user could participate in class discussions by printing his comments on the CRT display. With this approach the switching mechanism is connected to the display by low-power *radio signals.* The switching mechanism is used to activate a radio transmitter that is located next to it. The resulting signals are transmitted to a radio receiver that is located next to the display and connected to it. There are low-power radio transmitters available which are usable for this purpose. (Such a transmitter is described in Appendix D.)

Supplying Electrical Power. All of the displays used in electronic gestural-assisted communication systems require electrical power to function. The same is true of computers and other devices containing electronic circuits that are used in these systems. The power source can be batteries or an electrical outlet.

Batteries differ with regard to (1) their voltage, (2) the electrochemical process by which they generate their power, and (3) whether they are rechargeable. They are made in a number of voltages (the most frequently used is 1.5 volts). If batteries are connected in series (the "positive" terminal of one contacting the "negative" terminal of the next), the resulting voltage will be the sum of the individual voltages. Thus, four 1.5-volt batteries connected in series will generate six volts. There is no theoretical limit to the number of batteries that can be combined in series, but there is obviously a practical limit.

Several types of chemical processes can be used in a battery to generate electrical energy. The process used partially determines the length of time a battery will continue to deliver its nominal (specified) voltage. Among the types that tend to deliver their nominal voltages the longest are those referred to as *alkaline* batteries. Though they are more expensive than most other types of batteries that cannot be recharged, their relatively long life makes them desirable for use in communication systems; they have been reported to last as much as 10 times longer than conventional batteries.

The types of batteries described in the previous paragraph have to be replaced when they no longer generate their nominal voltage. There is a type of battery that can be recharged when it no longer generates this voltage, by plugging the unit in which it is mounted into an electrical outlet for a specified number of hours. If these batteries are used in a communication system, they can be recharged at night while the user is sleeping. An auxillary battery pack can be included in the system if it is apt to require more power during the day than can be supplied by a single set of batteries. While rechargable batteries initially are more expensive than disposable ones, they tend to cost less to use over their lifetime.

If the power source for a communication system is from an electrical outlet, it is important to determine whether the outlets that are to be used will provide the voltage required by the system. If they do not supply this voltage, an adapter will have to be used. This would be particularly important to check if some electrical components of the system were manufactured outside of the United States.

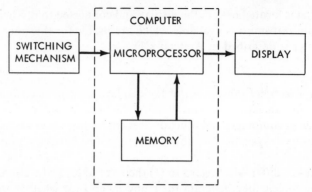

FIGURE 5.45. *Installation of a computer in a gestural-assisted communication system.*

Transforming User's Activations of a Switching Mechanism into a Form That Can Control a Particular Display. This ordinarily is done by means of a small computer, the switching mechanism being connected to its input and the display to its output (see Figure 5.45). Gestural-assisted communication systems that have a computer as a component of their control electronics include those which (1) use a Morse code input to control a CRT display, strip printer, or teletypewriter or (2) contain a speech synthesizer.

Computer systems consist of two types of components: *hardware* and *software*. The hardware includes the mechanical and electrical components of the system, and the software the programs which control the functioning of the hardware.

The *hardware* of a small computer system consists of four things: input, output, memory, and microprocessor. *Input* is a switching mechanism (usually a keyboard) through which messages are sent to the *microprocessor* (see Figure 5.45). The microprocessor follows the instructions in the *program* (software), and stores the instructions and resulting data (phonemes, letters, words, phrases, etc.) in the *memory*. After the operations in the program have been performed, the data can be retrieved from memory and displayed on an *output device* (CRT display, strip printer, teletypewriter, speech generator, etc.).

The *software* of a computer system consists of a detailed set of instructions, or program, that tells the computer's microprocessor how to perform the desired function. The program is written in a computer language such as FORTRAN or BASIC and is entered into the computer's memory by means of a keyboard. Programming a computer for a particular function (e.g., decoding Morse code) can be done by a computer specialist. (The company from which you purchase a computer should be able to recommend a local person who can program it for your application.)

Small computers that probably would be adequate for most applications in gestural-assisted communication systems could be purchased in 1979 for less than $800.00. Such computers are likely to cost even less in the future, judging by dramatic reduction in their price between 1972 and 1979.

Remembering the Components of a Message. A microprocessor can be programmed to store some or all of the components of a message (phonemes, letters, digits, punctuation marks, words, phrases, etc.) in *memory* from which they can be retrieved and displayed whenever the user wishes. A microprocessor also can be programmed to display message components that have been encoded (assigned a number) and stored in memory. The user would input the digit code of the message component that he or she wanted displayed, and the microprocessor would retrieve that component from memory and display it.

Preventing the Switching Mechanism from being Activated Accidentally. If a user of a gestural-assisted communication system has a neuromuscular disorder, he may accidentally activate the switching mechanism because of involuntary movement or poor motor control. This is particularly apt to be a problem in systems which use a keyboard-type switching mechanism because the individual switches tend to be in close proximity to each other.

A circuit can be incorporated into the control electronics of a communication system which requires that the gesture used to activate a switch (e.g., pressing, sucking, phonating, or tilting the arm) be *maintained* for a predetermined period of time (e.g., 3 seconds) before the switch will activate. Its duration would be positively related to the degree of disturbance in the control of the musculature used to perform the gesture; the greater the disturbance, the longer the gesture has to be maintained. This delay time, of course, should be kept as short as a user's neuromuscular functioning will allow.

REFERENCES

ARCHER, L. Blissymbolics—A non-verbal comunication system. *Journal of Speech and Hearing Disorders,* 42, 568-579 (1977).

BLISS, C.K. *Semantography (Blissymbolics)* (2nd ed.). Sydney, Australia: Semantography (Blissymbolics) Publications, 2 Vicar Street, Coogee (1965).

————. *Syntax Supplement no. 1.* Toronto: Blissymbolics Communication Institute, 862 Eglinton Avenue E (1975).

Braille. *Encyclopaedia Britannica* (15th Edition), Volume 3, p. 110 (1974).

CARLSON, F.L. *An adapted communication project for a nonspeaking child.* Paper presented at the 51st annual meeting of the American Speech and Hearing Association, Houston (1976).

CARRIER, J.K., Jr. Application of functional analysis and a non-speech response mode to teaching language. In L.V. McReynolds (Ed.), *Developing Systematic Procedures for Training Children's Language,* ASHA Monograph No. 18 (1974a).

————— . Application of a nonspeech language system with the severely language handicapped. In Lyle L. Lloyd (Ed.), *Communication Assessment and Intervention Strategies,* Baltimore: University Park Press, pp. 523-547 (1976).

————— . Nonspeech noun usage training with severely and profoundly retarded children. *Journal of Speech and Hearing Research, 17,* 510-517 (1974b).

CARRIER, J.K., Jr., and PEAK, T. *Program Manual for Non-SLIP (Non-Speech Language Initiation Program).* Lawrence, Kansas: H & H Enterprises, Inc., Box 3342 (1975).

CLARK, C.R., DAVIES, C.O., & WOODCOCK, R.W. *Standard Rebus Glossary.* Minneapolis: American Guidance Service (1974).

CLARK, C. R., MOORES, D.F., & WOODCOCK, R.W. *Minnesota Early Language Development Sequence.* Minneapolis: Research, Development, and Demonstration Center in Education of Handicapped Children, University of Minnesota (1973).

COLLINS, D.W. Patient initiated light operated telecontrol (PILOT). In Keith Copeland (Ed.), *Aids for the Severely Handicapped.* New York: Grune & Stratton, pp. 31-41 (1974).

COPELAND, K. (Ed.) *Aids for the Severely Handicapped.* New York: Grune & Stratton (1974).

DUNN, L.M. *Peabody Picture Vocabulary Test.* Minneapolis: American Guidance Service (1959).

EHRLICH, M.D. The Votrax Voice Synthesizer as an aid for the blind. *Proceedings of the 1974 Conference on Engineering Devices in Rehabilitation,* Boston (1974).

EICHLER, J.H., *Instructions for the ETRAN Eye Signaling System.* Ridgefield, Connecticut: Jack H. Eichler, 5 Beaver Brook Road (1973).

FEALLOCK, B. Communication for the nonverbal individual. *American Journal of Occupational Therapy, 12,* 60-63, 83 (1958).

GARDNER, H., ZURIF, E.B., BERRY, T., & BAKER, E. Visual communication in aphasia. *Neuropsychologia, 14,* 275-292 (1976).

GERTENRICH, R.L. A simple mouth-held writing device for use with cerebral palsy patients. *Mental Retardation, 4,* 13-14 (August, 1966).

GLASS, A.V., GAZZANIGA, M.S., & PREMACK, D. Artificial language training in global aphasia. *Neuropsychologia, 11,* 95-103 (1973).

GOLDBERG, H.R., & FENTON, J. *Aphonic Communication for Those with Cerebral Palsy: Guide for the Development and Use of a Conversation Board.* New York: United Cerebral Palsy of New York State (no date).

Handicapped youth "talks" with eyes. *News Journal* (Mansfield, Ohio) (October 22, 1974).

HARRIS-VANDERHEIDEN, D. Blissymbols and the mentally retarded. In Gregg C. Vanderheiden & Kate Grilley (Eds.), *Non-vocal Communication Techniques and Aids for the Severely Physically Handicapped* Baltimore: University Park Press, pp. 120-131 (1976).

HOLT, C., BUELOW, D., & VANDERHEIDEN, G. *Interface Switch Profile and Annotated List of Commerical Switches.* Madison, Wisconsin: Trace Research and Development Center for the Severely Communicatively Impaired, University of Wisconsin-Madison (1976).

HOLT, C., & VANDERHEIDEN, G. *Master Chart of Communication Aids.* Madison, Wisconsin: Trace Research and Development Center for the Severely Communicatively Impaired, University of Wisconsin, Madison (1974).

KATES, B., & MCNAUGHTON, S. *The First Application of Blissymbols as a Communication Medium for Non-speaking Children: History and Development, 1971-1974.* Toronto: Blissymbolics Communication Institute, 862 Eglinton Avenue East, (1975).

KORZYBSKI, A. *Science and Sanity: An Introduction to Non-Aristotelian Systems and General Semantics.* Lakeville, Connecticut: Institute of General Semantics (1933).

MAYBERRY, R. If a chimp can learn sign language, surely my nonverbal client can too. *Asha, 18,* 223-228 (1976).

MCDONALD, E.T. Design and application of communication boards. In Gregg C. Vanderheiden & Kate Grilley (Eds.), *Non-vocal Communication Techniques and Aids for the Severely Physically Handicapped.* Baltimore: University Park Press, pp. 105-119 (1976).

MCDONALD & SCHULTZ, A.R. Communication boards for cerebral palsied children. *Journal of Speech and Hearing Disorders, 38,* 73-88 (1973).

MCNAUGHTON, S. Blissymbolics—An alternative symbol system for the non-vocal pre-reading child. In Gregg C. Vanderheiden & Kate Grilley (Eds.), *Non-vocal Communication Techniques and Aids for the Severely Physically Handicapped.* Baltimore: University Park Press, pp. 85-104 (1976a).

————— . Symbol Communication Programme at OCCC. In Gregg C. Vanderheiden & Kate Grilley (Eds.), *Non-vocal Communication Techniques and Aids for the Severely Physically Handicapped.* Baltimore: University Park Press, pp. 132-143 (1976b).

————— . *Symbol Secrets.* Toronto: Blissymbolics Communication Institute, 862 Eglinton Avenue East (1975).

MCNAUGHTON, S., & KATES, B. *Visual symbols: Communication system for the pre-reading physically handicapped child.* Paper presented at the annual meeting of the American Association on Mental Deficiency,

Toronto, Ontario (1974).

Microprocessor based voice synthesizer puts speech at its user's fingertips. *Digital Design,* 15-16 (March, 1977).

NEWELL, A.F., & BRUMFITT, P.J. 'Talking brooch' communication aid. In Keith Copeland (Ed.), *Aids for the Severely Handicapped.* New York: Grune and Stratton, pp. 104-108 (1974).

OLSON, T. Return of the nonverbal. *Asha, 18,* 823 (1976).

Ontario Crippled Children's Centre Symbol Communication Programme. Toronto: Ontario Crippled Children's Centre, 350 Rumsey Road (1976).

PARKEL, D.A., WHITE, R.A., & WARNER, H. Implications of the Yerkes technology for mentally retarded human subjects. In Duane M. Rumbaugh (Ed.), *Language Learning by a Chimpanzee: The LANA Project.* New York: Academic Press (1977).

PREMACK, A.J., & PREMACK, D. Teaching language to an ape. *Scientific American, 277,* 92-99 (1972).

PREMACK, D. A functional analysis of language. *Journal of Experimental Analysis of Behavior, 14,* 107-125 (1970).

———. Language in chimpanzee? *Science, 172,* 808-822 (1971).

PREMACK, D., and PREMACK, A.J. Teaching visual language to apes and language-deficient persons. In Richard L. Schiefelbusch & Lyle L. Lloyd (Eds.), *Language Perspectives — Acquisition, Retardation, and Intervention.* Baltimore: University Park Press, 347-376 (1974).

RAHIMI, M.A., & EYLENBERG, J.B. *A computer terminal with synthetic speech output.* Paper presented at the National Conference on the Use of On-Line Computers in Psychology, St. Louis (1973).

RALSTON, A., & MEEK, C.L. (Eds.) *Encyclopedia of Computer Science.* New York: Petrocelli/Charter (1976).

Record-player "voice" for mutes. *NASA Tech Briefs,* 97-98 (Spring, 1977).

REUTER, D.B. Speech synthesis under APL. *Proceedings of the Sixth International APL Users Conference,* pp. 585-596 (1974).

RUMBAUGH, D.M. (Ed.) *Language Learning by a Chimpanzee: The LANA Project.* New York: Academic Press (1977).

SAYRE, J.M. Communication for the non-verbal cerebral palsied. *CP Review, 24,* 3-8 (November/December, 1963).

SCHURMAN, J.A. Custom designing communication board frames: The role of the occupational therapist. In Beverly Vicker (Ed.), *Nonoral Communication System Project 1964/1973,* Iowa City, Iowa: Campus Stores, The University of Iowa, pp. 177-211 (1974).

SILVERMAN, E.M., & SILVERMAN, F.H. Attitudes toward the adoption of an international language. In William C. McCormack & Stephen A. Wurm (Eds.), *Language and Society: Anthropological Issues.* The Hague and Paris: Mouton Publishers (1979).

SILVERMAN, H., MCNAUGHTON, S., & KATES, B. *Handbook of Blissymbolics for Instructors, Users, Parents and Administrators,* Toronto: Blissymbolics Communication Institute (1) 1978.

VANDERHEIDEN, D.H., BROWN, W.P., MACKENZIE, P., REINEN, S., & SCHEIBEL, C. Symbol communication for the mentally handicapped. *Mental Retardation, 13,* 34-37 (1975).

VANDERHEIDEN, D.H., and GRILLEY, K. (Eds.) *Non-vocal Communication Techniques and Aids for the Severely Physically Handicapped.* Baltimore: University Park Press (1976).

VANDERHEIDEN, G.C. *Design and construction of a laptray: Preliminary notes.* Madison, Wisconsin: Trace Research and Development Center for the Severely Communicatively Impaired, University of Wisconsin-Madison (1977).

————— . Providing the child with a means to indicate. In Gregg C. Vanderheiden and Kate Grilley (Eds.), *Non-vocal Communication Techniques and Aids for the Severely Physically Handicapped.* Baltimore: University Park Press, pp. 20-76 (1976).

VICKER, B. *Nonoral Communication System Project 1964/1973.* Iowa City, Iowa: Campus Stores, The University of Iowa (1974).

VONGLASSERSFELD, E. The Yerkish Language and its automatic parser. In Duane M. Rumbaugh (Ed.), *Language Learning in a Chimpanzee: The LANA Project.* New York: Academic Press, pp. 91-130 (1977).

WARNER, H., BELL, C.L., & BROWN, J.V. The conversation board. In Duane M. Rumbaugh (Ed.), *Language Learning in a Chimpanzee: The LANA Project.* New York: Academic Press, pp. 263-271 (1977).

WEPMAN, J.M. *Recovery from Aphasia.* New York: The Ronald Press (1951).

WOODCOCK, R.W. An experimental test for remedial readers. *Journal of Educational Psychology, 49,* 23-27 (1958).

————— . Rebuses as a medium in beginning reading instruction. *IMRID Papers and Reports, 5* (4) (1968).

————— . (Ed.) *The Rebus Reading Series.* Nashville, Tennessee: Institute on Mental Retardation and Intellectual Development, George Peabody College (1965).

————— . CLARK, C.R., & DAVIES, C.O. *The Peabody Rebus Reading Program.* Circle Pines, Minnesota: American Guidance Service (1968).

————— . *The Peabody Rebus Reading Program—Teacher's Guide.* Circle Pines, Minnesota: American Guidance Service (1969).

6 Neuro-assisted Modes

Almost all speechless children and adults can learn to communicate by the use of one or more gestural systems (see Chapter 4); gestural-assisted systems (see Chapter 5); or a combination of the two. There are a few, however, who are so involved motorically that they either are unable to gesturally activate a switching mechanism *reliably* or cannot due so without becoming unduly fatigued. At least some of these persons may be able to use the communication systems that are described in this chapter. These systems, however, should be viewed as *last resorts* because they have several limitations when compared to electronic gestural-assisted ones.

1. Neuro-assisted systems tend to *cost more* than gestural-assisted ones intended to perform the same function (e.g., to control an electric typewriter).
2. Neuro-assisted systems tend to *transmit messages at a slower rate* than gestural-assisted ones intended to perform the same function.
3. Neuro-assisted systems are *more likely to malfunction* than gestural-assisted ones intended to perform the same function because they tend to be more complex than them electronically.
4. It is necessary with a neuro-assisted system to *attach something to the user* (surface electrodes). The only gestural-assisted systems for which this is necessary are those in which a tilt switch or a headstick is used.
5. The *state of the art* for neuro-assisted communication systems is *not as highly developed* as that for gestural-assisted ones intended to perform the same function. The literature describing these systems is relatively small.

Neuro-assisted communication systems only differ from gestural-assisted systems intended to perform the same function in one way: they are activated, or controlled, by electrical signals generated by the body rather than by muscle gestures or movements. Users of a neuro-assisted system activate it by *willfully* varying *in an agreed upon manner* an aspect (or attribute) of some electrical signals emanating from their bodies. They may, for example, vary the *intensity* or *frequency* of such signals. A change in the frequency or intensity of a particular set of electrical signals emanating from a user's body can be detected by electrodes attached to his or her skin at a particular location. This location is determined by the *type* of electrical activity used to control, or activate, the system. If it is *brain waves,* the electrodes are mounted on the user's head; if it is *muscle action potentials,* they are attached to his or her skin over the muscle group (or groups) whose activity level (or activity levels) is (are) being used to control the system.

Any electrical signals generated by the body *theoretically* can be used to control a communication system so long as

> the user can learn to reliably willfully vary an aspect of it (e.g., its intensity or frequency) in an agreed upon manner;
> learning to do this would not be detrimental to his or her health; and
> the aspect of the signal varied can be monitored by electrodes attached to the user's skin.

Two types of biological electrical signals capable of being partially brought under voluntary control through *biofeedback* techniques are *muscle action potentials* and *brain waves.* (Biofeedback techniques are dealt with later in this chapter.) Both can be monitored by electrodes attached to the skin (surface electrodes); and both can be controlled well enough by *some* persons (with no reported detrimental effects on their health) to reliably activate, or control, an electric typewriter or teletypewriter (Combs, 1969; Rice & Combs, 1972; Torok, 1974; Dewan, 1966; Writing made possible for cerebral palsy victim, 1976). Since the *patterns* of bioelectric signals that would be used to control a CRT display, rotary scanning display, rectangular matrix display, LED display, strip printer, and a speech generator that operates in a scanning mode are the *same* as those that would be used to control a typewriter or teletypewriter, it seems reasonable to assume that muscle action potentials and brain waves could be controlled well enough by some persons to also reliably activate these displays.

The remainder of this chapter deals with the use of muscle action potentials and brain waves to control communication systems. While the literature concerned with this use of muscle action potentials and brain waves is limited, there is a relatively large literature dealing with their control by *biofeedback* techniques. Both the *instrumentation* and *teaching techniques* that are used in EMG and EEG biofeedback research (for monitoring and modifying muscle action potentials and brain waves, respectively) probably can be adapted for controlling most of the displays described in Chapter 5.

Use of Muscle Action Potentials for Controlling Communication Systems

Muscle action potentials are electrical signals that are associated with the *contraction* of muscle fibers. They do not arise from the contraction itself, but from the electrical signals conducted along the axons of lower motor neurons (anterior horn cells) to the muscle fibers they innervate, which causes them to contract. The process by which they arise can be summarized as follows:

> The striated muscle of man is composed functionally of motor units in which the axons of single motor (anterior horn) cells innervate many muscle fibers. Hundreds of muscle fibers may be innervated by a single axon. All of the fibers innervated by a single motor unit respond immediately in an "all-or-none" pattern, to adequate stimulation. The interactions of many motor units can produce relatively smooth motor performance. Increased motor power results from activation of a greater number of motor units or from repeated activation of a given number of motor units. The action potential of a muscle consists of the sum of the action potentials of many motor units. The action potential of normal muscle fibers originates at the motor end plates and is triggered by an incoming nerve impulse at the myoneural junction. It then spreads along muscle fibers, exciting contraction. (Chusid & McDonald, 1960, p. 209)

Note particularly that (1) when normal muscle is *at rest,* there are *no* action potentials and when it is in a *state of contraction,* there *are* action potentials and (2) the greater the number of motor units (in a muscle) that are activated, the greater the magnitude of the action potential. Both phenomena have been utilized in the control of communication systems.

A muscle's action potentials can be detected by *surface electrodes* that are in contact with the skin covering it. (They also can be detected by needle electrodes, but these do not appear to be practical for use with communication systems because they have to be inserted into the muscle.) A surface electrode consists of a small metal disc (sometimes silver) that has an insu-

FIGURE 6.1. *Surface electrode, with insulated electrical wire and connectors attached.*

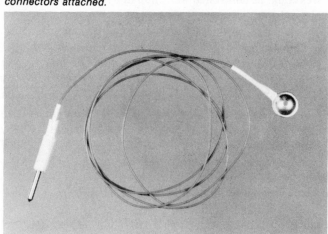

lated electrical wire soldered to it (see Figure 6.1). This wire usually has a male connector attached to its other end so that it can be plugged into, or interfaced with, an amplifier. These electrodes usually are used in pairs and are attached to the skin over the muscle being monitored, approximately one inch apart. A third, or ground, electrode also may be used.

Care must be taken in attaching surface electrodes to the skin. According to Smorto and Basmajian,

> It is extremely important in applying surface electrodes to ensure that the electric insulation between the muscle and the electrode is reduced to a minimum. Since a poor contact must be avoided, continued pressure is obviously important. Fortunately, the pressure provided by the adhesive strips used for securing the electrodes is usually adequate. Electrical contact is greatly improved by the use of a saline "electrode jelly"; this is retained between the electrode and the skin by making the silver disc of the elect- rode slightly concave on the aspect to be applied to the skin. The dead surface layer of the skin along with its protective oils must be removed to lower the electrical resistance to practical levels of about 3,000 ohms. This is best done by light abrasion of the skin at the site chosen for electrode application. In recent years we have found that it is best produced by "rubbing in" those types of electrode jelly that have powered abrasive included in their formula (Smorto & Basmajian, 1977, pp. 10-11).

Muscle action potentials are very weak electrical signals. To be usable for controlling a communication system, they have to be *amplified* sufficiently to activate a display (e.g., a tone generator) and trigger a switching mechanism (e.g., a relay). An amplifier intended for *low-level bioelectric signals* is used for this purpose (see Figure 6.2). It should contain isolation and filtering circuits in addition to those circuits required for amplification. *Isolation circuits* prevent the user from receiving an electrical shock (through the electrodes) if the equipment malfunctions. High-pass and low-pass *filtering circuits* that restrict the frequency range of signals the unit will detect to that within which muscle action potentials fall. Without these filtering circuits, the unit may respond to other bioelectric signals as well, such as those associated with heart activity.

After the bioelectric signals detected by the electrodes *that are muscle*

FIGURE 6.2. *Components of a myoswitch.*

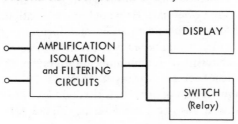

action potentials are amplified, they can be used to activate a display and a switching mechanism (Figure 6.2). The purpose of the display, which can be an oscilloscope, an oscillographic recorder, a meter, a light, or a sound generator, is to make the user aware of the pattern of muscle action potentials detected by the electrodes so that he or she can learn to produce them in the manner necessary for.activating the communication system. There is considerable evidence in the biofeedback literature which suggests that if a covert bioelectric process (such as the generation of muscle action potentials) can be made overt, a person is likely to be able to gain some degree of voluntary control over it (Karlins & Andrews, 1972). Such a process can be made overt in several ways, including:

1. displaying it on an oscilloscope screen;
2. having it cause a *light* to *go on* when it is the appropriate magnitude;
3. having it cause a *light* to *increase in intensity* as it increases in magnitude;
4. having it cause a *sound* to *be generated* when it is the appropriate magnitude;
5. having it cause a *sound* to *increase in volume* as it increases in magnitude;
6. having it cause a *sound* to *increase in frequency* as it increases in magnitude;
7. having it cause the *needle* on a meter to *move in a particular direction;* and;
8. having it drawn by an oscillographic recorder on a strip of paper.

Accordingly, the user would be instructed to look at or listen to the display and attempt to cause *one* of the following to occur:

1. an increase in the "height" of the electrical signals displayed on the oscilloscope screen;
2. a light to turn on (or off);
3. a light to increase in intensity;
4. a sound to be generated;
5. a sound to increase in volume;
6. a sound to increase in frequency;
7. the needle on a meter to move in a particular direction; or
8. an increase in the "height" of the electrical signals being drawn on paper by an oscillographic recorder.

The user would know when he observed one of these occurring that he had been successful in varying the bioelectric signal in the manner necessary for controlling the communication system. He may not be aware *on a conscious level* of specifically what he did to vary it (awareness of the control process on this level usually is not essential). He would practice with the display until he could cause light, tone, needle position, or wave-form changes to occur *whenever he wished*. He then would be ready to use the bioelectric signal to activate the switching mechanism of a communication system. (For further information about biofeedback see Karlins & Andrews, 1972.)

Amplified muscle action potentials that will activate a display also can be used to activate a switching mechanism (Figure 6.2). Switching mec-

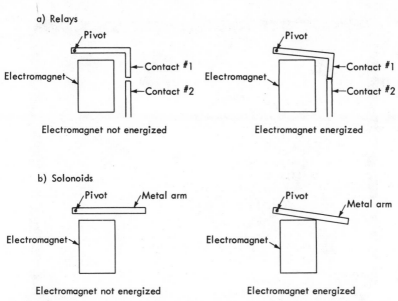

a) Relays

Pivot

Electromagnet

←—Contact #1

←—Contact #2

Electromagnet not energized

Pivot

Electromagnet

←—Contact #1

←—Contact #2

Electromagnet energized

b) Solonoids

Pivot   Metal arm

Electromagnet

Electromagnet not energized

Pivot

Metal arm

Electromagnet

Electromagnet energized

FIGURE 6.3. Function of the electromagnets in relays and solenoids.

hanisms that can be activated in this manner are likely to contain one of two electrical components: a *relay* or a *solenoid.*

A *relay* has three parts that allow it to function as a switch: two strips of metal that serve as electrical contacts, and an electromagnet (see Figure 6.3). The two strips of metal are mounted perpendicular to each other so that their ends are slightly separated when the electromagnet mounted beneath the horizontal one is not energized. When the electromagnet is energized (by the amplified muscle action potentials) it pulls the horizontal strip downward, causing its end to contact that of the vertical one. This "closes the bridge" (see Figure 5.19), or activates the switch. The electromagnet would not be energized until the muscle action potentials were of sufficient magnitude to cause a display to function in one of the ways described in this section.

A *solenoid* consists of an electromagnet and a pivoted metal strip, or arm, that is mounted in close proximity to it (Figure 6.3). When the electromagnet is energized, the part of the arm that is in close proximity to it is pulled toward it. This causes the end of the arm to move a fraction of an inch. If a push switch such as a lever microswitch (see Chapter 5) is mounted slightly below the arm, the arm will depress it when the electromagnet is energized.

Some small, relatively inexpensive, battery-operated electromyographs intended for biofeedback can be adapted to function as myoswitches (see Figure 6.4). These units come equipped with surface electrodes, amplifiers, and displays. A switching mechanism containing a relay or a solenoid can be attached to the output terminal of the unit that is intended for an oscillo-

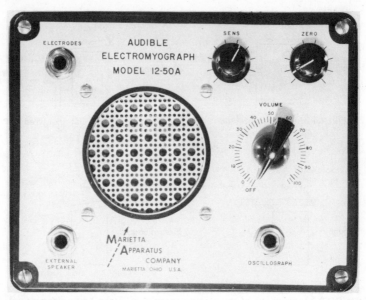

FIGURE 6.4. *A representative EMG (electromyography) biofeedback unit.*

graphic recorder (Figure 6.4) by an electrical cable that has an appropriate male connector attached to its end. An electrical engineer (possibly one on the faculty of a local college or university) should be able to design and fabricate the circuitry needed in the switching mechanism to activate a relay or solenoid in the required manner with the particular electromyograph being used.

There are two basic types of muscle action potential patterns that have been used for controlling neuro-assisted communication systems. The first is an increase in magnitude when a user wishes to activate a switch followed by a decrease. A myoswitch used in this manner can perform any of the functions of a switching mechanism containing a single switch. It can control a speech generator that operates in a scanning mode, a rotary scanning display, or a rectangular matrix scanning display (see Chapter 5). It also can be used *in conjunction with the latter* to control a CRT display, a strip printer, a typewriter, or a teletypewriter.

The second type of pattern consists of alternating periods of increase and decrease that correspond to patterns of "dots and dashes" in Morse code (see Table 4.3). There are several ways these patterns can be produced. A relatively *short* muscle contraction can stand for a dot and a longer one for a dash. Or a relatively *weak* muscle contraction can stand for a dot and a stronger one for a dash. It is crucial if these systems are used that the dots do not overlap the dashes (with regard to duration of contraction or strength of contraction). If it is likely that a user would be unable to keep dots and dashes from overlapping, there is another way that these Morse code patterns can be produced: *two myoswitches* are used. Each monitors the activity of a different muscle (e.g., one on the right arm and one on the left arm). The user would contact one muscle when he wished to produce a dot and the other when he wished to produce a dash. The Morse code patterns produced would be translated into letters, digits, etc, by a computer (see Chapter 5). Myoswitch generated Morse code patterns can be used to directly control CRT displays, strip printers, and teletypewriters.

What factors should be considered when deciding whether a particular muscle (or muscles) can be used for activating a myoswitch? There are several, including:

1.   the ease with which the muscle (or muscles) can be contracted (the greater the ease, the more usable the muscle, or muscles, for the purpose);

2.   whether or not the muscle contracts involuntarily (if a muscle contracts involuntarily because of a neuromuscular disorder, it may activate the communication system and interfere with message transmission);

3.   the ease with which electrodes can be attached to the skin over the muscle without interfering with ongoing, or daily, activity (some electrode locations are likely to interfere more with ongoing activities than are others);

4.   the electrical resistance of the skin (there are some locations on the body at which it is easier to lower the resistance of the skin to an acceptable level than it is at others); and

5.   the closeness of the muscle to the skin (the closer a muscle to the skin, the more successful one is likely to be in monitoring its action potentials by surface electrodes).

It is desirable, but not essential, that the muscle (or muscles) used to activate a myoswitch function normally. If a person can contract *some* of the fibers in a muscle whenever he wishes to, and none of the fibers in it contract involuntarily, it may be usable for activating a myoswitch.

All of the symbol systems described in Chapter 5 that are usable with electronic gestural-assisted communication systems are usable with communication systems that can be controlled by myoswitches. Also, the components of the control electronics for gestural-assisted communication systems that are described in Chapter 5 are usable with the type described here.

For further information about communication systems that can be controlled by muscle action potentials, see Combs (1969), Dewan (1966), Rice and Combs (1972), Torok (1974), and "Writing made possible for cerebral palsy victim" (1966). Also, the literature on EMG (electromyography) biofeedback and that (in physical medicine and physical therapy) on the use of muscle action potentials to control such devices as wheelchairs provide useful information about designing and fabricating myoswitches and teaching people how to use them.

Use of Brain Wave Patterns for Controlling Communication Systems

There is some suggestion in the literature (Dewan, 1966) that the alpha rhythm of the brain, as detected by surface electrodes attached to the scalp over the occipital lobe, can be controlled sufficiently well to generate a Morse code pattern that can be used to spell out messages on a CRT display (that can be typed by a teletypewriter). Alpha rhythm can be enhanced or reduced to form dots and dashes by *controlling eye function* (Dewan, 1966; Mulholland & Evans, 1965). According to Dewan,

> if the subject becomes alert or focuses his eyes with his eyes open (or, with practice, even with them closed) this rhythm tends to disappear, whereas it tends to be enhanced when the subject relaxes with his eyes closed and with minimal concentration or "visualization." Recently, T. Mulholland and the present author independently noticed that eye position can also play an important role, the upward position tending to enhance alpha activity (Dewan, 1966, p. 349).

Dewan trained three persons (who were normal neurologically) to send alpha dots and dashes "by altering their eye position, focusing muscles, and in some cases, by opening and closing the eyes" (1966, p. 349) accurately enough to type out messages character by character on a teletypewriter. The time needed for sending each character was over ½ minute. He was able to rule out the possibility that the EEG Morse code actually was being sent by neck muscle contractions.

The *components* of an *alphaswitch* are the same as those of a myoswitch (see Figure 6.2). The same types of surface electrodes, displays, and switching mechanisms would be used. The same type of amplifier also could be used, but would be adjusted somewhat differently. The biofeedback training procedures used would be the same as for EMG biofeedback. (For further information on EEG biofeedback procedures and instrumentation, see Karlins & Andrews, 1972.)

Since it appears that messages can be transmitted at a faster rate by EMG than by EEG Morse code (Dewan, 1966), the former probably would be preferable in most instances.

REFERENCES

Chusid, J.G., & McDonald, J.J. *Correlative Neuroanatomy and Functional Neurology.* Los Altos, California: Lange Medical Publications (1960).

Combs, R.G. Myocom: Communication for non-verbal handicapped. *Transactions of the Missouri Academy of Science, 3,* 102 (1969).

DEWAN, E.M. Communication by voluntary control of the electroencephalogram. *Proceedings of the Symposium on Biomedical Engineering, 1,* 349-351 (1966).

KARLINS, M., & ANDREWS, L.M. *Biofeedback.* Philadelphia: J.B. Lippincott (1972).

MULHOLLAND, T., & EVANS, C.R. An unexpected artifact in the human electroencephalogram concerning the alpha rhythm and the orientation of the eyes. *Nature, 207,* 36 (1965).

RICE, O.M., & COMBS, R.G. Practical aids for non-verbal handicapped. *Proceedings of the 1972 Carnahan Conference on Electronic Prosthetics* (1972).

SMORTO, M.P., & BASMAJIAN, J.V. *Electrodiagnosis: A Handbook for Neurologists.* New York: Harper & Row (1977).

TOROK, Z. A typewriter operated by electromyographic potentials (GMMI). In Keith Copeland (Ed.), *Aids for the Severely Handicapped.* New York: Grune & Stratton, pp. 77-82 (1974).

Writing made possible for cerebral palsy victim. *Pacific Review, 10* (4) 3 (February, 1976).

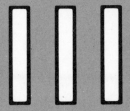

CLINICAL
CONSIDERATIONS

7 Selecting a Nonspeech Communication Mode (or Modes)

Many nonspeech communication modes (systems) are described in Chapters 4, 5, and 6. This Chapter provides guidelines for selecting from among them the one (or ones) most likely to be *optimal* for a particular child or adult. The optimal communication mode (or combination of modes) for a person is the one (or ones) from among those he *could use* that would *come closest* to meeting his communication needs at a *relatively low cost.* Cost refers here not only to the expense of purchasing and maintaining components (switching mechanisms, displays, etc.), but also to the time investments required of both client and clinician.

An evaluation procedure is outlined in this chapter for selecting the optimal nonspeech communication system (or combination of such systems) for a person, which requires six questions to be answered.

1. What is the cause of the person's communicative disorder?
2. How does the person communicate at present?
3. What are his communication needs?
4. What is his inner, receptive, and expressive language status?
5. Of the existing nonspeech communication systems, which would it be possible for him to use?
6. Of the systems he could use, which system (or combination of systems) would be *optimal* for meeting his communication needs?

Types of information are indicated that usually have to be obtained to answer these questions. Those mentioned, of course, are not the only ones that ever would be needed for this purpose. They are, however, ones that would be needed to answer these questions for almost all speechless children and adults. A form that can be used for recording the information obtained is reproduced in *Appendix E.*

What Is the Cause of the Person's Communicative Disorder?

Before beginning the evaluation it would be important to know the nature of the condition (or conditions) responsible for the person being speechless. Certain aspects of this information, including those below, could influence the choice of a communication mode.

Whether the condition is progressive. If a person has a progressive neurological condition, it would be important to consider how long he would be likely to be able to use each of the various modes that could be selected. *Ideally,* a mode (or modes) should be selected that he can use for a relatively long period of time.

The impact of the condition on the functioning of the musculature of the extremities, trunk, face, and neck. The impact of the condition on the total external body musculature can influence the selection of a communication mode. If the musculature of one or both upper extremities functions normally, a manual gestural system might be considered. And if some trunk muscle groups functioned normally, they might be usable for activating a switching mechanism. Hence, this information can be helpful in identifying nonspeech communication systems that it would be possible for a person to use.

The impact of the condition on cognitive and sensory functioning. If either cognitive or sensory functioning is disturbed, this of course can influence both the choice of a symbol system and the approach used to indicate (or generate) message components.

The permanence of the impact of the condition on speech. If the impact on speech could be temporary (which could be the case for a person seen shortly after a stroke before there has been much opportunity for spontaneous recovery), a different system might *initially* be selected than if it were likely to be permanent.

The prognosis for ambulation. If a person is likely to be confined to a bed or wheelchair, some systems (e.g., a large communication board) tend to be more practical than if he is likely to be ambulatory.

Whether there is litigation pending. If the condition resulted from trauma and there is litigation pending, this might reduce a person's motivation to improve his ability to communicate by any means.

Information about a client's condition and its impact on his motor, sensory, and cognitive functioning can be obtained from his physician and from his physical and occupational therapists if he is receiving or has received these services. It also could be important to obtain information about the impact of the condition on the person's *emotional* status. If he is very depressed, it *may* be difficult to get him to accept any nonspeech communication mode.

How Does The Person Communicate at Present?

Almost all functionally speechless persons can communicate in at least a limited way. Their communication may be limited to yes and no gestures which they use for answering questions. Information about how a functionally speechless person communicates can influence the choice of a communication system (or systems) for him in several ways.

The information can suggest communication systems that it would be possible for him to use: if he were using mime (pantomime) or a nonstandard manual gestural system, it probably would be possible to teach him to use Amerind or Ameslan signs. In addition, it can indicate whether a system is needed to *augment* speech and normal nonverbal communication or serve as an *alternative to* or substitute for them. This information also provides a *baseline* for assessing the impact of intervention with a particular communication system (or combination of systems) on a person's ability to communicate.

You should investigate both speech and nonspeech channels when you are attempting to determine how a person communicates. Nonspeech channels include normal nonverbal (gestural) aspects of oral communication, writing, typing, and the systems described in Chapters 4, 5, and 6. (It is conceivable that a person being evaluated has been taught to use a system described in these chapters or has learned to use it on his own.) The kinds of information that are needed to describe how a child or adult communicates include those below.

His use of speech. The focus here is on the person's ability to *successfully* use words, word approximations, and other vocal sounds (including inflection patterns) for communication. If he uses word approximations or "sounds" generated by the vocal tract *that are intelligible to others,* these can be considered to be part of his speech communication.

His use of writing. It is, of course, important to determine how well the person can encode and transmit messages by writing or printing with a pen or pencil. If he is a hemiplegic and his dominant side is involved, his ability to write with both right and left hands should be evaluated.

His ability to type. It would be particularly important to determine how well the person could type if he was unable to print or write intelligibly. If he cannot use a manual typewriter because he is unable to press the keys hard enough to activate them, an electric one should be tried.

His ability to communicate by gesture. Of interest here would be face and body gestures that accompany attempts at speech, pointing to desired objects, mime (pantomime), and use of the types of gestural systems described in Chapter 4. It is particularly important to determine whether the person has reliable yes and no gestures, and if he has, what they are.

His ability to understand speech and to read. The focus here is on how well the person can do these in his environment—how well he seems to understand what people say and what he reads.

His comprehension of gesture. The focus here would be on gestures that most people can understand, such as facial and body gestures accompanying speech, shaking the head yes or no, shrugging the shoulders, and simple mime (pantomime).

His knowledge of Morse code. It would only be important to determine this is the person were so involved motorically that a system might be considered for him in which Morse code is used to control a typewriter or other display. A person might have learned it in Boy Scouts, or in the army, or while meeting the requirements for an FCC "ham" radio license.

In addition to determining *how* the person communicates it also is important to determine *how often* he attempts to communicate in various ways. If he makes relatively little attempt to communicate, this could have one of several implications with regard to his probable acceptance of a non-speech communication system. First, it could indicate that he probably would accept it. If he is not communicating very much because he is being un-successful or because the approaches he is using are too fatiguing, he is likely to accept a system that will allow him to communicate more efficiently.

Second, his failure to communicate often could indicate that he would be unwilling to accept a nonspeech communication system. It could have this implication if he is not communicating very much because he is *depressed*. If his depression is specifically related to not being able to communicate, it is unlikely to interfere with his acceptance of a nonspeech communication system. If, however, it is primarily related to his reaction to the condition that caused him to be speechless (or something else other than not being able to communicate), it may have to be reduced before he will accept any communication system.

Another reason why he may not be communicating much is that he has relatively *little need* or *opportunity* to communicate. This is likely to be a reason if he lives alone or is a resident of an institution such as a nursing home or a facility for the mentally retarded. By increasing his need and opportunity to communicate, the likelihood he would accept a nonspeech communication system can be increased.

Finally, in addition to determining *how* and *how often* the person communicates, it is important to determine *what messages* he is able to communicate and by what means. What words and ideas has he been successful in communicating by speech, gesture, or a combination of the two? Persons with whom he communicates (such as his spouse or parents) should be asked to make a list of the words and ideas he has communicated to them and to indicate how he communicated each.

What Are His Communication Needs?

Before you can select a communication system for a person, you must first determine his communication needs. These can range from being able to communicate a few basic needs to the staff in a hospital or nursing home to being able to function as a professional including using a telephone and a typewriter.

It is necessary to consider *face-to-face* communication, *telephone* communication, and *written* communication when defining a person's communication needs. Some persons will require nonspeech communication systems for all three, and others will require them for only one or two. A single system may be usable for two or three of them (e.g., one containing a teletypewriter), or different systems may be used for each.

The *ultimate goal* of intervention with a nonspeech communication system (or systems) is meeting a person's communication needs. This goal is attainable in some cases, while in others it can only be approached. When it is not attainable, the goal should be to select the system (or systems) that comes closest to allowing him to meet his communication needs.

The clinician should make a judgment concerning the extent to which the person's communication ability meets his communication needs. A person is encountered occasionally who, though limited in ability to communicate, can communicate well enough to meet these needs. Such a person probably would not be a good candidate for a nonspeech communication system. One, of course, would have to be quite confident that a person's communication ability was adequate for his needs before ruling out a nonspeech communications system on this basis.

What is His Inner, Receptive, and Expressive Language Status?

A person's *inner language status* is partially a function of his ability to make sense out of his sensory environment (Myklebust, 1954). If he does not abstract the *"units of experience"* that are symbolized in his community by words, gestures, etc., he will not understand these symbols or be able to use them. He will also be unable to learn other symbols for them (e.g., Blissymbols).

Inner language can be *partially evaluated* by determining the extent to which a person is aware of how things are organized in his environment. If his use of his upper extremities is reasonably good, the following objects can be arranged randomly on a table in front of him: a doll house table, four chairs that will fit around it, and a doll family that can be positioned to sit in the chairs. If with little hesitation he places the chairs around the table and attempts to seat the dolls in the chairs, this would suggest his inner language functioning was at least at a two-year-old level (Weber, 1972). (For further information about evaluating inner language, see Myklebust, 1954.)

To determine a person's *receptive language status* it is necessary to assess his ability to understand speech and nonverbal (gestural) communication and to read. If a person experiences difficulty understanding speech because of a hearing loss, auditory agnosia, or receptive aphasia, this can interfere with his use of any nonspeech communication system described in this book. The extent to which it is likely to interfere is *partially* a function of the type and severity of the auditory impairment. Of course, even with a severe auditory impairment (e.g., deafness) it is possible to use a nonspeech communication system.

There are a number of test and parts of tests that can be used for estimating how well a person understands speech. Almost all aphasia tests contain items usable for this purpose. Also, there are a number of tests intended for assessing child language (e.g., the Peabody Picture Vocabulary Test—Dunn, 1959) that contain such items.

Either a rotary scanning display or a rectangular matrix display can be used for assessing the speech comprehension of persons who are unable to point, by a multiple-choice format. A set of stimuli consisting of photographs, drawings, words, or other symbols (see Chapter 5) can be mounted temporarily on one of these displays. The person being tested can indicate the member of the set he thinks is the correct response by manipulating a switching mechanism. If the Peabody Picture Vocabulary Test (Dunn, 1959) were administered in this manner, the four drawings presented for each stimulus word would be mounted temporarily on the display, one set at a time, and the person would indicate the drawing he thought illustrated a particular one by manipulating a switching mechanism. This approach also could be used for assessing reading ability and, possibly, comprehension of gestures.

Persons who have difficulty understanding nonverbal, or gestural, communication also are likely to have difficulty learning to use nonspeech communication systems, particularly the gestural type described in Chapter 4. A person's ability to understand gestural communication can be better than, the same as, or worse than his ability to understand speech. It would tend to be better than speech for the deaf, and the same as or worse than speech for some brain-damaged persons (Duffy, Duffy, & Pearson, 1975).

Procedures for evaluating comprehension of gestures are not as well standardized as those for evaluating speech comprehension. One task that could be used for the purpose would be instructing the person by mime (pantomime) how you wished him to manipulate some objects (e.g., put a ball in a cup). If he responded appropriately, this would suggest that he understood the gestural instructions. It is of course important before using a mime to make certain that a "normal" person of the examinee's age can understand it, particularly if the examinee is a child. If a mime is ambiguous or developmentally inappropriate, it is unusable for assessing comprehension of gestural communication.

Persons who have difficulty reading English *may* be unable to use an English-language symbol system (see Chapter 5) with either a gestural-assisted or neuro-assisted communication mode. Whether they could would depend on several factors, including their ability to read English, the prognosis for improving this ability, and the complexity of the symbol system they need to meet their communication needs.

There are a number of achievement tests that can be used for determining how well a child can read. Items that can be used for determining this in adults are included in most aphasia tests. If items have a multiple-choice response format, they can be adapted for presentation to severely motorically involved persons by mounting the possible responses on a rotary scanning display or rectangular scanning display (see Chapter 5).

Expressive language includes the abilities to speak, to produce symbolic gestures, and to write. A person's *speech* level, as already indicated, is important to determine because no matter what nonspeech system (or systems) is (are) selected for him, he is encouraged to use what speech he has along with it (them). A person's speech level also is important to determine because it can influence the choice of a communication system for him. If he has some usable speech, he may not require as flexible a system as he would if he had little or no intelligible speech. In the latter case, he would need a system to serve as an *alternative* to speech; in the former, he would need a system to *augment* it. There are items for determining speech level in almost all aphasia tests and in tests of children's language development.

A person's ability to communicate by gesture can have an impact on the choice of a communication system for him. If he uses mime, it probably would be worthwhile to try to teach him a formal gestural system such as Amerind or Ameslan. Items for evaluating a person's abilty to communicate by gesture can be found in several language tests, including the Parson's Language Sample (Spradlin, 1963), the Illinois Test of Psycholinguistic Abilities (Kirk, McCarthy, & Kirk, 1968), and the Porch Index of Communicative Ability (Porch, 1971).

Communicating by writing can *partially* compensate for the inability to communicate by speech. It is, of course, useless for communicating in certain situations (e.g., on the telephone). All functionally speechless persons (except, possibly, young children) should be provided with a system for generating permanent messages—ones that are typed—if they are unable to write or print them. Items for assessing an adult's writing ability can be found on most aphasia tests. A child's writing ability can be assessed by standardized achievement tests.

Of The Existing Nonspeech Communication Systems, Which Would It Be Possible For Him To Use?

When selecting a nonspeech communication system for a child or adult, all existing types (see Chapters 4, 5, and 6) initially should be regarded as possibilities. Doing so maximizes the probability that *at least one* system will be identified that the person could use. It also maximizes the probability that the *optimum* existing nonspeech communication system (or combination of such systems) for a person will be among those identified.

There are *three general aspects of functioning* that should be considered when you are attempting to determine whether it would be possible for a person to use a particular system: *motor, sensory,* and *cognitive.* Approaches are described in this section for evaluating each for the purpose of determining whether it is sufficiently intact for a person to use a particular communication mode.

Motor Functioning

It is necessary to evaluate motor functioning if the person has or is suspected of having an apraxia or a neuromuscular disorder (see Darley, Aronson, & Brown, 1975, for descriptions of these conditions). A person's motor status is one of the primary determiners of the communication systems he can use. The less impaired his motor functioning, the *greater the number* of systems and the *more efficient* the systems which it would be possible for him to use. Almost any message can be transmitted faster and with less energy drain by a manual gestural system such as Ameslan or Amerind (see Chapter 4) than by a system controlled by a myoswitch (see Chapter 6).

There are two basic strategies that can be used for evaluating motor functioning. The first is to attempt to elicit *all* overt bodily movements that could be used for interfacing a person with a communication system. Since almost any movement could be used for this purpose, the functioning of almost the entire motor system would have to be evaluated, including that of the four extremities, the trunk, and the face and neck. Such an evaluation could take a great deal of time.

The alternative strategy is to attempt to elicit only *certain* overt bodily movements that could be used for interfacing a person with a communication system. Selection of this subset of movements could be based on a *series of assumptions* such as those below.

1. If a person does not have (or is not suspected of having) an apraxia or a neuromuscular disorder, it is unnecessary to evaluate his motor functioning.
2. The muscle groups that are most desirable to use for interfacing a person with a nonspeech communication system are those of the *upper extremities.* Thus, these would be the muscle groups evaluated *first.* If the functioning of the musculature of one or both upper extremities appeared either normal or adequate to interface the person with a communication system that would meet his needs, further evaluation of muscle functioning would be unnecessary.
3. The musculature of the face or neck is the most desirable for interfacing a person with a communication system *if* that of the upper extremities is inadequate for the purpose. Thus, these would be the muscle groups evaluated second. If the functioning of a portion of this musculature appeared adequate to interface the person with a communication system that would meet his needs, further evaluation of muscle functioning would be unnecessary.
4. The musculature of the lower extremities or trunk (particularly the latter) is almost always the *least desirable* for interfacing a person with a communication system. Thus, these would be the muscle groups evaluated last.

Note that with this strategy it only is necessary to evaluate all overt bodily movements when the musculature of the upper extremities, face, and neck appears inadequate to interface the person with a communication system that will meet his needs. The organization of the summary form for motor functioning in Appendix E is based on this set of assumptions.

Several factors should be considered when assessing the adequacy of a particular gesture (or movement) for interfacing a person with (or allowing him to use) a particular communication system, including

the *accuracy* with which it can be produced;
the *speed* with which it can be produced;
the *force* (pressure) it can exert;
the presence of *hyperactive stretch reflexes* or other abnormal reflexes associated with spasticity;
the presence of *tremor* or other involuntary movement; and
the extent to which doing it *fatigues* the person.

The greater the potential accuracy, speed, and force of the movement and the less it tends to fatigue the person, the more useful it probably would be for interfacing him with (or allowing him to use) a communication system. The presence of hyperactive reflexes or involuntary movement can reduce its usefulness for the purpose. (For descriptions of these aspects of motor functioning, see Darley, Aronson, & Brown, 1975).

There are *two* approaches that can be used for assessing the adequacy of a particular muscle gesture for interfacing a person with a particular communication system. The first, or *direct approach,* is to have the person use the gesture in the context of the system. To determine his ability to produce a particular hand gesture necessary for Amerind or Ameslan, he would be asked to imitate an Amerind or Ameslan sign containing that gesture. To evaluate his ability to produce the gesture needed for activating a particular switching mechanism, he could be observed while attempting to activate that switching mechanism.

While the direct method provides highly reliable information about the adequacy of a particular gesture for a particular communication system, it has several *limitations.* First, it may not be possible to have all or even most of the communication systems available that the person could use. Few clinical facilities could afford to keep on hand the hardware for the variety of communication systems that might be needed by their clients.

A second limitation of the direct method is that it may be more time and energy consuming than necessary. Several communication systems that a person could use may all require the same gesture; a given gesture, for example, may be usable for acitvating more than one switching mechanism.

The *second approach* that can be used for determining the adequacy of particular muscle gestures for interfacing a person with particular communication systems is systematically evaluating the gestures that could be used for the purpose. The examinee is asked to imitate these gestures, and their adequacy is described. The assumption is made that if the examinee can produce the gesture (or gestures) required for him to use a particular communication system, he will be able to use that system. With this approach, then, the adequacy of a person's gestures is *inferred* rather than observed (as it is with the first approach). Such inferences usually can be made quite reliably if the examiner is acquainted with the motor requirements of the communication systems being considered. This approach usually tends to be more efficient than the first. A procedure for systematically implementing it is outlined in this section. The primary source for gestures was Daniels and Worthingham's (1972) book, *Muscle Testing.* (This book contains a detailed description of each gesture.)

The gestures evaluated are divided into three groups: (1) upper extremities, (2) neck and face, and (3) lower extremities and trunk. Each gesture, if possible, should be evaluated first *against gravity.* If the person is unable to produce it normally under this condition, it is then evaluated with *gravity eliminated.* A gesture that can be performed reasonably well with gravity eliminated but not against gravity can be used for some purposes in interfacing a person with a communication system.

For persons who are so severely involved motorically that they are unable to produce the gestures needed to interface them with a communication system *even with gravity eliminated,* the examiner should note whether there is any evidence of muscle contraction when they attempt to produce each gesture. If there is contraction under this condition, the gesture *might* be usable for activating a myoswitch (see Chapter 6).

Gestures Involving the Upper Extremities. Twenty-seven gestures are described in this section. Each should be evaluated for accuracy, speed, force, presence of abnormal reflexes, presence of involuntary movement, and fatigue level for both right and left extremities. The primary source for this discussion (as well as those for the face, neck, trunk, and lower extremities) is Daniels and Worthingham's (1972) book, *Muscle Testing.* There are drawings in it which illustrate how each gesture is tested.

1. *Scapular Abduction and Upward Rotation.* To test *against gravity,* the person lies on his back, with the arm being evaluated flexed to 90 degrees with slight abduction and the elbow in extension. He attempts to move the arm upward by abducting the scapula. To test *without gravity,* the person sits with the arm being evaluated resting on a table, flexed to 90 degrees. He attempts to move the arm forward by abducting the scapula.

2. *Scapular elevation.* To test *against gravity,* the person sits, with his arms at his sides, and attempts to raise his shoulders as high as possible. To test *without gravity,* the person lies on his stomach with his forehead touching the surface on which he is lying and his shoulders supported by the examiner. He attempts to move his shoulders toward his ears. (Obviously, a person would not lie on his stomach to communicate. This posture is only used for testing.)

3. *Scapular adduction.* To test *against gravity,* the person lies on his stomach, with the arm being evaluated abducted to 90 degrees and laterally rotated and with the elbow flexed to a right angle. The examiner stabilizes his thorax. He attempts to raise the arm in horizontal abduction. To test *without gravity,* the person sits with the arm being evaluated resting on a table, midway between flexion and abduction. The examiner stablizes his thorax. He attempts to horizontally abduct the arm and, if successful, adducts the scapula.

4. *Scapular depression and adduction.* To test *against gravity,* the person lies on his stomach, with his forehead resting on the surface on which he is lying and with the arm being tested extended overhead. The patient attempts to raise the arm and move scapula upward.

5. *Shoulder flexion to 90 degrees.* To test *against gravity,* the person sits, with the arm being tested at his side and with the elbow slightly flexed. The examiner stabilizes his scapula. He attempts to flex (raise) his arm to 90 degrees. To test *without gravity,* the person lies on the side not being tested, with the arm being tested at his side and the elbow slightly flexed. The examiner stabilizes his scapula. He attempts to bring his arm forward to 90 degrees of flexion.

6. *Shoulder extension.* To test *against gravity,* the person lies on his stomach, with the arm being tested medially rotated and adducted (at side). The examiner stabilizes his scapula. He attempts to extend (raise) the arm. To test *without*

gravity, the person lies on the side not being tested, with the arm being tested flexed (at his side) and resting on a smooth board. The examiner stabilizes his scapula. He attempts to extend the arm (i.e., to slide it backward on the surface of the board).

7. *Shoulder abduction to 90 degrees.* To test *against gravity*, the person sits, with the arm being tested at his side in midposition between medial and lateral rotation and the elbow slightly flexed. The examiner stabilizes his scapula. He attempts to abduct (raise) the arm to 90 degrees. To test *without gravity*, the person lies on his back, with the arm being tested at his side in midposition between medial and lateral rotation. The examiner stabilizes his scapula. He attempts to abduct the arm to 90 degrees.

8. *Shoulder horizontal abduction.* To test *against gravity*, the person lies on his stomach, with the shoulder being tested abducted to 90 degrees, the upper arm resting on the surface on which he is lying, and the lower arm hanging vertically over the edge. The examiner stabilizes his scapula. He attempts to abduct (raise) the upper arm. To test *without gravity*, the person sits with the arm being tested supported (e.g., on a table top) in a position of 90 degrees of flexion. The examiner stabilizes his scapula. He attempts to horizontally abduct the arm (i.e., move it backward on the surface).

9. *Shoulder horizontal adduction.* To test *against gravity*, the person lies on his back, with the arm being tested abducted to 90 degrees. He attempts to adduct the arm (i.e., move it toward the midline of the body). To test *without gravity*, the person sits with the arm being tested resting on a table in 90 degrees of abduction. The examiner stabilizes his trunk. He attempts to bring the arm forward.

10. *Shoulder lateral rotation.* To test *against gravity*, the person lies on his stomach, with the shoulder being tested abducted to 90 degrees, upper arm resting on the surface on which he is lying (e.g., a table), and the lower arm hanging vertically over the edge. The examiner stabilizes the scapula. He attempts to swing his lower arm forward and upward and to laterally rotate his shoulder. To test *without gravity*, the person lies on his stomach with the entire arm being tested hanging over the surface on which he is lying (e.g., a table) in medially rotated position. The examiner stabilizes his scapula. He attempts to laterally rotate the arm.

11. *Shoulder medial rotation.* To test *against gravity*, the person lies on his stomach, with the shoulder being tested abducted to 90 degrees, upper arm supported on the surface on which he is lying, and the lower arm hanging vertically over the edge. The examiner stabilizes the scapula. He attempts to swing his lower arm backward and upward and medially rotate the shoulder. To test *without gravity*, the person lies on his stomach, with the arm of the extremity being tested hanging over the edge of the surface on which he is lying in lateral rotation. The examiner stabilizes the scapula. He attempts to medially rotate the arm.

12. *Elbow flexion.* To test *against gravity*, the person sits, with the arm being tested at his side and forearm supinated. The examiner stabilizes his upper arm. He attempts to flex the elbow. To test *without gravity*, the person lies on his back, with the shoulder of the extremity being tested abducted to 90 degrees and laterally rotated. The examiner stabilizes his upper arm. He attempts to flex the elbow by sliding his forearm along the table.

13. *Elbow extension.* To test *against gravity*, the person lies on his back, with the shoulder of the extremity being tested flexed to 90 degrees and elbow flexed. The examiner stabilizes his arm. He attempts to extend the elbow. To test

without gravity, the person lies on his back, with the arm being tested abducted to 90 degrees and laterally rotated, with the elbow flexed. The examiner stabilizes his arm. He attempts to extend the elbow by sliding his forearm along the table.

14. *Forearm supination.* The person sits, with the arm being tested at his side, elbow flexed to 90 degrees, and forearm pronated. The examiner stabilizes his arm. He attempts to supinate the forearm.

15. *Forearm pronation.* The person sits, with the arm being tested at his side, elbow flexed to 90 degrees, and forearm supinated. The examiner stabilizes his arm. He attempts to pronate the forearm.

16. *Wrist flexion.* The person sits, with the forearm of the extremity being tested resting on a table supinated. The examiner stabilizes his forearm. He attempts to flex the wrist.

17. *Wrist extension.* The person sits, with the forearm of the extremity being tested resting on a table pronated. The examiner stabilizes his forearm. He attempts to extend the wrist.

18. *Flexion of metacarpophalangeal joints of fingers.* The person sits, with the hand of the extremity being tested resting on a surface (e.g., a tabletop). The examiner stabilizes his metacarpals. He attempts to flex the fingers (all four together) at their metacarpophalangeal joints, keeping the interphalangeal joints extended.

19. *Flexion of interphalangeal joints of fingers.* To test flexion of the *proximal interphalangeal joints,* the person sits, with the hand of the extremity being tested resting (on a table) on the dorsal surface, palm upward with wrist and fingers extended. The examiner stabilizes the proximal phalanx of the finger being tested. The person attempts to flex the middle phalanx of this finger. To test flexion of the *distal interphalangeal joints,* the person sits, with the hand of the extremity being tested resting palm upward on a table with fingers extended. The examiner stabilizes the middle phalanx of the finger being tested. The person attempts to flex the distal phalanx of this finger.

20. *Extension of metacarpophalangeal joints of fingers.* The person sits, with the arm being tested resting on a table, with the hand supported by the examiner, wrist in midposition, fingers flexed. The examiner stabilizes his metacarpals. He attempts to extend the proximal row of phalanges (all four) with the interphalangeal joints partially flexed.

21. *Finger abduction.* The person sits, with the hand being tested supported by the examiner, palm downward with fingers adducted. The examiner stabilizes his metacarpals. He attempts to abduct the fingers.

22. *Finger adduction.* The person sits, with the hand being tested supported by the examiner, palm downward, fingers abducted. He attempts to adduct the fingers.

23. *Flexion of joints of thumb.* To test flexion of the *metacarpophalangeal joint* of a thumb, the person sits, with the hand being tested resting palm upward on a table. The examiner stabilizes the first metacarpal of his thumb. He attempts to flex the first phalanx of the thumb. To test flexion of the *interphalangeal joint* of a thumb, the person sits, with the hand being tested resting palm upward on a table. The examiner stabilizes the first phalanx of his thumb. He attempts to flex the distal phalanx of the thumb.

24. *Extension of joints of thumb.* To test extension of the *metacarpophalangeal joint* of a thumb, the person sits, with the hand being tested resting on a table. The examiner stabilizes the first metacarpal of his thumb. He attempts to extend the first phalanx of the thumb. To test extension of the *interphalangeal*

joint of a thumb, the person sit, with the hand being tested resting on a table on the ulnar border. The examiner stabilizes the first phalanx of his thumb. He attempts to extend the distal phalanx of the thumb.

25. *Thumb abduction.* The person sits, with the hand being tested supported by the examiner. The examiner stabilizes the four metacarpals of the fingers and the wrist of this hand. He attempts to abduct the thumb by raising it vertically.

26. *Thumb adduction.* The person sits, with the hand being tested supported by the examiner. The examiner stabilizes the medial four metacarpals of the fingers of this hand. He attempts to adduct the thumb.

27. *Opposition of thumb and fifth finger.* The person sits, with the hand being tested resting palm upward on a table. He attempts to bring the palmar surfaces of the distal phalanges of the thumb and fifth finger together.

Gestures Involving the Face and Neck. Fourteen gestures are described in this section. Each should be evaluated for accuracy, speed, force, presence of abnormal reflexes, presence of involuntary movement, and fatigue level. The primary source for this section is Daniels and Worthingham's (1972) book, *Muscle Testing.*

1. *Neck flexion.* The person lies on his back. The examiner stabilizes his lower thorax. He attempts to flex the cervical spine (neck).

2. *Neck extension.* The person lies on a table on his stomach, with his head over the edge (neck in flexion). The examiner stabilizes the upper thoracic area and scapulae. He attempts to extend the cervical spine (neck).

3. *Moving head from side to side.* The person sits on a chair. The examiner stabilizes his shoulders. He attempts to turn his head to one side and then to the opposite side.

4. *Raise eyebrows.* The person, while in a sitting position, attempts to raise his eyebrows, which, if successful, forms horizontal wrinkles in the forehead.

5. *Close eyes.* The person, while in a sitting position, attempts to close both eyes tightly.

6. *Direct gaze to the right.* The person, while in a sitting position, attempts to move his eyes to the right.

7. *Direct gaze to the left.* The person, while in a sitting position, attempts to move his eyes to the left.

8. *Compress lips.* The person, while in a sitting position, attempts to approximate and compress his lips.

9. *Smile.* The person, while in a sitting position, attempts to raise the lateral angle of the mouth upward and lateralward.

10. *Suck.* The person, while in a sitting position, attempts to suck water through a straw.

11. *Blow.* The person, while in a sitting position, attempts to blow out a candle or a match.

12. *Phonate.* The person, while in a sitting or lying position, attempts to produce a speech or a nonspeech sound (e.g., a sustained vowel or a voluntary cough).

13. *Extend and retract tongue.* The person, while in a sitting position, attempts to protrude his tongue between the central incisors and then retract it.

14. *Close jaws.* The person, while in a sitting position, attempts to close his jaws tightly.

Gestures Involving the Trunk and Lower Extremities. Seven gestures are described in this section. Each should be evaluated for accuracy, speed, force, presence of abnormal reflexes, presence of involuntary movement, and fatigue level. The primary source for this section (as it was for the previous ones) is Daniels and Worthingham's (1972) book, *Muscle Testing.*

1. *Trunk flexion.* The person lies on his back, with his arms at his sides. The examiner stabilizes his legs firmly. He attempts to flex (elevate) his thorax.
2. *Trunk rotation.* The person lies on his back, with his arms at his sides. The examiner stabilizes his legs firmly. He attempts to rotate his thorax to one side and then to the opposite side.
3. *Hip flexion.* The person sits on a table, with his legs dangling over the edge. The examiner stabilizes his pelvis. He attempts to flex his hip on one side and then on the opposite side.
4. *Hip lateral rotation.* The person sits on a table, with his legs dangling over the edge. He grasps the edge of the table to stabilize his pelvis and attempts to laterally rotate his thigh on one side and then on the opposite side.
5. *Hip medial rotation.* The person sits on a table, with his legs dangling over the edge. He grasps the edge of the table to stabilize his pelvis and attempts to medially rotate his thigh on one side and then on the opposite side.
6. *Knee flexion.* The person sits on a table, with his legs dangling over the edge. He grasps the edge of the table to stabilize his pelvis and attempts to flex his knee on one side and then on the opposite side.
7. *Knee extension.* The person sits on a table, with his legs dangling over the edge. He grasps the edge of the table to stabilize his pelvis and attempts to extend his knee on one side and then on the opposite side.

Implications of Motor Functioning Data. The results of a motor evaluation such as the one outlined here are relevant when you are attempting to identify gestural, gestural-assisted, and neuro-assisted communication systems that it would be possible for a person to use. Some implications that they have for this purpose are indicated here.

1. If the musculature of *one* upper extremity functioned essentially normally, the person would have the motor capability for learning a manual gestural system such as Amerind (see Chapter 4). If the musculature of *both* upper extremities functioned normally, he probably would have the motor capability for learning any of the gestural systems described in Chapter 4.
2. If the musculature of an upper extremity functioned sufficiently well that he could touch with a finger (or another part of the hand) any point he wished on a communication board that was mounted on his wheelchair (or elsewhere within the range of motion of that extremity), he probably would have the motor capability for using a communication board with a direct-selection response mode (see Chapter 5).
3. If a person can produce certain gestures with an upper extremity reasonably normally (see Table 7.1), he probably has the motor capability for activating certain switching mechanisms that can interface him with an electronic gestural-assisted communication system (see Chapter 5). He *should* be able to activate a switching mechanism that is marked with an *X* in Table 7.1 with the gesture

TABLE 7.1. Switching mechanisms that can be activated by particular gestures of the upper extremities.

Switch Type	Scapular Abduction and Upward Rotation	Scapular Elevation	Scapular Adduction	Scapular Depression	Shoulder Flexion to 90°
Push Button					
Push Plate					
Paddle					?
Sliding Handle or Foot Trolley					
Wobblestick					?
Pillow, Pad, or Squeeze Bulb	?	?	?	?	?
Tip, or Tilt, Switch					X
Magnetic Reed Switch					
Suck or Blow Switch					
Touch Switch					
Sound-Controlled Switch					
Light-Controlled Switch					
Myoswitch	?	?	?	?	X
(Location of Electrodes)	Over Serratus Anterior	Over Trapezius (Superior Fibers)	Over Trapezius (Middle Fibers)	Over Trapezius (Lower Fibers)	Over Deltoideus (Anterior Fibers)

TABLE 7.1. *(Continued)*

Switch Type	Shoulder Extension	Shoulder Abduction to 90°	Shoulder Horizontal Abduction	Shoulder Horizontal Adduction	Shoulder Lateral Rotation
Push Button			?	?	?
Push Plate	?		X	?	
Paddle	?		?	?	
Sliding Handle or Foot Trolley					
Wobblestick	?	?	X	X	X
Pillow, Pad, or Squeeze Bulb	X	?	X	X	?
Tip, or Tilt, Switch		X			
Magnetic Reed Switch			?	?	
Suck or Blow Switch					
Touch Switch	X	?	?	?	X
Sound-Controlled Switch	?	X	?	?	
Light-Controlled Switch	?	?	?	?	
Myoswitch (Location of Electrodes)	Over Latissimus Dorsi	Over Deltoideus	Over Deltoideus (Posterior Fibers)	Over Pectoralis Major	Over Infraspinatus

TABLE 7.1. (Continued)

Switch Type	Shoulder Medial Rotation	Elbow Flexion	Elbow Extension	Forearm Supination	Forearm Pronation
Push Button					
Push Plate	?		X	?	?
Paddle			X		
Sliding Handle or Foot Trolley					
Wobblestick			X		
Pillow, Pad, or Squeeze Bulb	X	X	X	X	X
Tip, or Tilt, Switch	?	X	X	?	?
Magnetic Reed Switch					
Suck or Blow Switch					
Touch Switch	X		X	X	X
Sound-Controlled Switch					
Light-Controlled Switch			X		
Myoswitch	?	?	?	?	?
(Location of Electrodes)	Over Subscapularis	Over Biceps Brachii	Over Triceps Brachii	Over Biceps Brachii	Over Pronator Teres

TABLE 7.1. *(Continued)*

Switch Type	Wrist Flexion	Wrist Extension	Flexion of Metacarpo-phalangeal Joints of Fingers	Flexion of Interphalangeal Joints of Fingers
Push Button	X	X	?	
Push Plate	X	?		
Paddle				
Sliding Handle or Foot Trolley				
Wobblestick		X		
Pillow, Pad, or Squeeze Bulb	X	X	X	?
Tip, or Tilt, Switch				
Magnetic Reed Switch	?	?		
Suck or Blow Switch				
Touch Switch	X	X	?	X
Sound-Controlled Switch				
Light-Controlled Switch				
Myoswitch (Location of Electrodes)	? Over Flexor Carpi Radalis	? Over Extensor Carpi Radialis Longus		? Over Flexor Digitorum Superficialis

TABLE 7.1. (Continued)

Switch Type	Extension of Metacarpophalangeal Joints of Fingers	Finger Abduction	Finger Adduction	Flexion of Joints of Thumb
Push Button		?	?	?
Push Plate		?		
Paddle				
Sliding Handle or Foot Trolley				
Wobblestick				
Pillow, Pad, or Squeeze Bulb		?	?	?
Tip, or Tilt, Switch				
Magnetic Reed Switch		?		
Suck or Blow Switch				
Touch Switch		?	X	X
Sound-Controlled Switch				
Light-Controlled Switch				
Myoswitch (Location of Electrodes)	? Over Extensor Digitorum Communis		?	Over Flexor Pollicis

TABLE 7.1. *(Continued)*

Switch Type	Extension of Joints of Thumb	Thumb Abduction	Thumb Adduction	Opposition of Thumb and Fifth Finger
Push Button		?	?	
Push Plate		?		
Paddle				
Sliding Handle or Foot Trolley				
Wobblestick				
Pillow, Pad, or Squeeze Bulb		?	?	?
Tip, or Tilt, Switch				
Magnetic Reed Switch				
Suck or Blow Switch				
Touch Switch		?	X	X
Sound-Controlled Switch				
Light-Controlled Switch				
Myoswitch (Location of Electrodes)	? Over Extensor Pollicis	? Over Abductor Pollicis	? Over Adductor Pollicis	

TABLE 7.2. Switching mechanisms that can be activated by particular gestures of the face and neck.

Switch Type	Neck Flexion	Neck Extension	Moving Head from Side to Side	Raise Eyebrows	Close Eyes
Push Button	With Headstick				
Push Plate	With Headstick				
Paddle					
Sliding Handle or Foot Trolley					
Wobblestick					
Pillow, Pad, or Squeeze Bulb	X	X			
Tip, or Tilt, Switch					
Magnetic Reed Switch			With Headstick		
Suck or Blow Switch					
Touch Switch	X		With Headstick		
Sound-Controlled Switch					
Light-Controlled Switch			X		X*
Myoswitch (Location of Electrodes)	? Over Sternocleido-mastoideus	? Over Trapezius (Superior Fibers)		? Over Occipito-frontalis	

*Small light sources in an eyeglass frame shine on the white of the eye. If the eye is open a different amount of light is reflected than if it is closed.

196

TABLE 7.2. *(Continued)*

Switch Type	Direct Gaze to Right	Direct Gaze to Left	Compress Lips	Smile	Suck
Push Button					
Push Plate					
Paddle					
Sliding Handle or Foot Trolley					
Wobblestick					
Pillow, Pad, or Squeeze Bulb			?		
Tip, or Tilt, Switch					
Magnetic Reed Switch					
Suck or Blow Switch					X
Touch Switch			?		
Sound-Controlled Switch					
Light-Controlled Switch	X**	X**			
Myoswitch			?	?	
(Location of Electrodes)			Over Orbicularis Oris	Over Zygomaticus Major	

**Small light sources in an eyeglass frame shine on the eye. If gaze is directed, a different amount of light is reflected than if it isn't.

TABLE 7.2. *(Continued)*

Switch Type	Blow	Extend and Retract Tongue	Phonate	Close Jaws
Push Button				With Mouthstick
Push Plate				With Mouthstick
Paddle		?		
Sliding Handle or Foot Trolley				
Wobblestick				
Pillow, Pad, or Squeeze Bulb		?		?
Tip, or Tilt Switch				
Magnetic Reed Switch				
Suck or Blow Switch	X			
Touch Switch				
Sound-Controlled Switch	X		X	?
Light-Controlled Switch				
Myoswitch	?			?
(Location of Electrodes)	Over Buccinator			Over Temporalis

indicated; he *may* be able to activate that marked with a *?* with this gesture. The switching mechanisms listed in Table 7.1, of course, may not be the only ones that can be activated by a particular gesture, and there may be switching mechanisms in this Table not marked with an *X* or *?* for a particular gesture that can be activated with it. All of the switching mechanisms in the Table are described in Chapter 5.

4. If the musculature of the neck functioned essentially normally, the person probably would have the motor capability for using a communication board with a direct-selection response mode, indicating message components with a headstick (see Chapter 5).

5. If the musculature of the mandible and neck functioned essentially normally, the person probably would have the motor capability for using a communication board with a direct-selection response mode, indicating message components with a mouthstick (see Chapter 5).

6. If the musculature of the eyes functioned normally, the person probably would have the motor capability for using a communication board, such as the ETRAN or ETRAN-N (see Chapter 5), with a direct-selection or encoding response mode, indicating message components by directing gaze, or eyepointing (see Chapter 5).

7. If the person can produce certain gestures with the face or neck (see Table 7.2) reasonably normally, he probably has the motor capability for activating certain switching mechanisms that can be used to interface him with an electronic gestural-assisted communication system. (See comment number 3 above for information relevant to interpreting Table 7.2.)

8. If the person can produce certain gestures with the trunk or lower extremities (see Table 7.3) reasonably normally, he probably has the motor capability for activating certain switching mechanisms that can be used to interface him with an electronic gestural-assisted communication system. (See comment number 3 above for information relevant to interpreting Table 7.3.)

9. If the person can produce certain gestures with the upper extremities (see Table 7.1), face and neck (see Table 7.2), or trunk and lower extremities (see Table 7.3) at least partially, he *may* have the motor capacity for activating a *myoswitch* that can be used to interface him with an electronic neuro-assisted communication system (see Chapter 6). Electrode placements that may be usable for activating a myoswitch are indicated in Tables 7.1, 7.2, and 7.3.

Sensory Functioning

The degree of intactness of a person's auditory, visual, and tactile-kinesthetic-proprioceptive systems partially determines the nonspeech communication modes it is possible for him to use. If he has difficulty understanding speech, his ability to benefit from any of the communication systems described in Chapters 4, 5, or 6 may be reduced *unless* his auditory problem can be compensated for *visually* (this could be done by transmitting messages to him in a manual sign language or by improving his ability to speechread).

If a person has difficulty understanding visual symbols (e.g., words or Blissymbols), there are many gestural-assisted and neuro-assisted communication systems (see Chapters 5 and 6) he will be unable to use unless his visual problem can be compensated for by tactile means. The reason, of course, is

TABLE 7.3. Switching mechanisms that can be activated by particular gestures of the trunk and lower extremities.

Switch Type	Trunk Flexion	Trunk Rotation	Hip Flexion	Hip Lateral Rotation
Push Button				
Push Plate				
Paddle				
Sliding Handle or Foot Trolley				
Wobblestick				
Pillow, Pad, or Squeeze Bulb	Under Head or Shoulders	Under Shoulder on Side Rotated Toward		
Tip, or Tilt, Switch			With Person in Sitting Position	With Person in Sitting Position
Magnetic Reed Switch				
Suck or Blow Switch				
Touch Switch				
Sound-Controlled Switch	Squeeze Bulb Noise Generator	Squeeze Bulb Noise Generator		
Light-Controlled Switch				
Myoswitch	?	?	?	
(Location of Electrodes)	Over Rectus Abdominis	Over Obliquus Externus Abdominis		

TABLE 7.3. *(Continued)*

Switch Type	Hip Medial Rotation	Knee Flexion	Knee Extension
Push Button			
Push Plate		With Person in Sitting Position	With Person in Sitting Position
Paddle			
Sliding Handle or Foot Trolley		?	?
Wobblestick			
Pillow, Pad, or Squeeze Bulb		With Person in Sitting Position	With Person in Sitting Position
Tip, or Tilt, Switch	With Person in Sitting Position	With Person in Sitting Position	With Person in Sitting Position
Magnetic Reed Switch			
Suck or Blow Switch		?	?
Touch Switch			
Sound-Controlled Switch			
Light-Controlled Switch	?	?	?
Myoswitch			

that if he cannot understand the visual symbols on a display (either because he does not see them or he sees them but cannot understand them), he would have difficulty using them to encode messages. It sometimes is possible to compensate for a visual deficit by making it possible to identify visual message components by Braille (see Chapter 5). A communication board could be constructed on which the Braille equivalent of each visual message component appeared below it. A user could locate the components of his messages by scanning the board with his fingertips.

A disturbance in a person's use of tactile, kinesthetic, or proprioceptive sensation could have a detrimental effect on his ability to use gestural and possibly gestural-assisted communication systems. It can impede his ability to produce muscle gestures needed for implementing them. A given deficit of this type would tend to affect a person's use of some systems more than others. The more precise (or refined) the gestures needed to implement a system, the greater the probable impact of such a disability.

Kinds of information relevant to auditory, visual, and tactile-kines-thetic-proprioceptive functioning that can influence decisions about communication systems a person can use are indicated in this section. A form that can be used for summarizing this information is included in Appendix E.

Audition. It is necessary to determine whether the person has a hearing loss, and if he has, how much it interferes with speech comprehension. Hopefully, if he is experiencing some difficulty understanding speech, this can be partially compensated for by a hearing aid and/or by auditory training and speechreading instruction. The status of his hearing can be determined by audiometric testing.

It also is necessary to determine whether the person has auditory agnosia (or any other auditory perceptual or memory problem) or receptive aphasia; and if so how much it interferes with speech comprehension. Most aphasia tests contain items that are usable for this purpose.

Vision. It is necessary to determine whether the person has a loss of visual acuity or a visual field problem, and if he has, how much it interferes with (or probably would interfere with) reading, typing, indicating message components on a communication board, or activating an electronic switching mechanism. While it would be best for his vision to be evaluated by an ophthalmologist or an optometrist, there are simple tests that can be used to *screen* for visual acuity and visual field problems. A chart containing letters or other symbols of different sizes can be used to screen visual acuity, and moving the tip of the finger laterally through the visual field (upper and lower halves separately) can be used to screen for visual-field disturbances such as homonymous hemianopsia.

It also is necessary to determine whether the person manifests visual agnosia (or other visual perceptual or memory problems) or dyslexia and if

TABLE 7.4. Data summary worksheet for identifying the optimal system or combination of systems for meeting a person's communication needs.

Name_____ Date_____ Examiner_____

System	Could Person Use it?	Selection Criteria 1 2 3 4 5 6 7 8
Pantomime		
Amerind		
Ameslan		
Left-Hand Manual Alphabet		
Limited Manual Systems		
Gestures for "Yes" and "No"		
Eye Blink Encoding		
Gestural Morse Code		
Pointing		
Direct-Selection Communication Board		
Encoding Communication Board		
Scanning Communication Board		
Direct-Selection Electronic System		
Encoding Electronic System		
Scanning Electronic System		

A "grade" is assigned to each criterion for each system a person could use (which would be marked "yes" in the second column). In the grading system *A* signifies "excellent," *B* "good," *C* "satisfactory." The selection criteria are described in the text.

he does, how much it interferes with or would be likely to interfere with reading, typing, indicating message components on a communication board, or activating an electronic switching mechanism. Most aphasia tests contain items that can be used for evaluating these areas.

Tactile-Kinesthetic-Proprioceptive Functioning. It is necessary to determine whether there are disturbances in any of these areas that could interfere with manual signing, writing, typing, indicating message components on a communication board, or activating electronic switching mechanisms. A neurological examination should provide information about functioning in these areas. Of course, if the person could perform these activities normally, it would be safe to assume that tactile-kinesthetic-proprioceptive functioning is adequate.

Cognitive Functioning

Any disturbance in the person's ability to solve problems and see relationships can influence the choice of a communication system. Children diagnosed as mentally retarded and adults having such conditions as cerebral arteriosclerosis or Huntington's chorea show this type of disturbance.

A disturbance in cognitive functioning can influence the choice of a symbol system in several ways. First, it can make it difficult or impossible for him to use relatively abstract symbols, those that are *not pictographic* (see Chapter 4). He would be likely to experience far more difficulty using English words than Blissymbols or photographs and drawings (see Chapter 5). And second, it can influence the *size* of the symbol set the person can manage and the complexity of its *syntax*. Because a disturbance in cognitive functioning is almost always accompanied by a *learning deficit,* a person who has such a disturbance probably would be unable to learn as many symbols (message components) and as many ways of combining them as would his cognitively normal peer.

A standardized intelligence test can be used to assess cognitive functioning. One that is relatively "language free" such as the Leiter International Performance Scale (Arthur, 1952) is preferable because it assesses cognitive ability relatively independently of receptive and expressive oral language ability. Many speechless children and adults have a language deficit; if a relatively language-free test of cognitive functioning is not used, *they may appear to have a severe deficit in this area when they do not have one.*

Of The Systems He Could Use, Which Would Be Optimal For Meeting His Communication Needs?

Once the communication systems that it would be possible for the person to use have been identified, the next task is to select the system or combination of systems that would be *optimal* for meeting his communication needs. That system or combination of systems would be optimal that came closest to allowing him to meet these needs at a *relatively low cost.* Cost here refers not only to the expense of acquiring and maintaining system components, but also to the time and energy investment required for him to learn to use the system or systems.

A worksheet that can be useful when attempting to identify the optimal system (or combination of systems) for a person is reproduced in Table 7.4.

Various types of nonspeech communication systems are listed in the first column of Table 7.4. (Gestural-assisted and neuro-assisted communications systems, of course, could have been listed individually. A "yes" or "no" would be recorded beside each system (column two) to indicate whether the person should be able to use it (based on the results of the evaluation outlined in this chapter). For those systems he probably could use, a "grade" is assigned for each selection criterion (columns numbered 1 to 8). In the grading system used, *A* signifies excellent, *B* good, *C* satisfactory, and *F* unsatisfactory. The criteria on which each system is graded are the following:

1. The extent to which the system would allow the person to meet his communication needs.
2. The cost of components (i.e., hardware) and their maintenance; the higher this cost, the lower the grade.
3. The length of time it probably would take the person to learn to use the system well enough to meet his communication needs; the longer this time period, the lower the grade.
4. The portability of the system; the more portable the system, the higher the grade.
5. The extent to which using the system is likely to interfere with ongoing activity e.g., that involving the use of the hands; the greater the probable interference, the lower the grade.
6. The intelligibility of messages communicated by it to untrained observers; the higher their intelligibility, the higher the grade.
7. The amount of training likely to be necessary to learn to interpret messages communicated by it; the more training necessary, the lower the grade.
8. The acceptability of the system to users and interpreters; the more acceptable the system, the higher the grade.

The optimal system or combination of systems for a person can be inferred from the grades assigned to the systems he probably would be able to use. That system (or combination of systems) would be optimal which came closest to allowing him to meet his communication needs and which —

would be acceptable to him and those in his environment;
would be highly intelligible to observers who were not trained (or were only minimally trained) to interpret messages transmitted by it;
would interfere little, if at all, with his ongoing acitivity;
would be sufficiently portable for his needs;
would not take a great deal of time to learn to use; and
would not exceed available funding to purchase and maintain.

REFERENCES

ARTHUR, G. *The Arthur Adaptation of the Leiter International Performance Scale.* Washington, D.C.: Pyschological Service Center Press (1952).
DANIELS, L., & WORTHINGHAM, C. *Muscle Testing: Techniques of Manual Examination* (3rd ed.) Philadelphia: W.B. Saunders (1972).

DARLEY, F.L., Aronson, A.E., & Brown, J.R. *Motor Speech Disorders.* Philadelphia: W.B. Saunders (1975).

DUFFY, R.J., DUFFY, J.R., & PEARSON, K.L. Pantomime recognition in aphasics. *Journal of Speech and Hearing Research, 18,* 115-132 (1975).

DUNN, L.M. *Peabody Picture Vocabulary Test.* Minneapolis: American Guidance Service (1959).

KIRK, S., McCARTHY, J., & Kirk, W. *Illinois Test of Psycholinguistic Abilities.* Urbana: University of Illinois Press (1968).

MYKLEBUST, H.R. *Auditory Disorders in Children.* New York: Grune & Stratton (1954).

PORCH, B. *Porch Index of Communicative Ability.* Palo Alto, California: Consulting Psychologists Press (1971).

SPRADLIN, J. Assessment of speech and language of retarded children: The Parsons Language Sample. *Journal of Speech and Hearing Disorders,* Monograph Supplement *10,* 8-31 (1963).

WEBER, S.C. *Preliminary norms pertaining to the inner language construct in children.* Unpublished Essay, Marquette University (1972).

⑧ Intervention Strategies for Nonspeech Communication Modes

Once the system or combination of systems is identified that comes closest to being optimal for a person, the next step is intervention with it. Such intervention typically has a number of aspects. Some are necessary *regardless* of the system or systems selected and others only are necessary for intervention with particular systems. The discussion in this chapter is devoted primarily to aspects of intervention that are necessary regardless of the systems selected. Those necessary for particular systems are discussed in papers and books dealing with them in the bibliography (Appendix A). Sources of teaching materials and hardware components for intervention with them are indicated in Appendices B and C, respectively. Also, instructions for constructing several gestural-assisted systems are included in Appendix D.

Aspects of the intervention process that are dealt with in this chapter include the following:

gaining the acceptance of potential users and those with whom they communicate for using such a system (or systems) to augment or serve as a substitute for speech;

generating motivation for communication;

increasing awareness of the nature of communication;

periodically reassessing communication needs;

funding communication system components;

gaining administrative support for the use of nonspeech intervention programs;

training persons in a user's environment to interpret messages transmitted by nonspeech communication systems;

assessing the impacts of nonspeech intervention programs on users;

preventive maintenance of components of gestural-assisted and neuro-assisted systems; and

utilizing gestural-assisted electronic systems and neuro-assisted systems for environmental control.

Gaining Acceptance for a System From Potential Users and Those With Whom They Communicate

A necessary prerequisite for successful intervention with any nonspeech communication system is its acceptance by the user and those with whom he communicates. If he has reservations about using a system, this tends to limit his use of it, which in turn reduces its potential for benefiting him. And if persons with whom he communicates have reservations about his using such a system, they are likely to communicate it to him verbally, nonverbally, or both. Obviously, any negative reactions to his attempts to use a nonspeech system are likely to discourage his future use of that system (since it would function as response-contingent adversive reinforcement) and thereby reduce its potential for benefiting him.

It probably is reasonable to assume that both the potential user and those with whom he communicates will have some reservations about his using any nonspeech system. Such reservations could arise from several sources, including the feeling that

the clinician has given up on improving (or developing) the person's speech; intervention with a nonspeech communication system will reduce the person's motivation to improve his speech
using a nonspeech communication system will call adverse attention to him (i.e., make him appear abnormal);
he is a "failure" if he has to communicate by means of a nonspeech system; or intervention with such a system will not significantly improve his ability to communicate.

Strategies are outlined in this section for dealing with each of these attitudes.

"The Clinician has Given up on Improving (or Developing) the Person's Speech"

One of the most common causes of resistance to the use of nonspeech communication systems is the belief held by the family of a potential user (particularly that of a child) or by the user himself that the clinician has given up on improving (or developing) speech. Here are two arguments that may be useful in dealing with this belief:

1. The clinician will continue to work on speech. However, it is unlikely that his speech will be adequate to meet his communication needs in the near future. He needs a way to meet these needs now. He will be encouraged to use what speech he has along with the nonspeech system (i.e., he will be encouraged to use "total" communication). If his speech improves, he will be encouraged to rely more on it and less on the nonspeech system.
2. Learning a nonspeech system seem to facilitate speech production in some

speechless children and adults (see Table 2.2). Intervention with these systems can, thus, be viewed as *speech therapy.*

"Intervention with a Nonspeech Communication Mode Will Reduce the Person's Motivation to Improve His Speech"

There is considerable evidence (see Table 2.2) that intervention with a nonspeech communication mode is highly unlikely to reduce verbal output. If such intervention does have an impact on verbal output, it is to increase it (see Table 2.2).

"Using a Nonspeech Communication System Will Call Adverse Attention to the Person (i.e., Make Him Appear Abnormal)"

The persons attitude toward using a communication system probably is the main determiner of how those in his environment will react to him when he uses it. If he has an *objective attitude,* it is unlikely to call adverse attention to him. An objective attitude in this context would be one of both intellectual and emotional acceptance of having to use the system. If he is embarrassed, ashamed, or uncomfortable about having to use it, he is likely to communicate this attitude to persons in his environment, which in turn will tend to make them uncomfortable when he uses it. In such a case, using the system would call adverse attention to the person, not because of reactions to the systems *per se,* but because of reactions to his being uncomfortable while using it.

Approaches for developing an objective attitude toward using a nonspeech communication system are essentially the same as those for developing an objective attitude toward wearing a hearing aid. Some people refuse to wear a hearing aid because they feel it calls adverse attention to them. Suggestions in the audiology and hearing-aid-dealer literature relevant to gaining acceptance for a hearing aid probably would be applicable for developing an objective attitude toward using a nonspeech communication system.

"He is a 'Failure' if He Has to Communicate by Means of a Nonspeech System"

If the person believes (or those with whom he communicates believe) that he should be able to learn to communicate by speech and that the nonspeech system is a "last resort," he (or they) may reject the system because it symbolizes "failure." The attitude of the clinician toward the system can have a profound impact on that of the person and those with whom he communicates. If the clinician views it as a "last resort," they probably will also. A clinician is less likely to communicate such an attitude if he has a *communication* orientation rather than a speech orientation (see Chapter 1).

*"Intervention with Such a System Will Not Significantly
Improve His Ability to Communicate"*

There is a high probability that intervention with a nonspeech system
will significantly improve a speechless child's or adult's ability to communicate. The outcome research summarized in Table 2.1 should be useful for
convincing a potential user of a nonspeech system, and his family, that it
could facilitate communication for him.

Generating Motivation for Communication

If a person does not have a need to communicate, he is unlikely to be helped
by any intervention with any communication system. Not perceiving a need to
communicate can arise from several sources, including the following:

> having everything done for one (i.e., not being expected to make decisions);
>
> having little, or no, opportunity to communicate (i.e., limited opportunity for
> interpersonal relationships);
>
> not understanding the benefits of communicating (i.e., how gratification can
> come from it); and
>
> not wishing to communicate (because of depression, withdrawal, pending litiga-
> tion, or some other reason).

How one would deal with a motivation problem would, of course, depend on
its source. Several strategies are outlined in this section that may be helpful in
dealing with motivation problems arising from these sources.

A child or adult who was not expected to make decisions probably
would have little motivation to communicate. If a person has a difficult time
communicating, it tends to take less time for the family or the staff at the
institution to *anticipate* his needs than to wait for them to be communicated.
Anticipating needs rather than waiting for them to be communicated is
particularly likely to occur in hospitals, nursing homes, and institutions for
the mentally retarded. Persons in such institutions may in fact be *discouraged*
from attempting to communicate because it makes their care more time-
consuming for the staff. If a person were to sense that those with whom he
interacted responded negatively to his attempts at communication, he probably would make fewer attempts to communicate, which would be likely to
result in a *vicious circle:* reduced attempts to communicate would lead to
reduced practice in communicating, which in turn would lead to lack of
improvement (or regression) in communication ability, which in turn would
lead to discouragment of attempts to communicate, and so on (see Figure
8.1).

Lack of motivation to communicate resulting from not being encour-

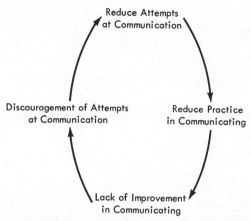

Reduce Attempts
at Communication

Discouragement of Attempts
at Communication

Reduce Practice
in Communicating

Lack of Improvement
in Communicating

FIGURE 8.1. *Vicious circle resulting from discouragement of attempts at communication.*

aged to make decisions can be dealt with, in part, by expecting the person to participate in decision making to the extent allowed by his communication ability. If he is able to understand speech reasonably well and signal "yes" and "no," he can be expected to indicate choices by answering questions. By explaining the serious consequences of his not being encouraged to communicate to those responsible for his care, it should be possible to obtain at least their partial cooperation.

Another reason why a person may not feel a need to improve his ability to communicate is that he doesn't have much opportunity to communicate. This is particularly apt to be a cause of lack of motivation to communicate for persons over the age of fifty who live alone and have limited opportunity for interpersonal relationships. Such persons could be motivated to improve their abilities to communicate by increasing their opportunities for interpersonal relationships (e.g., by getting them involved with groups such as "golden age" clubs), or by convincing them that even with their present opportunities for interpersonal relationships it would be advantageous for them to be able to communicate more effectively, or both of these.

A third reason why a person (particularly a child) may not be motivated to learn to communicate better is that he may be unaware of the benefits he could receive from doing so. He may not be aware that communicating better would give him greater control over what happens to him. Strategies for increasing awareness of the nature of communication and of the benefits that can be derived from it are described in the next section of this chapter.

A fourth reason why a person may not be motivated to learn to communicate better is that he either does not enjoy communicating or feels that it would be disadvantageous to learn to do it better. Naturally, persons who are depressed or withdrawn do not tend to be highly motivated to communicate. Also, persons whose communicative disorders resulted from trauma and who are in the process of suing the party responsible for injuring them probably would not be highly motivated to learn to communicate better until litigation is completed. The approach used to motivate such persons would, of course, depend on the reason why they do not choose to communicate better.

Increasing Awareness
of the Nature of Communication

Before a person would be capable of communicating with any system, he would have to understand how being able to communicate would permit him to manipulate (or control to some extent) his environment. If a person is taught a communication system and is unaware of how he can use it to manipulate his environment, knowing the system probably will have little or no impact on him. While adults who have little or no speech because of dysarthria, verbal apraxia, dysphonia, or glossectomy are likely to understand the nature of communication, *children* who are speechless because of mental retardation, childhood autism, congenital aphasia, or dysarthria may not understand this process if they are not made aware of it. Hence, increasing awareness of the nature of communication would be a necessary component of an intervention program for many speechless persons, particularly children.

Understanding communication as a process requires several kinds of awareness including the awareness (1) that gestures, sounds, and printed (visual) configurations can represent, or symbolize, objects and events; and (2) that transmission of an appropriate symbol (or sequence of symbols) at an appropriate time can cause a desired event to occur. Both of these are dealt with in this section.

Developing Awareness that Gestures, Sounds, and Printed (Visual) Configurations Can Symbolize Objects and Events

An initial step in any nonspeech intervention program is making certain the client realizes that gestures (manual movements, etc.) sounds (both speech and other), and printed configurations (words, Blissymbols, drawings, photographs, manipulatable tokens, etc.) can represent objects and events. To develop this awareness he must be able to do the following (Carrier, Jr. & Peak, 1975, pp. 6-7):

1. Discriminate among the various members of the symbol set . . .
2. Discriminate among various classes of environmental stimuli that call for different symbolic responses.

3. Discriminate among various sequential arrangements of stimuli (declarative sentences, interrogative sentences, etc.)
4. Associate symbols and environmental stimuli (meanings)
5. Associate sequential arrangements and meanings

The client has to be able to discriminate among the various gestures, sounds, and printed configurations that are being used as symbols (i.e., the various members of the symbol set). He has to be made aware of the differences between them. Strategies for developing such awareness for a symbol set consisting of manipulatable tokens are included in the Non-SLIP Program (Carrier, Jr. & Peak, 1975). These strategies are adaptable for other types of symbol sets.

The client also has to be able to discriminate among the various *classes* of objects or events ("units of experience") that can be represented by the symbols in the set he will be using. To do this he must be aware of both how they are similar and how they differ. Specifically, he must be aware of the attribute or attributes on the basis of which individual objects and events are assignable to a class (or category) that can be represented by a given symbol. An apple, a sucker, a hamburger, and ice cream, for example, all have the attribute of being edible. They are thus assignable to a class (or category) that can be represented by a symbol such as the word "food," a gesture in which a finger is pointed to the mouth, or a drawing of someone eating. The client also must be able to discriminate objects and events for which the use of the symbol would be appropriate from those for which it would be inappropriate (because they do not possess the attribute, or attributes, necessary for assignment to the category symbolized). While an apple, a sucker, a hamburger, and ice cream appropriately can be symbolized by the word "food," a pipe, a hammer, and a chair can not. Strategies for discriminating among various classes of environmental stimuli that call for different symbol responses are included in the Non-SLIP Program (Carrier, Jr. & Peak, 1975).

A third competency the client must have if his communication is to be more complex than the presentation of single symbols is the ability to discriminate among various sequential arrangements of symbols. He has to be able to discriminate among the various types of permutations and combinations (orderings) of the symbols in the set that are usable for encoding messages. Tasks for providing such training are included in the Non-SLIP Program (Carrier, Jr. & Peak, 1975).

Once the client can discriminate among the environmental stimuli (objects and events) that he will be taught to symbolize and the symbols he will use to represent them he can be taught how symbols and environmental stimuli are *associated*. That is, he can be taught that symbols can *represent* environmental stimuli *even when they are not present*. A person has to intuitively understand this relationship between symbol and referent before he can learn to use any symbol system. The Non-SLIP Program (Carrier, Jr. & Peak, 1975) includes tasks for developing this awareness.

After the client understands how *individual* symbols and environmental stimuli are related, he can be taught how *combinations* of symbols are related to environmental stimuli. Both the symbols with which a particular symbol is combined and its location in a series (of symbols) can influence its meaning. Ordered combinations of symbols, of course, can encode messages which would not be possible to encode using single symbols. The Non-SLIP Program (Carrier, Jr. & Peak, 1975) also includes tasks that are usable for developing an understanding of this concept.

A source of strategies for developing these competencies is the research of Premack (1970, 1971), Premack and Premack (1972, 1974), Rumbaugh and Associates (Rumbaugh, 1977), and Gardner and Gardner (1969) on teaching symbol systems to subhuman primates. The approaches used by these investigators to teach the *concept of symbol* to such primates can be adapted for teaching this concept to mentally retarded children. Indeed, the Non-SLIP Program (Carrier, Jr. & Peak, 1975) which was developed for teaching this general concept to mentally retarded children is based upon primate research by the Premacks.

Developing Awareness
of the Pragmatics of Communication

Once the client (1) understands that gestures, sounds, and printed configurations singly and in combination can represent (or symbolize) objects and events and (2) is able to produce (or point to) at least one such symbol, he is ready to learn that *transmission of an appropriate symbol (or combination of symbols) at an appropriate time can cause a desired event to occur (i.e., can allow him to manipulate his environment.)* It is desirable that the first symbols he is taught allow him to ask for things that he needs or wants often. Specific symbols that should be among the first taught are those for hunger, thirst, more, and wanting to go to the bathroom (particularly important for children who are not toilet trained.)

To help the client become aware of how symbols can be used to manipulate his environment, it is desirable that you use tasks in which he receives immediate reinforcement for producing or indicating a symbol, the reinforcement being successful manipulation of his environment. If, for example, he knows a symbol for "more," he can be given a *small amount* of a food he likes. He can then be shown that producing (or indicating) his symbol for "more" results in his receiving more of it. (It is desirable, incidentally, when teaching this symbol to use a number of different foods, liquids, and other objects as reinforcers. Otherwise, the client might interpret it as meaning more of a *specific* thing.)

Some of the strategies used in the subhuman primate research of the Premacks, the Gardners, and Rumbaugh and his associates (cited previously) for teaching pragmatics of communication can be adapted for teaching this concept to speechless children and adults. The language program developed by Kent (1974) also contains some tasks that can be used for this purpose.

Periodically Reassessing Communication Needs

After a person has been taught or interfaced with a nonspeech communication system, it is necessary to periodically reevaluate the ability of it to meet his communication needs. Both his symbol set and the manner in which he uses it to encode and transmit messages may have to be modified from time to time. Such modification may be necessary for one or both of the following reasons: (1) the symbol set is no longer appropriate, and / or (2) the approach used to encode and transmit messages is no longer appropriate.

The symbol set that a person is initially provided with probably will have to be *added to* from time to time because the things he will need to communicate about are likely to change. It also may be necessary to delete some symbols from this set when new ones are added if he uses a communication board or an electronic display (e.g., a rectangular matrix display), since the number of symbols that can be used with such devices is finite. Because of the need to be able to change symbols on communication boards and electronic displays, it is desirable to design them so that symbols can be changed relatively easily.

The symbol set that a person is using also may have to be changed for another reason: he may improve in his ability to use symbols or regress in this ability to the point that he needs a *different* symbol set. A young child who uses a communication board may begin with a symbol set that consists of pictures, then improve to the point that he can handle one consisting of Blissymbols and words. An adult who has a degenerative central nervous system condition may begin with one consisting of printed words, then regress to the point where he becomes so dyslexic that he needs one consisting of pictures.

The approach that a person uses for encoding and transmitting messages also may have to be changed periodically. One reason why it may be necessary to make such a change is either (1) the person becomes capable of using a more *efficient* strategy for indicating message components than previously or (2) he can no longer use a strategy he used previously because of further central nervous system damage. He may progress from a scanning to a direct-selection response mode or regress from a direct-selection to a scanning one.

Another reason why the approach a person uses for encoding and transmitting messages may have to be changed periodically is either (1) he may become able to use a display containing a larger number of message components or (2) he may not be able to utilize as large a display as he did previously because of additional central nervous system damage. He may be able to go from a communication board or rectangular matrix display (see Chapter 5) containing 100 message components to one containing a significantly greater number. Or he may be unable to use as large a display as he could previously because of additional strokes that affected his motor, sensory, or cognitive functioning.

A third reason for the approach used to encode and transmit messages having to be changed periodically is the person's changing communication needs. When a child who lacks normal use of his upper extremities reaches the point in school that he is expected to do written assignments, he may have to be interfaced with a system (or have components added to his present system) that will allow him to control an electric typewriter, teletypewriter, or strip printer (see Chapter 5). It is desirable, when designing a system for a person, to anticipate his future communication needs and make provisions for components to be added to the system at a later date to meet them. A system containing an electronic rectangular matrix display usually can be adapted to control a CRT display (see Chapter 5) alone or in conjunction with an electric typewriter, teletypewriter, or strip printer.

Funding Communication System Components

The components for an electronic communication system may cost more than a potential user or his family can afford. There are sources from which it may be possible to obtain funding in such cases, including the following:

1. the school system in which a child is enrolled (Public Law 94-142, for example, mandates that the school system has to provide a nonvocal communication system for a child who needs one to meet his educational objectives.);

2. the vocational rehabilitation commission in the person's state (if it can be argued that providing him with such a system will make him more employable);

3. a community service organization such as the Kiwanis Club or Sertoma International;

4. an insurance company (if the cause of the person becoming speechless was trauma);

5. Medicare, Medicaid, or other state or federal health insurance program;

6. the State Bureau for Crippled Children (or other state agency that performs its function);

7. United Cerebral Palsy, the National Easter Seal Society for Crippled Children and Adults, or some other voluntary organization which assists persons who have the condition that caused the client's communicative disorder;

8. "title funds" available from state departments of education;

9. trust funds administered by local banks or foundations that are intended for helping crippled children or adults; and

10. the Telephone Pioneers of America (see Howard, 1974).

The use of the term *Communication Prosthesis* to label such systems *may* be helpful when seeking funding from private, state, and federal insurance programs.

Gaining Administrative Support For The Use Of Nonspeech Intervention Programs

Your supervisor and other administrators of the institution where you are employed *initially* may not be very enthusiastic about your using nonspeech intervention programs with your clients. This lack of enthusiasm is likely to be due to their not understanding (1) the positive impacts that such intervention programs can have on speechless persons and (2) that intervention with such programs does not reduce motivation for learning speech. The outcome data summarized in Chapter 2 should be useful to you when you are attempting to convince administrators that these programs are of value.

Training Persons in A User's Environment to Interpret Messages Transmitted by Nonspeech Communication Systems

If the person is using a symbol system that is unfamiliar to those with whom he has to communicate, it is necessary to train them to interpret messages encoded using the symbols. It also is necessary to train them *how* to communicate with him if he is using a device (for example, how to "scan" his communication board so that he can encode and transmit messages).

It is important that such training be both as *brief* and as *readily* available as possible. The less time and effort necessary to learn to use the system and to interpret messages transmitted by it, the more likely those in his environment are to take the time to learn to use and interpret it. This is particularly likely to be true if the person lives in an institution such as a residential facility for the mentally retarded or a nursing home. Also, the more readily available such training, the more likely those interacting with the person are to take it. If he is in a hospital or nursing home, and training in using the system is available on the ward, nurses who interact with him probably are more likely to take the time to learn to use the system than they would be if they had to go elsewhere to receive the training.

How can persons in a user's environment be trained to assist him in transmitting messages and in interpreting the messages he transmits? There are several general approaches that can be used singly or in combination.

1. *Typewritten instructions* (with drawings or photographs) can be prepared on how to assist the person in transmitting messages, or on how to interpret the symbols he uses, or both of these. One Xerox copy of the instructions should be

kept near the user (e.g., it could be attached to his bed, or wheelchair, or communication device). Other copies could be given to persons who will be communicating with him often. The writing should be as clear as possible; no technical jargon should be used and the level of vocabulary and syntax should be no higher than sixth grade (because it is important that the instructions be understandable to members of the user's family, including older children).

2. *Videotaped* or *audiotaped instructions* can be prepared on how to assist the person in transmitting messages and/or how to interpret the symbols he uses. This approach using videotape can be quite effective for teaching interpretation of manual gestural signs (Bady & Silverman, 1978). For such an approach to be practical it would, of course, be necessary to have an appropriate audiotape or videotape player readily available to those who would be communicating with the person.

3. *Training sessions* can be conducted by the user's clinician (or someone trained by him or her) on how to assist him in transmitting messages and/or on how to interpret the symbols he uses. This approach is the least desirable of the three because of the demands it tends to place on the clinician's time and because this training can only be available at certain times. These times would not necessarily coincide with occasions during which an untrained person would have to communicate with the user.

Assessing the Impact of Nonspeech Intervention Programs On Users

One aspect of every nonspeech intervention program should be a *periodic systematic assessment* of its impact on the user. This information is needed for at least two reasons. The first is to periodically inform the clinician whether the program is having the desired impact on the client. If it does not appear to be achieving the clinician's goals, it may, of course, have to be modified.

Another reason why such information is needed is to add to our knowledge concerning the impact of particular nonspeech systems on populations of children and adults who are speechless, for various reasons. The more outcome data available, the better able we will be as clinicians to select the optimal system or combination of systems for each of our clients.

Several kinds of information are needed to systematically assess the impact of intervention with nonspeech communication systems on clients. This information can be abstracted from observations that are made to answer questions such as the following (Silverman, 1977, pp. 250-251):

1. What are the effects of the therapy upon specific behaviors that contribute to a client's communicative disorder?

2. What are the effects of the therapy upon other attributes of a client's communicative behavior?

3. What are the effects of the therapy upon the client other than those directly related to communicative behavior?

4. What are the client's attitudes toward the therapy and its effects upon his communicative and other behaviors?

5. What are the attitudes of a client's clinician, family, friends, and others toward the therapy and toward its effects upon the client's communicative behavior and other attributes of behavior?

6. What investment is required of client and clinician?

7. What is the probability of relapse following termination of the therapy?

These questions can be used to assess the impacts of any therapy on persons who have a communicative disorder. Their application to the assessment of the impacts of nonspeech intervention programs is illustrated in Chapter 2. Methodology that can be used for generating the observations needed to answer each question is described in Chapter 11 of *Research Design in Speech Pathology and Audiology* (Silverman, 1977).

Preventive Maintenance for Components of Gestural-Assisted and Neuro-Assisted Communication Systems

If a person will be using a gestural-assisted or neuro-assisted system, it is necessary to make some provision for the maintenance of the components of that system. Such a maintenance program may include the following:

1. arranging to have the batteries checked periodically and replaced before they fail;

2. arranging to have electronic components checked periodically so that malfunctions (and, hence, periods of time during which the person cannot communicate) can be reduced to a minimum;

3. periodically checking the electrical cables used for interconnecting the components of the system for signs of wear, and replacing them when necessary; and

4. cleaning the surfaces of communication boards and other displays.

Someone in a user's environment (e.g., a parent or spouse) should be trained to perform as many of these maintenance functions as possible. He should be taught how to test the batteries (if the device contains these) with a voltmeter and to check the electrical cables for signs of wear. It also may be possible to train him to troubleshoot problems with the switching mechanism, display, and control electronics and to do some repairs on them. The electronics of most components are mounted on circuit boards. For this reason, a component often can be repaired merely by replacing a circuit board. (It might be advisable to keep spare circuit boards on hand, particularly if they are not available locally.)

Utilizing Gestural-Assisted Electronic Systems and Neuro-Assisted Systems for Environmental Control

A switching mechanism used for activating a communication system also may be usable for controlling other electrical devices as well. Such devices could include a nurse call system (in a hospital or nursing home), a television set, a book-page turner, a thermostat (to make the room warmer or colder), and an automatic telephone dialer. (See Copeland, 1974, for further information about devices that could be controlled in this manner.)

Adapting an electronic communication system for environmental control requires some modification of its control electronics (see Chapter 5). An electronics technician or electrical engineer should be able to make the necessary modifications.

REFERENCES

BADY, J.A., & SILVERMAN, F.H. A videotape approach to teaching interpretation of Amerind Signs. *Perceptual and Motor Skills, 47,* 530 (1978).

CARRIER, J.K., Jr. and PEAK, T. *Program Manual for Non-SLIP.* Lawrence, Kansas: H & H Enterprises (1975).

COPELAND, K. (Ed.) *Aids for the Severely Handicapped.* New York: Grune & Stratton (1974).

GARDNER, R., & GARDNER, B. Teaching sign language to a chimpanzee. *Science, 165,* 664-672 (1969).

HOWARD, G. (Ed.). *Helping the Handicapped.* New York: Telephone Pioneers of America, 195 Broadway (1974).

KENT, L. *Language Acquisition Program for the Severely Retarded.* Champaign, Illinois: Research Press (1974).

PREMACK, A.J., & PREMACK, D. Teaching language to an ape. *Scientific American, 277,* 92-99 (1972).

PREMACK, D. A. Functional analysis of language. *Journal of Experimental Analysis of Behavior, 14,* 107-125 (1970).

———. Language in chimpanzee? *Science, 172,* 808-822 (1971).

PREMACK, D., and PREMACK, A.J. Teaching visual language to apes and language-deficient persons. In Richard L. Schiefelbusch and Lyle L. Lloyd (Eds.), *Language Perspectives — Acquisition, Retardation, and Intervention.* Baltimore: University Park Press, pp. 347-376 (1974).

RUMBAUGH, D.M. (Ed.) *Language Learning by a Chimpanzee: The LANA Project.* New York: Academic Press (1977).

SILVERMAN, F.H. *Research Design in Speech Pathology and Audiology.* Englewood Cliffs, New Jersey: Prentice-Hall (1977).

APPENDICES

Comprehensive Bibliography Relevant to Nonspeech Communication Modes

Note

This bibliography includes almost all published and unpublished papers which to my knowledge contain information relevant to nonspeech communication modes for children and adults with one or more of the following conditions: (1) dysarthria, (2) aphasia, (3) dysphonia, (4) verbal apraxia, (5) glossectomy, (6) mental retardation, or (7) childhood autism. The papers are categorized by type of mode—that is, gestural, gestural-assisted, or neuro-assisted. A number of sources were consulted in compiling this bibliography including *dsh Abstracts, Index Medicus,* the MEDLINE data base, bibliographies published by the Trace Center, and the reference lists of the papers located. A few of the references obtained from the latter source are not complete. I nevertheless decided to inlcuce them to make this bibliography as complete as possible. It was compiled during the second quarter of 1978.

Preparation of this bibliography was supported by a Faculty Grant from the Marquette University Graduate College. An earlier version was published in the *Ohio Journal of Speech and Hearing.*

Gestural Modes

ABRAMS, P. *Simultaneous Language Program for Non-Verbal Pre-School Children.* Chicago: Dysfunctioning Child Center, Michael Reese Medical Center (1975).

American Indian Sign: Gestural Communication for the Speechless. A series of four videotapes (VC 1 PT. 1 - PT. 4) distributed by the Learning Resources Center, Veterans Administration Hospital, St. Louis, Missouri (1974).

Amerind Dictionary Part One: Action Words. Kenosha, Wisconsin: Speech

& Hearing Program, Columbus Special Education Center (1977).

Amerind Video Dictionary. A series of four videotapes (VC 76 PT. 1 - PT. 4) distributed by the Learning Resources Center, Veterans Administration Hospital, St. Louis, Missouri (1975).

ANDERSON, K., & NEUMAN, S. *Total communication for mentally retarded children.* Videotape presented at the 52nd annual meeting of the American Speech and Hearing Association, Chicago (1977).

ASSAL, G., & BUTTET, J. Non-verbal vocal expression in aphasics. *Review of Otoneuroophthalmology, 48,* 373-379 (1976).

BADY, J., & SILVERMAN, F.H. A videotape approach to teaching interpretation of Amerind signs. *Perceptual and Motor Skills, 47,* 530 (1978).

BALICK, S., SPIEGEL, D., & GREENE, G. Mime in language therapy and clinician training. *Archives of Physical Medicine and Rehabilitation, 57,* 35-38 (1976).

BARNES, S. *The use of sign language as a technique for language acquisition in autistic children: An applied model bridging verbal and nonverbal theoretical systems.* Unpublished doctoral dissertation, California School of Professional Psychology, San Francisco (1973).

BARON, N., ISENSEE, L., & DAVIS, A. *Iconicity and learnability: Teaching sign language to autistic children.* Paper presented at the Second Boston University Conference on Language Development, Boston (1977).

BARTAK, L., RUTTER, M., & COX, A. A comparative study of infantile autism and specific developmental receptive language disorders: 1. The children. *British Journal of Psychiatry, 126,* 127-145 (1975).

BATTISON, R., & MARKOWICZ, H. *Sign Aphasia and Neurolinguistic Theory.* Washington, D.C.: Linguistics Research Laboratory, Gallaudet College (1976).

BATTISON, R., & PADDEN, C. *Sign language aphasia: A case study.* Paper presented at the 49th annual meeting of the Linguistic Society of America, New York (1974).

BELL, D.J., *et al, Let Your Fingers Do the Talking: A Teaching Manual for Use with Non-Verbal Retardates.* Sonyea, N.Y.: Craig Development Center (1976). (Copies can be obtained from the ERIC Document Reproduction Service, P.O. Box 190, Arlington. Virginia.)

BENAROYA, S., WESLEY, S., OGILVIE, H., KLEIN, L.S., & MEANEY, M. Sign language and multisensory input training of children with communication and related developmental disorders. *Journal of Autism and Childhood Schizophrenia, 7,* 23-31 (1977).

BICKER, D.D. Imitative sign training as a facilitator of word-object association with low-functioning children. *American Journal of Mental Deficiency, 76,* 509-516 (1972).

BONVILLIAN, J.D., & NELSON, K.E. Sign language acquisition in a mute autistic boy. *Journal of Speech and Hearing Disorders, 41,* 339-347 (1976).

BORNSTEIN, H. Signed English: A manual approach to English language development. *Journal of Speech and Hearing Disorders, 39,* 330-343 (1974).

BROOKNER, S.P., & HARRIS, C.A. *Interactive techniques to facilitate communication in non-vocal children.* Poster presentation at the 52nd annual meeting of the American Speech and Hearing Association, Chicago (1977).

BROOKNER, S.P., & MURPHY, N.O. The use of a total communication approach with a nondeaf child: A case study. *Language, Speech, and Hearing Services in Schools, 6,* 131-137 (1975).

BROWN, W.P., VANDERHEIDEN, G.C., & HARRIS, D. *1977 Bibliography on Non-Vocal Communication Techniques and Aids.* Madison, Wisconsin: Trace Research and Development Center for the Severely Communicatively Handicapped. University of Wisconsin (1977).

CARLSON, F. L. *An adapted communication project for a nonspeaking child.* Paper presented at the 51st annual meeting of the American Speech and Hearing Association, Houston (1976).

CHEN, L.Y. Manual communication by combined alphabet and gestures. *Archives of Physical Medicine and Rehabilitation, 52,* 381-384 (1971).

———. "Talking hands" for aphasic patients. *Geriatrics, 23,* 145-148 (1968).

CHESTER, S.L., & EGOLF, D.B. *Nonverbal communication and aphasia therapy.* Paper presented at the 47th annual meeting of the American Speech and Hearing Association, San Francisco (1972).

CLARK, T.A. *American sign language and the recently devised sign systems.* Paper presented at the 51st annual meeting of the American Speech and Hearing Association, Houston (1976).

COHEN, L.K. *Communication Aids for the Brain Damaged Adult.* Minneapolis: Sister Kenny Institute (1976).

CREEDON, M.P. (Ed.) *Appropriate Behavior Through Communication: A New Program in Simultaneous Language.* Chicago: Dysfunctioning Child Center, Michael Reese Medical Center (1975).

DEVILLIERS, J.G., & NAUGHTON, J.M. Teaching a symbol language to autistic children. *Journal of Consulting and Clinical Psychology, 42,* 111-117 (1976).

DUFFY, R.J., DUFFY, J.R., & PEARSON, K.L. *Impairment of gestural ability in aphasics.* Paper presented at the 48th annual meeting of the American Speech and Hearing Association, Detroit (1973).

———. Pantomime recognition in aphasics. *Journal of Speech and Hearing Research, 18,* 115-132 (1975).

DUNCAN, J.L., & SILVERMAN, F.H. *Impacts of learning Amerind sign language on mentally retarded children.* Paper presented at the 52nd annual meeting of the American Speech and Hearing Association, Chicago (1977). (Paper is printed in James R. Andrews and Martha S. Burns [Eds.]. *Remediation of Language Disorders,* Evanston, Illinois:

Institute for Continuing Professional Education, 1978.)

————— . Impacts of learning American Indian Sign Language on mentally retarded children: A preliminary report. *Perceptual and Motor Skills, 44,* 1138 (1977).

EAGLESON, H.M., VAUGHN, G.R., & KNUDSON, A.B. Hand signals for dysphasia. *Archives of Physical Medicine and Rehabilitation, 51,* 111-113 (1970).

EGAN, J.J., ANTHONY, G.M., & HONKE, L.E. *Joan: A case study of manual communication with a severe cerebral palsied dysarthric.* Paper presented at the 51st annual meeting of the American Speech and Hearing Association, Houston (1976).

ELLSWORTH, S., & KOTKIN, R. If only Jimmy could speak. *Hearing and Speech Action, 43,* 6-10 (November/December, 1975).

ENGLISH, S.T., & PRUTTING, C.A. Teaching American Sign Language to a normally hearing infant with tracheostenosis: A case study. *Clinical Pediatrics* (Philadelphia), *14,* 1141-1145 (1975).

FEALLOCK, B. Communication for the nonverbal individual. *American Journal of Occupational Therapy, 12,* 60-63, 83 (1958).

FENN, G., & ROWE, J.A. An experiment in manual communication. *British Journal of Disorders of Communication, 10,* 3-16 (1975).

FLETCHER, E.C., & HAVEMEYER, S. *Teaching sign language to severely retarded adults: Three case studies.* Paper presented at the 52nd annual meeting of the American Speech and Hearing Association, Chicago (1977).

FOLDI, N., GARDNER, H., ZURIF, E., & DAVIS, L. *Pragmatic use of gesture in aphasic communication.* Paper presented at the Conference on Neurolinguistics and Sign, Rochester, New York (1976).

FREIMAN, R., & SCHLANGER, P.H. *Using pantomime therapy with aphasics.* Paper presented at the 52nd annual meeting of the American Speech and Hearing Association, Chicago (1977). (Based on an M.A. thesis by R. Freiman, Herbert H. Lehman College, 1977).

FRISTOE, M. *Language Intervention Systems for the Retarded.* Decatur, Alabama: L.B. Wallace Developmental Center (1976).

FRISTOE, M., & LLOYD, L.L. Manual communication for the retarded and others with severe communication impairments: A resource list. *Mental Retardation, 15,* 18-19 (1977).

FULWILER, R.L., & FOUTS, R.S. Acquisition of American Sign Language by a noncommunicating autistic child. *Journal of Autism and Childhood Schizophrenia, 6,* 43-51 (1976).

GITLIS, K.R. *Rationale and precedents for the use of simultaneous communication as an alternate system of communication for non-verbal children.* Paper presented at the 50th annual meeting of the American Speech and Hearing Associaton, Washington, D.C. (1975).

GOLDOJARB, M.F. *The use of video confrontation in teaching AMERIND to aphasic adults.* Videotape presented at the 51st annual meeting of the American Speech and Hearing Association, Houston (1976).

GOLDSTEIN, H., & CAMERON, H. New method of communication for the aphasic patient. *Arizona Medicine, 8,* 17-21 (1952).

GOODMAN, L., WILSON, P.S., & BORNSTEIN, H. *Sign system questionnaire report.* Report of a committee of the Division of Speech Pathology and Audiology, American Association of Mental Deficiency (1977).

GORDON, K.C., & HYTA, M.B. *Assessment of nonverbal gestures in language-disabled children.* Paper presented at the 52nd annual meeting of the American Speech and Hearing Associaton, Chicago (1977).

GRAHAM, L.W. Language programming and intervention. In Lyle L. Lloyd (Ed.), *Communication Assessment and Intervention Strategies.* Baltimore: University Park Press, pp. 371-422 (1976).

GRECCO, R.V. *Manual Language Program.* Mansfield Depot, Connecticut: Mansfield Training School (1972).

————. *Results of a manual language program for non-verbal hearing and hearing impaired retarded.* Paper presented at the annual meeting of the Connecticut Speech and Hearing Association (1974).

GREEN, L.C. *Acquisition of words versus signs in receptive language therapy with severely retarded, institutionalized children.* Paper presented at the 50th annual meeting of the American Speech and Hearing Association, Washington, D.C. (1975).

GRIMMEL, M., DELAMORE, K., & LIPPKE, B. Sign it successfully—Manual English encourages expressive communication. *Teaching Exceptional Children,* 123-124 (Spring, 1976).

HAIGHT, C. Modification of signs to maximize the learning of concepts. In M.P. Creedon (Ed.), *Appropriate Behavior Through Communication: A New Program in Simultaneous Language.* Chicago: Dysfunctioning Child Center, Michael Reese Medical Center, pp. 74-84 (1975).

HALL, S.M., & TALKINGTON, L.W. Evaluation of a manual approach to programming for deaf retarded. *American Journal of Mental Deficiency, 75,* 378-380 (1970).

HANSON, W.R. *Measuring gestural communication in a brain-injured adult.* Videotape presented at the 51st annual meeting of the American Speech and Hearing Association, Houston (1976).

HAYES, H.T.P. The pursuit of reason. *The New York Times Magazine* (June 12, 1977).

HELFRICH, K.R. *Total communication with an oral apractic child.* Videotape presented at the 51st annual meeting of the American Speech and Hearing Association, Houston (1976).

HOFFMEISTER, R.J., & FARMER, A. The development of manual sign language in mentally retarded deaf individuals. *Journal of Rehabilitation of the Deaf, 6,* 19-26 (1972).

HOLLANDER, F.M., & JUHRS, P.D. Orff-Schulwerk, an effective treatment tool for autistic children. *Journal of Music Therapy, 11,* 1-12 (1974).

HOLLIS, J.H., & CARRIER Jr., J.K. Research implications for communication deficiencies. *Exceptional Children, 41,* 405-412 (1975).

HOLLIS, J.H., CARRIER, Jr., J.K., & SPRADLIN, J.E. An approach to remediation of communication and learning deficiencies. In Lyle L. Lloyd (Ed.), *Communication Assessment and Intervention Strategies.* Baltimore: University Park Press, pp. 265-294 (1976).

HUGHES, J. Acquisition of a non-verbal "language" by aphasic children. *Cognition, 3,* 41-55 (1974/5).

IRWIN, D.L. Amerind. *Asha, 19,* 746 (1977).

KAHN, J.V. A comparison of manual and oral training with mute retarded children. *Mental Retardation, 15* (3), 21-23 (1977).

KENT, L. *Language Acquisition Program for the Severely Retarded.* Champaign, Illinois: Research Press (1974).

KIERNAN, C. Alternatives to speech: A review of research on manual and other forms of communication with mentally handicapped and other noncommunicating populations. *Journal of Mental Subnormality, 23,* 6-28 (1977).

KIESOW, J. *Effective Communication Training for the Profoundly Retarded.* Chippewa Falls, Wisconsin: Northern Wisconsin Center for the Developmentally Disabled (no date).

KIMBLE, S.L. *A language teaching technique with totally nonverbal, severely mentally retarded adolescents.* Paper presented at the 50th annual meeting of the American Speech and Hearing Association, Washington, D.C. (1975).

KIRSCHNER, A.E. A comparison of two manual communication systems: Implications for training the nonverbal mentally retarded. Unpublished M.A. thesis, University of Florida (1977).

Koko: The signs of language. *Science News, 111,* 172 (1977).

KOLLER, J.J., SCHLANGER, P.H., & GEFFNER, D.S. *Identification of action words and activity pantomimes by aphasics.* Paper presented at the 50th annual meeting of the American Speech and Hearing Association, Washington, D.C. (1975).

KONSTANTAREAS. M., OXMAN, J., WEBSTER, C., FISCHER, H., & MILLER, K. *A Five Week Simultaneous Communication Programme for Severely Dysfunctional Children: Outcome and Implications for Future Research.* Toronto, Ontario, Canada: Clarke Institute of Psychiatry (1975).

KOPCHICK, G.A., Jr., and LLOYD, L.L. Total communication programming for the severely language impaired—A 24-hour approach. In Lyle L. Lloyd (Ed.), *Communication Assessment and Intervention Strategies.* Baltimore: University Park Press, pp. 501-521 (1976).

KOPCHICK, G.A., Jr., ROMBACK, D.W., & SMILOVITZ, R. A total communication environment in an institution. *Mental Retardation, 13* (3), 22-23 (1975).

KOSELKA, M.J., HANNAH, E.P., GARDNER, J.O., & REAGAN, W. *Total communication therapy for a nondeaf child and his family.* Paper presented at the 50th annual meeting of the American Speech and Hearing Association, Washington, D.C. (1975).

LAKE, S.J. *The Hand-Book.* Tucson, Arizona: Communication Skill Builders (1976).

LARSON, T. *Communication for the Non-Verbal Child.* Johnstown, Pennsylvania: Mafex Associates (1975).

LARSON, T. Communications for the nonverbal child. *Academic Therapy Quarterly, 6,* 305-312 (1971).

LEBEIS, S., and LEBEIS, R.F. The use of signed communication with the normal-hearing, nonverbal mentally retarded. *Bureau Memorandum* (Wisconsin Department of Public Instruction), *17* (1), 28-30 (1975).

LEIBL, J., PETTET, A., & WEBSTER, C.D. *Two Behavior Modification Approaches to the Treatment of Autistic Children: Simultaneous Communications vs. Vocal Imitation* (Substudy 74-7). Toronto, Ontario, Canada: Clarke Institute of Psychiatry (1974).

LEVETT, L.M., Discovering how mime can help. *Special Education, 60,* 17-19 (1971).

———— . A method of communication for non-speaking, severely subnormal children. *British Journal of Disorders of Communication, 4,* 64-66 (1969).

———— . A method of communication for non-speaking severely subnormal children—Trial results. *British Journal of Disorders of Communication, 6,* 125-128 (1971).

LINVILLE, S.E. Signed English: A language teaching technique with totally nonverbal mentally retarded adolescents. *Language, Speech, and Hearing Services in Schools, 8,* 170-175 (1977).

LLOYD, L.L. (Ed.). *Communication Assessment and Intervention Strategies.* Baltimore: University Park Press (1976).

LUCAS, E.V., & DEAN, M.B. *An alternative approach to oral communication for an autistic child.* Videotape presented at the 51st annual meeting of the American Speech and Hearing Association, Houston (1976).

MAYBERRY, R. If a chimp can learn sign language, surely my nonverbal client can too. *Asha, 18,* 223-228 (1976).

MENYUK, P. The bases of language acquisition: Some questions. *Journal of Autism and Childhood Schizophrenia, 4,* 325-345 (1974).

MILLER, A., & MILLER, E.E. Cognitive-developmental training with elevated boards and sign language. *Journal of Autism and Childhood Schizophrenia, 3,* 65-85 (1973).

MOORES, D.F. Nonvocal systems of verbal communication. In Richard L. Schiefelbusch and Lyle L. Lloyd (Eds.), *Language Perspectives—Acquisition, Retardation, and Intervention.* Baltimore: University Park Press, pp. 377-417 (1974).

OFFIR, C.W. Visual speech: Their fingers do the talking. *Psychology Today,*
10 (1), 72-78 (1976).

OLSON, T. Return of the nonverbal. *Asha, 18,* 823 (1976).

OWENS, M., & HARPER, B. *Sign Language: A Teaching Manual for Cottage*
Parents of Non-Verbal Retardates. Pineville, Louisiana: Pinecrest
State School (1971).

PETERS, L. Sign language stimulus in vocabulary learning of a brain-injured
child. *Sign Language Studies, 3,* 116-118 (1973).

PRIOR, M.R. Psycholinguistic disabilities of autistic and retarded children.
Journal of Mental Deficiency Research, 21, 37-45 (1977).

RICHARDSON, T. Sign language for the SMR and PMR. *Mental Retardation,*
13 (3), 17 (1975).

RICKS, D.M., & WING, L. Language, communication, and use of symbols in
normal and autistic children. *Journal of Autism and Childhood*
Schizophrenia, 5, 191-221 (1975).

ROBBINS, N. *Selected sign systems for multi-handicapped students.* Paper
presented at the 51st annual meeting of the American Speech and
Hearing Association, Houston (1976).

SALVIN, A., ROUTH, D.K., FOSTER, R.E., & LOVEJOY, K.M. Acquisition of
modified American Sign Language by a mute autistic child. *Journal of*
Autism and Childhood Schizophrenia, 7, 359-371 (1977).

SANDERS, D.A. A model of communication. In Lyle L. Lloyd (Ed.), *Com-*
municaton Assessment and Intervention Strategies. Baltimore: University Park Press, pp. 1-32 (1976).

SARNO, J., SWISHER, L., & SARNO, M. Aphasia in a congenitally deaf man.
Cortex, 5, 398-414 (1969).

SCHAEFFER, B. Spontaneous language through signed speech. In Richard L.
Schiefelbusch (Ed.), *Nonspeech Language Intervention.* Baltimore:
University Park Press (1979).

SCHAEFFER, B., KOLINZAS, G., MUSIL, A., & McDOWELL, P. *Signed speech:*
A new treatment for autism. Paper presented at the annual meeting of
the National Society for Autistic Children, San Diego (1975).

SCHAEFFER, B., McDOWELL, P., MUSIL, A., & KOLLINZAS, G. Spontaneous
verbal language for autistic children through signed speech. *Research*
Relating to Children (ERIC Clearinghouse for Early Childhood
Education), Bulletin 37, 98-99 (1976).

SCHIEFELBUSCH, R.L. (Ed.). *Nonspeech Language Intervention.* Baltimore:
University Park Press (1979).

SCHLANGER, P.H. *Training the adult aphasic to pantomime.* Paper presented
at the 51st annual meeting of the American Speech and Hearing Association, Houston (1976).

SCHLANGER, P.H., GEFFNER, D.S., & DiCARRADO, C. *A comparison of*
gestural communication with aphasics: Pre- and post-therapy. Paper

presented at the 49th annual meeting of the American Speech and Hearing Association, Las Vegas (1974).

SCHLANGER, P.H., & SCHLANGER, B.B. Adapting role-playing activities with aphasic patients. *Journal of Speech and Hearing Disorders, 35,* 229-235 (1970).

SHAFFER, T.R., & GOEHL, H. The alinguistic child. *Mental Retardation, 12* (2), 3-6 (1974).

SHIPLEY, K.G., & JARROW, J.E. An experimental university clinic training program for a non-language child. *Journal of the National Student Speech and Hearing Association, 4,* 9-16 (1976).

SILVERMAN, F.H. A bibliography of literature relevant to nonspeech communication modes for the speechless. *Ohio Journal of Speech and Hearing, 12,* 83-102 (1977).

_____. Non-vocal communication systems: Implications for the neurosciences. *Trends in Neurosciences, 1,* 147-148 (1978).

_____. Why not Amerind. *Asha, 19,* 463 (1977).

SILVERMAN, F.H., and BADY, J. Need for including coursework on nonvocal communication systems: A survey. *Asha, 20,* 1023 (1978).

SKELLY, M. Amerind clarified. *Asha, 19,* 746-747 (1977).

_____. *Amer-Ind Gestural Code.* New York: Elsevier (1979).

SKELLY, M., SCHINSKY, L., SMITH, R., DONALDSON, R., & GRIFFIN, J. American Indian Sign: A gestural communication system for the speechless. *Archives of Physical Medicine and Rehabilitation, 56,* 156-160 (1975).

SKELLY, M., SCHINSKY, L., SMITH, R.W., & FUST, R.S. American Indian Sign (AMERIND) as a facilitator of verbalization for the oral verbal apraxic. *Journal of Speech and Hearing Disorders, 39,* 445-456 (1974).

SMITH, C.H. Total communication utilizing the simultaneous method. In M.P. Creedon (Ed.), *Appropriate Behavior Through Communication: A New Program in Simultaneous Language.* Chicago: Dysfunctioning Child Center, Michael Reese Medical Center (1975).

SUTHERLAND, G.F., & BECKETT, J.W. Teaching the mentally retarded sign language. *Journal of Rehabilitation of the Deaf, 2,* 56-60 (1969).

TAMAN, T., & WEBSTER, C.D. *Teaching Autistic-Retarded Children Through Simultaneous (Gestural and Verbal) Communications* (15 minute black and white moving film). Toronto, Ontario, Canada: Clarke Institute of Psychiatry (1973).

TENENBAUM, D., & SCHLANGER, B.B. *Gestural communication by aphasics in dyadic situations.* Paper presented at the 43rd annual meeting of the American Speech and Hearing Association, Denver (1968).

TOMKINS, W. *Indian Sign Language.* New York: Dover Publications (1969).

TOPPER, S.T. Gestural language for a non-verbal severely retarded male. *Mental Retardation, 13* (1), 30-31 (1975).

VAIL, J.L., & SPAS, D.L. *A Manual Communication Program for Non-*

Verbal Retardates. DeKalb, Illinois: MWSEARCH-Title 1, 145 Fisk Avenue (1974).

VANBIERVLIET, A. Establishing words and objects as functionally equivalent through manual sign training. *American Journal of Mental Deficiency, 82,* 178-186 (1977).

VAN HOOK, K.W., & STOHR, P.G. *The development of manual communication in a profoundly retarded hearing population.* Paper presented at the 48th annual meeting of the American Speech and Hearing Association, Detroit (1973).

WEBSTER, C.D., MCPHERSON, H., SLOMAN, L., EVANS, M.A., & KUCHAR, E. Communicating with an autistic boy by gestures. *Journal of Autism and Childhood Schizophrenia, 3,* 337-346 (1973).

WILBER, R.B. The linguistics of manual languages and manual systems. In Lyle L. Lloyd (Ed.), *Communication Assessment and Intervention Strategies.* Baltimore: University Park Press, pp. 423-500 (1976).

WILSON, P.S. *A manual language dialect for the retarded.* Paper presented at the 49th annual meeting of the American Speech and Hearing Association, Las Vegas (1974).

WILSON, P.S., GOODMAN, L., & WOOD, R.K. *Manual Language for the Child Without Language.* Hartford, Connecticut: Department of Mental Retardation Developmental Team, 79 Elm Street (1975).

ZWEIBAN, S.T. Indicators of success in learning a manual communication mode. *Mental Retardation, 15* (2), 47-49 (1977).

Gestural-Assisted Modes

ABELSON, C., & PFEIFFER, D. Communication aids for the non-verbal severely handicapped child — A multidimensional challenge. *Canadian Journal of Occupational Therapy, 42,* 141-144 (1975).

ADAMS, M.R. Communication aids for patients with amyotrophic lateral sclerosis. *Journal of Speech and Hearing Disorders, 31,* 274-275 (1966).

ALLEN, J.B. Nu-Life for amputees and paralyzed patients. *Congressional Record-Extensions of Remarks* (April 30, 1974).

ANDERSON, K. An eye position controlled typewriter. In P. Nelson (Ed.), *Proceedings of Workshop on Communication Aids.* Ottawa, Ontario, Canada: Canadian Medical and Biological Engineering Society, National Research Council (1978).

ARCHER, L.A. Blissymbolics—A nonverbal communication system. *Journal of Speech and Hearing Disorders, 42,* 568-579 (1977).

Astros aid quadraplegic. *Atlantic City Press* (Atlantic City, New Jersey) (March 21, 1974).

Australian News and Information Bureau. Blissymbolics. *Hearing and Speech News, 41* (5) 6-7 (1973).

BEESLEY, M. The importance of positioning and seating for the cerebral palsied child. In P. Nelson (Ed.), *Proceedings of the Workshop on Communication Aids.* Ottawa, Ontario, Canada: Canadian Medical and Biological Engineering Society, National Research Council (1978).

BLISS, C.K. *Sematography (Blissymbolics)* (2nd ed.). Coogee, Sydney, Australia: C.K. Bliss, 2 Vicar Street (1965).

BOBBY, B. *Say it with symbols* (Filmstrip). Toronto, Ontario, Canada: Blissymbolics Communication Institute, 862 Eglinton Avenue E. (1976).

BRALLEY, R.C., & ORMOND, T.F. *Communication for the Laryngectomized.* Danville, Illinois: Interstate Printers and Publishers (1970).

BROWN, W.P., VANDERHEIDEN, G.C. & HARRIS-VANDERHEIDEN, D. *1977 Bibliography on Non-Vocal Communication Techniques and Aids.* Madison, Wisconsin: Trace Research and Development Center for the Severely Communicatively Handicapped, University of Wisconsin (1977).

BRUNN, G., JARKLER, B., & SPELDT, P. Communication display/printout aid with a memory. In Keith Copeland (Ed.), *Aids for the Severely Handicapped.* New York: Grune & Stratton, pp. 116-118 (1974).

BULLOCK, A., DALRYMPLE, G.F., & DANCA, J.M. The Auto-Com at Kennedy Memorial Hospital: Rapid and accurate communication by a multi-handicapped student. *American Journal of Occupational Therapy, 29,* 150-152 (1975).

BUTLER, O., & FOULDES, J. Typing aid remote controlled (TARC). In Keith Copeland (Ed.), *Aids for the Severely Handicapped.* New York: Grune & Stratton, pp. 83-88 (1974).

CALCULATOR, S.N. *Design and Revision of Non-Oral Systems of Communication for the Mentally Retarded Physically Handicapped: A Discussion of the Unicolor Binary Visual Encoding Board with General Implications for Communication* (Working Paper 101). Madison, Wisconsin: Department of Communicative Disorders, University of Wisconsin (no date).

CARLSON, F.L. *An adapted communication project for a nonspeaking child.* Paper presented at the 51st annual meeting of the American Speech and Hearing Association, Houston (1976).

CARRIER, J.K., Jr. Application of functional analysis and non-speech response mode to teaching language. In L.V. McReynolds (Ed.), *Developing Systematic Procedures for Training Children's Language,* ASHA Monograph No. 18 (1974).

———. Nonspeech noun usage training with severely and profoundly retarded children. *Journal of Speech and Hearing Research, 17,* 510-517 (1974).

———. Application of a nonspeech language system with the severely language handicapped. In Lyle L. Lloyd (Ed.), *Communication Assess-*

ment and Intervention Strategies. Baltimore: University Park Press, pp. 523-547 (1976).

CARRIER, J.K., Jr. and PEAK, T., *Program Manual for Non-SLIP (Non-Speech Language Initiation Program).* Lawrence, Kansas: H & H Enterprises, Inc., P.O. Box 3342 (1975).

CHARBONNEAU, J.R., COTE, C., & ROY, O.Z. *NRC's "Comhandi" communication system technical description and application at the Ottawa Crippled Children's Treatment Center.* Paper presented at the seminar on Electronic Controls for the Severely Physically Handicapped, Vancouver, British Columbia (1974).

CLAPPE, C., GRANT, M., HAZARD, G., LANG, J., & TOMLINSON, R. *The Morse Code Visual Translator—A means of communication for the anarthric patient.* Paper presented at the 48th annual meeting of the American Speech and Hearing Association, Detroit (1973).

CLARKE, C.R., DAVIES, C.O., & WOODCOCK, R.W. *Standard Rebus Glossary.* Minneapolis: American Guidance Service (1974).

CLARK, C.R., & GRECO, J.A. *MELDS Glossary of Rebuses and Signs.* Minneapolis: Research, Development, and Demonstration Centre in Education of Handicapped Children, University of Minnesota-Minneapolis (1973).

CLARK, C.R., & WOODCOCK, R.W. Graphic systems of communication. In Lyle L. Lloyd (Ed.), *Communication Assessment and Intervention Strategies.* Baltimore: University Park Press (1976).

CLEMENT, M. Morse Code method of communication for the severely handicapped cerebral palsied child. *Cerebral Palsy Review,* 15-16 (September-October, 1961).

COHEN, L.K. *Communication Aids for the Brain Damaged Adult.* Minneapolis: Sister Kenny Institute (1976).

COLBY, K.M., CHRISTINOZ, D., & GRAHM, S. *A Personal, Portable, and Intelligent Speech Prosthesis* (Working Paper). Los Angeles: Department of Psychiatry, University of California School of Medicine (no date).

COLLINS, D.W. Patient initiated light operated telecontrol (PILOT). In Keith Copeland (Ed.), *Aids for the Severely Handicapped.* New York: Grune & Stratton, pp. 31-41 (1974).

Computerized device speaks for handicapped youngsters. *Journal of the Acoustical Society of America, 59,* 1520-1521 (1976).

COPELAND, K. (Ed.). *Aids for the Severely Handicapped.* New York: Grune & Stratton (1974).

——— . Simplified communication system for the aged infirm. In Keith Copeland (Ed.), *Aids for the Severely Handicapped.* New York: Grune & Stratton, pp. 99-103 (1974).

CRITCHER, C.G., CARRIER, J.K., Jr., & LaCROIX, Z.E. *Speech and language training using a nonspeech response mode.* Paper presented at the 48th annual meeting of the American Speech and Hearing Association, Detroit (1973).

CROCHETIERE, J.W., FOULDS, R.A., & STERNE, R.G. *Computer-aided motor communication.* Paper presented at the Conference on Engineering Devices in Rehabilitation, Boston (1974). (Paper is published in the conference proceedings volume.)

CULATTA, B., COLUCCI, S., CAPOZZI, M., & SCHMIDT, A. *Spontaneous use of trained language symbols in multihandicapped children.* Paper presented at the 52nd annual meeting of the American Speech and Hearing Association, Chicago (1977).

DAVIS, G.A. Linguistics and language therapy: The sentence construction board. *Journal of Speech and Hearing Disorders, 38,* 205-214 (1973).

DEPAPE, D.J., & HARRIS-VANDERHEIDEN, D. *Selecting Initial Vocabulary Elements: Preliminary Notes.* Madison, Wisconsin: Trace Research and Development Center for the Severely Communicatively Handicapped, University of Wisconsin (1977).

DEPAPE, D.J., & VANDERHEIDEN, G.C. *Initial and Secondary Approaches for Developing a Means of Response and Expression for Non-Vocal Severely Physically Handicapped Children and Adults: Preliminary Notes.* Madison, Wisconsin: Trace Research and Development Center for the Severely Communicatively Handicapped. University of Wisconsin (1977).

Devices speak English for laryngectomy cases. *Clinical Trends* (Ophthalmology, Otolaryngology, Allergy), *16* (8), 6 (1978).

DIXON, C. Electronic aids for the severely physically handicapped. *District Nursing* (August, 1971).

DIXON, C., & CURRY, B. Some thoughts on the communication board. *Cerebral Palsy Journal, 26,* 12-13 (1965).

EGERTON, S.W. Technical aids for the disabled. *The B.C. Professional Engineer, 27* (7), 25-27 (1976).

EHRLICH, M.D. *The Votrax Voice Synthesizer as an aid for the blind.* Paper presented at the Conference on Engineering Devices in Rehabilitation, Boston (1974). (Paper is published in the conference proceedings volume.)

ELDER, P.S. *Nonspeech visual symbol training.* Paper presented at the annual meeting of the American Association of Mental Deficiency, New Orleans, (1977).

ELDER, P.S., & BERGMAN, J.S. Visual symbol communication instruction with nonverbal, multiply-handicapped individuals. *Mental Retardation, 16,* 107-112 (1978).

Engineering a good deed. *We, 16* (5), 34 (1964).

ENGLEHART, T.W. *A computerized typing system for the handicapped.* M.S. Thesis, University of Alberta (1971).

FEALLOCK, B. Communication for the nonverbal individual. *American Jour-*

nal of Occupational Therapy, 12, 60-63, 83 (1958).

FISH, K. Trying to break into "Their Own World." *Democrat and Chronicle* (Rochester, New York) (May 27, 1969).

FOTHERGILL, J., VANDERHEIDEN, G.C., HOLT, C., & LUSTER, M.J. Illustrated digest of non-verbal communication and writing aids for severely physically handicapped individuals. In Gregg C. Vanderheiden (Ed.), *Non-Vocal Communication Resourcebook.* Baltimore: University Park Press (1978).

FOULDS, R.A. *The Tufts Interactive Communicator.* Paper presented at the Carnahan Conference on Electronic Prosthetics, Lexington, Kentucky (1972). (Paper is published in the conference proceedings volume, pp. 16-24.)

FOULDS, R.A., BALETSA, G., & CROCHETIERE, W.J. *The effectiveness of language redundancy in non-verbal communication.* Paper presented at the Seminar on Devices and Systems for the Disabled, Philadelphia (1975). (Paper is published in seminar proceedings volume, pp. 82-86.)

FOULDS, R.A., & GADDIS, W. *The practical application of an electronic communication device in a special needs classroom.* Paper presented at the Seminar on Devices and Systems for the Disabled, Philadelphia (1975). (Paper is published in seminar proceedings volume, pp. 77-80.)

GARDNER, H., ZURIF, E.B., BERRY, T., & BAKER, E. Visual communication in aphasia. *Neuropsychologia, 14,* 275-292 (1976).

General reference source on aids for the severely handicapped (bibliography). In Keith Copeland (Ed.), *Aids for the Severely Handicapped.* New York: Grune & Stratton, pp. 141-144 (1974).

GERTENRICH, R.L. A simple mouth-held writing device for use with cerebral palsy patients. *Mental Retardation, 4,* 13-14 (August, 1966).

GLASS, A.V., GAZZANIGA, M.S., & PREMACK, D. Artificial language training in global aphasics. *Neuropsychologia, 11,* 95-103 (1973).

GOLDBERG, H.R., & FENTON, J. *Aphonic Communication for Those with Cerebral Palsy: Guide for the Development and Use of a Conversation Board.* New York: United Cerebral Palsy of New York State (1960).

GOODWIN, M., & GOODWIN, T.C. In a dark mirror. *Mental Hygiene, 53,* 550-563 (1969).

GORDON, J. *Symbol communication system.* B.S. Thesis, University of Manitoba (1975).

GRAHAM, L.W. Language programming and intervention. In Lyle L. Lloyd (Ed.), *Communication Assessment and Intervention Strategies.* Baltimore: University Park Press, pp. 371-422 (1976).

GREEN, C.N. A signal system of communication. *Hearing and Speech Action, 45* (4), 22-23 (1977).

HAGEN, C., PORTER, W., & BRINK, J. Nonverbal communication: An alternative mode of communication for the child with severe cerebral palsy. *Journal of Speech and Hearing Disorders, 38,* 448-455 (1973).

HAMMOND, J., & BAILEY, P. An experiment with Blissymbolics. *Special Education Forward Trends, 3* (3), 21-22 (1976).

Handicapped youth "talks" with eyes. *News Journal* (Mansfield, Ohio) (October 22, 1974).

HARDING, P.J.R., KINGMAN, V.J., KOZAK, A.J., STROMORE, K.A., & VANELDIK, J.F. *Typewriter for teaching severely handicapped children.* Paper presented at the Carnahan Conference on Electronic Prosthetics, Lexington, Kentucky (1973). (Paper is published in conference proceedings volume, pp. 43-46).

HARRIS-VANDERHEIDEN, D. Blissymbols and the mentally retarded. In Gregg C. Vanderheiden and Kate Grilley (Eds.), *Non-vocal Communication Techniques and Aids for the Severely Physically Handicapped.* Baltimore: University Park Press, pp. 120-131 (1976).

————. Field evaluation of the Auto-Com. In Gregg C. Vanderheiden and Kate Grilley (Eds.), *Non-vocal Communication Techniques and Aids for the Severely Communicatively Handicapped.* Baltimore: University Park Press, pp. 144-151 (1976).

————. *A Survey of Critical Factors in Evaluating Communication Aids.* Madison, Wisconsin: Trace Research and Development Center for the Severely Communicatively Handicapped, University of Wisconsin (1975).

HARRIS-VANDERHEIDEN, D., & DEPAPE, D.J. *Review of Common Symbol Systems for Use with Communication Aids: Preliminary Notes.* Madison, Wisconsin: Trace Research and Development Center for the Severely Communicatively Handicapped, University of Wisconsin (1977).

HARRIS-VANDERHEIDEN, D., LIPPERT, J.C., YODER, D.E., & VANDERHEIDEN, G.C. Bliss Symbols: An augmentative symbol/communication system for non-vocal severely handicapped children. In R. York & E. Edgar (Eds.), *Teaching the Severely Handicapped* (Volume IV). Seattle, Washington: American Association for the Education of the Severely Physically Handicapped (1978).

HARRIS, VANDERHEIDEN, D., MCNAUGHTON, S., & MCDONALD, E.T. Some remarks on assessment. In Gregg C. Vanderheiden and Kate Grilley (Eds.), *Non-vocal Communication Techniques and Aids for the Severely Physically Handicapped.* Baltimore: University Park Press, pp. 152-158 (1976).

HARRIS-VANDERHEIDEN, D., SPEILMAN, M., VALLEY, V., & GEISLER, C. *A Preliminary Evaluation of the Auto-Com as an Aid to the Education and Communication of the Non-vocal Physically Handicapped Child.* Madison, Wisconsin: Trace Research and Development Center for the Severely Communicatively Handicapped, University of Wisconsin (1973).

HARRIS-VANDERHEIDEN, D., & VANDERHEIDEN, G. Basic considerations in the development of communicative and interactive skills for non-vocal severely handicapped children. In E. Sontag and N. Certo (Eds.), *Educational Programming for the Severely and Profoundly Handicapped.* Reston, Virginia: CEC Division on Mental Retardation (1977).

HARRIS-VANDERHEIDEN, D., & VANDERHEIDEN, G.C. Enhancing the development of communicative interaction in non-vocal severely physically handicapped children. In R. Schiefelbusch (Eds.), *Non-speech Language Intervention Processes.* Baltimore: University Park Press (1979).

HARTLEY, N. Symbols for diplomats used for children. *Special Education Canada, 4* (2), 5-7 (1974).

HEHNER, B. *Blissymbols to Use* (Dictionary). Toronto, Ontario, Canada: Blissymbolics Communication Institute, 862 Eglinton Avenue E. (in press).

Help for patients with language and visual problems. *Physical Therapy, 54,* 69 (1974).

HENKLE, J.E. *A micro-processor-based gesture entry non-vocal communication system.* Paper presented at the Fourth Annual Conference on Systems and Devices for the Disabled, Seattle, Washington (1977). (Paper is published in conference proceedings volume which is distributed by Continuing Medical Education, University of Washington School of Medicine.)

HILL, S.D., CAMPAGNA, J., LONG, D., MUNCH, J., & NAECHER, S. An explanation of the use of two response keyboard as a means of communication for the severely handicapped child. *Perceptual and Motor Skills, 26,* 699-704 (1968).

HOLBROOK, A., & HARDIMAN, C.J. *Nonverbal communication systems for the severely handicapped.* Paper presented at the 52nd annual meeting of the American Speech and Hearing Association, Chicago (1977).

HOLLIS, J.H., & CARRIER, J.K., Jr. Research implications for communication deficiencies. *Exceptional Children, 41,* 405-412 (1975).

HOLLIS, J.H., CARRIER, J.K., Jr., & SPRADLIN, J.E. An approach to remediation of communication and learning deficiencies. In Lyle L. Lloyd (Ed.), *Communication Assessment and Intervention Strategies.* Baltimore: University Park Press, pp. 265-294 (1976).

HOLMLAND, B.A., & KAVANAGH, R.N. Communication aids for the handicapped. *American Journal of Occupational Therapy, 21,* 357-361 (1976).

HOLT, C., BUELOW, D., & VANDERHEIDEN, G. *Interface Switch Profile and Annotated List of Commercial Switches.* Madison, Wisconsin: Trace Research and Development Center for the Severely Communicatively Handicapped, University of Wisconsin (1976).

HOLT, C.S., RAITZER, G.A., HARRIS-VANDERHEIDEN, D., & VANDERHEIDEN, G. *Formative Evaluation/Design of a Low Cost Scanning Aid.* Madison, Wisconsin: Trace Research and Development Center for the

Severely Communicatively Handicapped, University of Wisconsin (1976).

HOWARD, G. (Ed.). *Helping the Handicapped.* New York: Telephone Pioneers of America, 195 Broadway (1974).

ILES, G.H. *Interfaces for the C.P.* Paper presented at the Seminar on Electronic Controls for the Severely Handicapped, Vancouver, British Columbia (1974). (Paper is published in seminar proceedings volume, pp. 71-82.)

ISRAEL, B.L. *Responsive Environment Program, Brooklyn, New York.* Springfield, Virginia: United States Department of Commerce, Institute for Applied Technology (1969).

Jack, H. Eichler: Builds communication device. *Case Alumnus* (Publication of Case Institute of Technology Alumni Association, Cleveland, Cleveland, Ohio), 211 (June, 1973).

JEFCOATE, R. New independence for the disabled. In Keith Copeland (Ed.), *Aids for the Severely Handicapped.* New York: Grune & Stratton, 129-136 (1974).

————. Possum—Its significance to multiple sclerosis patients. *M. S. News* (December, 1970).

JENKINS, R. Possum, a new communication aid. *Special Education* (Great Britain), *56,* 9-11 (1967).

JOHNSTON, H.B., MANNING, R.P., & LAPPIN, J.S. *A communications prosthesis for a quadraplegic.* Paper presented at the Carnahan Conference on Engineering Devices in Rehabilitation, Lexington, Kentucky (1972). (Paper is published in conference proceedings volume.)

JONES, M.V. Electronic communication devices. *American Journal of Occupational Therapy, 15,* 110-111 (1961).

KAFAFIAN, H. *A Study of Man-Machine Communication Systems for the Handicapped* (3 Volumes). Washington, D.C.: Cybernetics Research Institute (1970-1973).

KATES, B., & MCNAUGHTON, S. *The First Application of Blissymbolics as a Communication Medium for Non-speaking Children: History and Development, 1971-1974.* Toronto, Ontario, Canada: Blissymbolics Communication Institute, 862 Eglinton Avenue East (no date).

KATES, B., MCNAUGHTON, S., & SILVERMAN, H. *Handbook for Instructors, Users, Parents, and Administrators.* Toronto, Ontario, Canada: Blissymbolics Communication Institute, 862 Eglinton Avenue East (1977).

KAVANAGH, R.N., HOLMLUND, B.A., & KRAUSE, A.E. *Communications systems for the physically handicapped.* Paper presented at the Canadian Medical and Biological Engineering Conference (1966). (Paper is published in conference digest volume.)

KEIRNAN, C. Alternatives to speech: A review of research on manual and other forms of communication with mentally handicapped and other noncommunicating populations. *Journal of Mental Subnormality, 23,* 6-28 (1977).

KLADDE, A.G. Nonoral communication techniques: Project Summary #1, August, 1967. In Beverly Vicker (Ed.), *Nonoral Communication System Project 1964/1973.* Iowa City, Iowa: Campus Stores, University of Iowa, pp. 57-104 (1974).

KOLSTOE, B.J. Assisting the non-verbal to 'talk.' *Journal of Physically Handicapped, Homebound, and Hospitalized, 3,* 18-21 (1976).

KUNTZ, J.B. *A nonvocal communication development program for severely retarded children.* Unpublished Doctoral Dissertation, Kansas State University (1974).

LAVOY, R.W. Ricks communicator. *Exceptional Child, 23,* 338-340 (1957).

LOWE, H., CHURCHILL, T., GOSLING, T., & BATTISON, D. Lightwriter. In Keith Copeland (Ed.), *Aids for the Severely Handicapped.* New York: Grune & Stratton, pp. 109-115 (1974).

LOWMAN, E.W., & KLINGER, J.L. *Aids to Independent Living: Self-Help for the Handicapped.* New York: McGraw-Hill (1969).

LLOYD, L.L. (Ed.). *Communication Assessment and Intervention Strategies.* Baltimore: University Park Press (1976).

LUSTER, M.J. *Preliminary Selected Bibliography of Articles, Brochures and Books Related to Communication Techniques and Aids for the Severely Handicapped.* Madison, Wisconsin: Trace Research and Development Center for the Severely Communicatively Handicapped, University of Wisconsin (1974).

LUSTER, M.J., & VANDERHEIDEN, G.C. *Preliminary Annotated Bibliography of Communication Aids.* Madison, Wisconsin: Trace Research and Development Center for the Severely Communicatively Handicapped, University of Wisconsin (1974).

———. *Preliminary Annotated Bibliography of Researchers and Institutions.* Madison, Wisconsin: Trace Research and Development Center for the Severely Communicatively Handicapped, University of Wisconsin (1974).

LYWOOD, D.W., & VASA, J.J. *A brief survey and classification of available systems.* Paper presented at the Seminar on Electronic Controls for the Severely Disabled, Vancouver, British Columbia (1974). (Paper is published in seminar proceedings volume, pp. 7-11.)

MCDONALD, E.T. Conventional symbols of English. In Gregg C. Vanderheiden and Kate Grilley (Eds.), *Non-vocal Communication Techniques and Aids for the Severely Physically Handicapped.* Baltimore: University Park Press, pp. 77-84 (1976).

———. Design and application of communication boards. In Gregg C. Vanderheiden and Kate Grilley (Eds.), *Non-vocal Communication Techniques for the Severely Physically Handicapped.* Baltimore: University Park Press, pp. 105-119 (1976).

_____ . Identification of children at risk. In Gregg C. Vanderheiden and Kate Grilley (Eds.), *Non-vocal Communication Techniques and Aids for the Severely Physically Handicapped.* Baltimore: University Park Press, pp. 12-15 (1976).

McDONALD, E.T., and SCHULTZ, A.R. Communication boards for cerebral palsied children. *Journal of Speech and Hearing Disorders, 38,* 73-88 (1973).

McNAUGHTON, S., *Symbol Secrets.* Toronto, Ontario, Canada: Blissymbolics Communication Institute, 862 Eglinton Avenue East (1975).

_____ . Symbol Communication Programme at OCCC. In Gregg C. Vanderheiden and Kate Grilley (Eds.), *Non-vocal Communication Techniques and Aids for the Severely Physically Handicapped.* Baltimore: University Park Press, pp. 132-143 (1976).

_____ . Blissymbolics — An alternative symbol system for the non-vocal pre-reading child. In Gregg C. Vanderheiden and Kate Grilley (Eds.), *Nonvocal Communication Techniques and Aids for the Severely Physically Handicapped.* Baltimore: University Park Press, pp. 85-105 (1976).

_____ . Electronic aids in Blissymbol communications. In P. Nelson (Ed.), *Proceedings of the Workshop on Communication Aids,* Ottawa, Ontario, Canada: Canadian Medical and Biological Engineering Society, National Research Council (1978).

McNAUGHTON, S., & KATES, B. *Visual symbols: Communication system for the pre-reading physically handicapped child.* Paper presented at the annual meeting of the American Association on Mental Deficiency, Toronto, Ontario (1974).

Machine turns handwriting into sound. *The Milwaukee Journal* (Milwaukee, Wisconsin) (December 1, 1976).

MALING, R. Control systems—Concept and development (POSSUM). In Keith Copeland (Ed.), *Aids for the Severely Handicapped.* New York: Grune & Stratton, pp. 22-30 (1974).

MALING, R., & CLARKSON, D.C. Electronic controls for the tetraplegic (Possum) (Patient Operated Selector Mechanisms—P.O.S.M.). *Paraplegia, 1,* 161-174 (1963).

Microprocessor based voice synthesizer puts speech at its user's fingertips. *Digital Design,* 15-16 (March, 1977).

MILLER, J., & CARPENTER, C. Electronics for communication. *American Journal of Occupational Therapy, 18,* 20-23 (1964).

MONTGOMERY, J. Review of "The L Board"—A language board for nonoral communication. *Asha, 19,* 379-380 (1977).

MOOGK-SOULIS, C.A. *An experimental evaluation of selected communication technical aids.* Paper presented at the Fourth Annual Conference on Systems and Devices for the Disabled, Seattle, Washington (1977). (Paper is published in the conference proceedings volume which can be obtained from Continuing Medical Education, University of Washington School of Medicine.)

MOORE, M.V. Binary communication for the severely handicapped. *Archives of Physical Medicine and Rehabilitation, 53,* 532-533 (1972).

NELSON, P.J. (Ed.). *Proceedings of Workshop on Communication Aids.* Ottawa, Ontario, Canada: Canadian Medical and Biological Engineering Society, National Research Council (1978).

————. *Speech synthesis for non-verbal children—A progress report.* Paper presented at the Fourth Annual Conference on Systems and Devices for the Disabled. Seattle, Washington (1977). (Paper is published in the conference proceedings volume which can be obtained from Continuing Medical Education, University of Washington School of Medicine.)

NEWELL, A.F. Morse code and voice control for the disabled (VOTEM). In Keith Copeland (Ed.), *Aids for the Severely Handicapped.* New York: Grune & Stratton, pp. 54-58 (1974).

NEWELL, A.F., BEYNON, J.D.E., BRUMFITT, P.J., & HOSSAIN, K.S. An alphanumeric display as a communication aid for the dumb. *Medical and Biological Engineering, 13,* 84-88 (1975).

NEWELL, A.F., & BOUR, J.S. Voice operated powered devices. *Biomechanics, 4,* 45-48 (1971).

NEWELL, A.F., & BRUMFITT, P.J. 'Talking brooch' communication aid. In Keith Copeland (Ed.), *Aids for the Severely Handicapped.* New York: Grune & Stratton, pp. 104-108 (1974).

NEWELL, A.F., & NABAUI, C.D. VOTEM: The voice operated typewriter employing Morse Code. *Journal of Scientific Instruments,* Series *2, 2* (1969).

NICOL, E. Breakthrough to communication. *Special Education, 61* (4), 25-28 (1972).

NUFFER, P.S. *Communication Bracelet Manual.* Tempe, Arizona: Ideas, P.O. Box 741 (no date).

NUGENT, C.L. Rehabilitative speech and language pathology and non-oral communication. *Resources* (Everest & Jennings, Inc., Los Angeles, California) (December, 1977).

OLSON, T. Return of the nonverbal. *Asha, 18,* 823 (1976).

Ontario Crippled Children's Centre Bliss Project Team, *Ontario Crippled Children's Centre Symbol Communication Research Project 1972-1973.* Toronto, Ontario, Canada: Ontario Crippled Children's Centre (1973).

PARISH, G. Prescription of remote-control devices for disabled adults. In Keith Copeland (Ed.), *Aids for the Severely Handicapped.* New York: Grune & Stratton, pp. 15-21 (1974).

PARKEL, D.A., WHITE, R.A., & WARNER, H. Implications of the Yerkes technology for mentally retarded subjects. In Duane M. Rumbaugh (Ed.), *Language Learning by a Chimpanzee: The LANA Project.* New York: Academic Press (1977).

PERRON, J.V. Typewriter control for an aphasic quadriplegic patient. *Canadian Medical Association Journal, 92,* 557 (1965).

Physically handicapped children learn to communicate. *Science Dimension,* 8-13 (April, 1973).

PREMACK, A.J., & PREMACK, D. Teaching language to an ape. *Scientific American, 277,* 92-99 (1972).

PREMACK, D. A functional analysis of language. *Journal of Experimental Analysis of Behavior, 14,* 107-125 (1970).

——. Language in chimpanzee? *Science, 172,* 808-822 (1971).

PREMACK, D., & PREMACK, A.J. Teaching visual language to apes and language-deficient persons. In Richard L. Schiefelbusch and Lyle L. Lloyd (Eds.), *Language Perspectives — Acquisition, Retardation, and Intervention.* Baltimore: University Park Press, pp. 347-376 (1974).

PRINCE, S. Something new. *Asha, 18,* 880 (1976).

Provisional Dictionary (Blissymbolics). Toronto, Ontario, Canada: Blissymbolics Communication Institute, 862 Eglinton Avenue East (1976).

RAHIMI, M.A., and EYLENBERG, J.B. *A computer terminal with synthetic speech output.* Paper presented at the National Conference on the Use of On-Line Computers in Psychology, St. Louis (1973).

——. *A computing environment for the blind.* Paper presented at the AFIPS National Computer Conference (1974). (Paper is published in conference proceedings volume.)

RAITZER, G.A., VANDERHEIDEN, G.C., & HOLT, C.S. *Interfacing computers for the physically handicapped—A review of international approaches.* Paper presented at the AFIPS National Computer Conference (1976). (Paper is published in conference proceedings volume, pp. 209-216.)

RANSAY, D.A., SNAPPER, A.G., & KOP, P.F.M. A foot-operated typewriter. *Archives of Physical Medicine and Rehabilitation, 53,* 190 (1972).

RATUSNIK, C.M., & RATUSNIK, D.L. A comprehensive communication approach for a ten-year-old nonverbal autistic child. *American Journal of Orthopsychiatry, 44,* 396-403 (1974).

Record-player "voice" for mutes. *NASA Tech Briefs,* 97-98 (Spring, 1977).

RICE, O.M., & COMBS, R.G. *Practical aids for non-verbal handicapped.* Paper presented at the Carnahan Conference on Electronic Prosthetics (1972). (Paper is published in conference proceedings volume.)

RINARD, G. An ocular-controlled video terminal. In P. Nelson (Ed.), *Proceedings of Workshop on Communication Aids.* Ottawa, Ontario, Canada: Canadian Medical and Biological Engineering Society, National Research Council (1978).

RING, N. Possum typewriter — Consumer experience. In Keith Copeland (Ed.), *Aids for the Severely Handicapped.* New York: Grune & Stratton, pp. 124-128 (1974).

———. Specification of interfaces for communication aids. In P. Nelson (Ed.), *Proceedings of Workshop on Communication Aids.* Ottawa, Ontario Canada: Canadian Medical and Biological Engineering Society, National Research Council (1978).

ROBENAULT, I.P. *Functional Aids for the Multiply Handicapped.* Evanston: Harper & Row (1973).

ROSEN, M., DRINKER, P., & DALRYMPLE, G. *A Display Board for Non-verbal Communication Encoded as Eye Movement.* Cambridge, Massachusetts: Department of Mechanical Engineering, Massachusetts Institute of Technology (1976).

ROSENBERG, G. *Assistive Devices for the Handicapped.* Atlanta: American Rehabilitation Foundation (1968).

ROSS, A., & FLANAGAN, K. *Communication system using Morse Code to printed English translation.* Paper presented at the Fourth Annual Conference on Systems and Devices for the Disabled, Seattle, Washington (1977). (Paper is published in conference proceedings volume which is available from Continuing Medical Education, University of Washington School of Medicine.)

ROY, O.Z. A communication system for the handicapped. *Medical Electronics and Biological Engineering, 3,* 427 (1965).

ROY, O.Z., & CHARBONNEAU, J.R. A communications system for the handicapped (COMHANDI). In Keith Copeland (Ed.), *Aids for the Severely Handicapped.* New York: Grune & Stratton, pp. 89-98 (1974).

RUMBAUGH, D.M. (Ed.). *Language Learning by a Chimpanzee: The LANA Project.* New York: Academic Press (1977).

SAARNIO, I. Typewriter control by dental palate key. In Keith Copeland (Ed.), *Aids for the Severely Handicapped.* New York: Grune & Stratton, pp. 59-62 (1974).

SAMPSON, D. A communication device for patients unable to speak. *Medical and Biological Engineering, 8,* 99-101 (1970).

SANDERS, D.A. A model for communication. In Lyle L. Lloyd (Ed.), *Communication Assessment and Intervention Strategies.* Baltimore: University Park Press, pp. 1-32 (1976).

SAYRE, J.M. Communication for the non-verbal cerebral palsied. *CP Review, 24,* 3-8 (November/December, 1963).

SCHIEFELBUSCH, R.L. (Ed.). *Nonspeech Language Intervention.* Baltimore: University Park Press (1979).

SCHMIDT, M.J., CARRIER, J.K., JR., & PARSONS, S.D. *Use of a nonspeech mode for teaching language.* Paper presented at the 46th annual meeting of the American Speech and Hearing Association, Chicago (1971).

SCHURMAN, J.A. Custom designing communication board frames: The role of the occupational therapist. In Beverly Vicker (Ed.), *Nonoral Communication System Project 1964/1973*. Iowa City, Iowa: Campus Stores, The University of Iowa, pp. 177-211 (1974).

SELIGMAN, J., & GANNON, R. *A new approach to communication for the severely physically handicapped child.* Paper presented at the 47th annual meeting of the American Speech and Hearing Association, San Francisco (1972).

SHANE, H., & MELROSE, J. *An electronic conversation board and an accompanying training program for aphonic expressive communication.* Paper presented at the 50th annual meeting of the American Speech and Hearing Association, Washington, D.C. (1975).

SHANE, H.C., & WILSON, M.S. Blissymbolics. *Asha, 19,* 223 (1977).

SHWEDYK, E., & GORDON, J. Communication aid for nonvocal handicapped people. *Medical and Biological Engineering and Computing, 15,* 189-194 (1977).

SILVERMAN, F.H. A bibliography of literature relevant to nonspeech communication modes for the speechless. *Ohio Journal of Speech and Hearing, 12,* 83-102 (1977).

SILVERMAN, F.H., & BADY, J., Need for including coursework on nonvocal communication systems: A Survey. *Asha, 20,* 1023 (1978).

SILVERMAN, H., & KELSO, D. *The Bliss-com: A portable symbol printing communication aid.* Paper presented at the Fourth Annual Conference on Systems and Devices for the Disabled, Seattle (1977). (Paper is published in the conference proceedings volume which can be obtained from Continuing Medical Education, University of Washington School of Medicine.)

SKLAR, M., & BENNETT, D.N. Initial communication chart for aphasics. *Journal of the Association of Physical and Mental Rehabilitation, 10,* 43-53 (1956).

SOEDE, M., & STASSEN, H.G. A light spot operated typewriter for severely disabled patients. *Medical and Biological Engineering, 11,* 641-644 (1973).

SOEDE, M., STASSEN, H.G., LUNTEREN, A.V., & LUITSE, W.J. A lightspot-operated typewriter (LOT). In Keith Copeland (Ed.), *Aids for the Severely Handicapped.* New York: Grune & Stratton, pp. 42-53 (1974).

SONTAG, E., SMITH, J., & CERTO, N. (Eds.). *Educational Programming for the Severely and Profoundly Handicapped.* Reston, Virginia: The Council for Exceptional Children (1977).

STEELE, D. Visual effect from muscular movement (Systems 7 and 9). In Keith Copeland (Ed.), *Aids for the Severely Handicapped.* New York: Grune & Stratton, pp. 63-71 (1974).

SUTHERLAND, D., & KATES, B. *Considerations in Assessing a Child's Communication Needs.* Toronto, Ontario, Canada: Blissymbolics Communication Institute, 862 Eglinton Avenue East (1975).

Symbols are Bliss. *Asha, 19,* 104 (1977).

Syntax Supplement No. 1 (for Bliss Symbols). Toronto, Ontario, Canada: Blissymbolics Communication Institute, 862 Eglinton Avenue East (no date).

Teaching Aids for Children with Cerebral Palsy. Albany, New York: State Department of Education (1966).

Teaching Guidelines (for Bliss Symbols). Toronto, Ontario, Canada: Blissymbolics Communication Institute, 862 Eglinton Avenue East (no date).

TOLSTRUP, I.M. *VIDIALOG: TV-based communication system for the motor handicapped.* Paper presented at the Third Nordic Meeting on Medical and Biological Engineering, Tampere, Finland (1975). (Paper is published in conference proceedings volume.)

TRAUB, D.A. *Training teachers to use communication boards with the mentally retarded.* Paper presented at the 52nd annual meeting of the American Speech and Hearing Association, Chicago (1977).

TRAYNOR, C.D. *A breath-controlled computer data system.* Paper presented at the Fourth Annual Conference on Systems and Devices for the Disabled, Seattle, Washington (1977). (Paper is published in conference proceedings volume which can be obtained from Continuing Medical Education, University of Washington School of Medicine.)

VANDERHEIDEN, D.H., BROWN, W.P., MACKENZIE, P., REINEN, S., & SCHEIBEL, C. Symbol communication for the mentally handicapped. *Mental Retardation, 13,* 34-37 (1975).

VANDERHEIDEN, G.C. *Design and Construction of a Laptray: Preliminary Notes.* Madison, Wisconsin: Trace Research and Development Center for the Severely Communicatively Handicapped, University of Wisconsin (1977).

————. *Evaluation and Further Development of the Automonitoring Communication Board as an Educational Aid for Severely Handicapped Children: Summary Final Report.* Madison, Wisconsin: Trace Research and Development Center for the Severely Communicatively Handicapped, University of Wisconsin (1975).

————. (Ed.) *Non-vocal Communication Resourcebook.* Baltimore: University Park Press (1978).

————. Providing the child with a means to indicate. In Gregg G. Vanderheiden and Kate Grilley (Eds.), *Non-vocal Communication Techniques and Aids for the Severely Physically Handicapped.* Baltimore: University Park Press, pp. 20-76 (1976).

————. *Synthesized Speech as a Communication Mode for Non-vocal Severely Handicapped Individuals.* Madison, Wisconsin: Trace Research and Development Center for the Severely Communicatively Handicapped, University of Wisconsin (1976).

VANDERHEIDEN, G.C., BROWN, W.P., & FOTHERGILL, J. Master chart of communication aids. In Gregg C. Vanderheiden (Ed.), *Non-vocal Communication Resourcebook*. Baltimore: University Park Press (1978).

VANDERHEIDEN, G.C. & GRILLEY, K. (Eds.), *Non-vocal Communication Techniques and Aids for the Severely Physically Handicapped*. Baltimore: University Park Press (1976).

VANDERHEIDEN, G.C., & HARRIS-VANDERHEIDEN, D. Communication techniques and aids for the nonvocal severely handicapped. In Lyle L. Lloyd (Ed.), *Communication Assessment and Intervention Strategies*. Baltimore: University Park Press (1976).

――――― . Developing effective modes of response and expression in nonvocal severely handicapped children. In P. Mittler (Ed.), *Research in Practice in Mental Retardation*. Baltimore: University Park Press (1977).

――――― . Field evaluation of the Auto-Com, An auto-monitoring communication board. *Research Relating to Children* (ERIC Clearinghouse for Early Childhood Education), Bulletin 37, 86-87 (1976).

VANDERHEIDEN, G.C., KELSO, D.P., HOLT, C.S., & RAITZER, G.A. Cost reduction in the development of new communication aids through use of a common control system: A case example, the Blisscom. In P. Nelson (Ed.), *Proceedings of Workshop on Communication Aids*. Ottawa, Ontario, Canada: Medical and Biological Engineering Society, National Research Council (1978).

――――― . *A Teacher Modifiable Portable Microprocessor Based Aid for Nonvocal Severely Physically Handicapped Individuals*. Madison, Wisconsin: Trace Research and Development Center for the Severely Communicatively Handicapped, University of Wisconsin (1976).

VANDERHEIDEN, G.C., LAMERS, D.F., VOLK, A.M., & GEISLER, C.D. *A Portable Non-vocal Communication Prosthesis for the Severely Physically Handicapped*. Madison, Wisconsin: Trace Research and Development Center for the Severely Communicatively Handicapped, University of Wisconsin (1975).

VANDERHEIDEN, G.C., & LUSTER, M.J. *Communication Techniques and Aids to Assist in the Education of Non-vocal Physically Handicapped Children: A State-of-the-Art Review*. Madison, Wisconsin: Trace Research and Development Center for the Severely Communicatively Handicapped, University of Wisconsin (1976).

VANDERHEIDEN, G.C., RAITZER, G.A., & KELSO, D.P *The Portable Auto-Com/ Wordmaster: A Portable Non-vocal Communications Prosthesis for the Severely Physically Handicapped*. Madison, Wisconson: Trace Research and Development Center for the Severely Communicatively Handicapped, University of Wisconsin (1976).

VANDERHEIDEN, G.C., RAITZER, G.A., KELSO, D.P., & GEISLER, C.D. *An Automated Technique for the Interpretation of Erratic Pointing*

Motions of Severely Cerebral Palsied Individuals. Madison, Wisconsin: Trace Research and Development Center for the Severely Communicatively Handicapped, University of Wisconsin (1974).

VANDERHEIDEN, G.C., VOLK, A.M., & GEISLER, C.D. *An alternative interface to computers for the physically handicapped.* Paper presented at the AFIPS National Computer Conference (1974). (Paper is published in conference proceedings volume, pp. 115-121.)

————. *The auto-monitoring technique and its application in the automonitoring communication board (Auto-Com), A new communication technique for the severely handicapped.* Paper presented at the Carnahan Conference on Electronic Prostheses, Lexington, Kentucky (1973). (Paper is published in conference proceedings volume, pp. 47-51.)

VASA, J.J., & LYWOOD, D.W. High-speech communication aid for quadriplegics. *Medical and Biological Engineering, 14,* 445-450 (1976).

————. *A typing aid for the severely handicapped.* Paper presented at the Canadian Medical and Biological Engineering Conference (1972). (Paper is published in the conference digest volume which is available from the Canadian Medical and Biological Engineering Society, National Research Council, Ottawa, Ontario, Canada, 1972).

VASA, J.J., & MANSELL, M. *Queen's communication aids.* Paper presented at the Seminar on Electronic Controls for the Severely Disabled, Vancouver, British Columbia (1974). (Paper is published in seminar proceedings volume, pp. 37-39.)

VICKER, B. Advances in nonoral communication system programming: Project Summary #2, August, 1973. In Beverly Vicker (Ed.), *Nonoral Communication System Project 1964/1973.* Iowa City, Iowa: Campus Stores, University of Iowa, pp. 105-175 (1974).

————. Communication board programming with a four-year-old child: A case report. In Beverly Vicker (Ed.), *Nonoral Communication System Project 1964/1973.* Iowa City, Iowa: Campus Stores, University of Iowa, pp. 213-261 (1974).

————. The communication process using a nonoral means. In Beverly Vicker (Ed.), *Nonoral Communication System Project 1964/1972.* Iowa City, Iowa: Campus Stores, University of Iowa, pp. 15-56 (1974).

————. *Nonoral Communication System Project 1964/1973.* Iowa City, Iowa: Campus Stores, University of Iowa (1974).

WALDO, L.J. *Functional communication board training for the severely handicapped.* Paper presented at the 52nd annual meeting of the American Speech and Hearing Association, Chicago (1977).

WARDELL, R. Development of the eyewriter. In P. Nelson (Ed.), *Proceedings of Workshop on Communication Aids.* Ottawa, Ontario, Canada:

Canadian Medical and Biological Engineering Society, National Research Council (1978).

WARRICK, A., *et al.* Synthesized speech as an aid in communication and learning for the non-verbal. In P. Nelson (Ed.), *Proceedings of Workshop on Communication Aids.* Ottawa, Ontario, Canada: Canadian Medical and Biological Engineering Society, National Research Council (1978).

WENDT, E., SPRAGUE, M.J., & MARQUIS, J. Communication without speech. *Teaching Exceptional Children,* 38-42 (Fall, 1975).

WHITE, S.D. A modular communication device for paralyzed patients. *Archives of Physical Medicine and Rehabilitation, 55* (2), 94-95 (1974).

ZISKIND, A., & ZISKIND, R. Remote control typewriter for paraplegics. *Journal of the American Medical Association, 169,* 459-460 (1959).

Neuro-Assisted Modes

COMBS, R.G. Myocom: Communication for non-verbal handicapped. *Transactions of the Missouri Academy of Science, 3,* 102 (1969).

DEWAN, E.M. Communication by voluntary control of the electroencephalogram. *Proceedings of the Symposium of Biomedical Engineering* (Marquette University), *1,* 349-351 (1966).

RICE, O.M., & COMBS, R.G. *Practical aids for non-verbal handicapped.* Paper presented at the Carnahan Conference on Electronic Prosthetics, Lexington, Kentucky (1972). (Paper is published in conference proceedings volume.)

TOROK, Z. A typewriter operated by electromyographic potentials (GMMI). In Keith Copeland (Ed.), *Aids for the Severely Handicapped.* New York: Grune & Stratton, pp. 77-82 (1974).

TOROK, Z., & HAMMOND, P.H. *On the performance of single motor units as sources of control signals.* Paper presented at the Conference of Human Locomotor Engineering, University of Sussex (1971). (Paper is published in conference proceedings volume, pp. 35-40.).

Writing made possible for cerebral palsy victim. *Pacific Review, 10* (4), 3 (February, 1976).

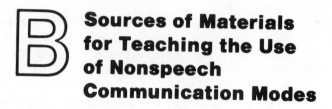

Sources of Materials for Teaching the Use of Nonspeech Communication Modes

Note

There are seven *organizations* listed in this appendix that publish or distribute books and other materials that can be useful when teaching certain nonspeech communication systems. The listing for each includes an address and a brief description of the kinds of materials it publishes and/or distributes. These organizations, of course, are not the only ones that publish or distribute materials that can be useful when teaching such systems.

The appendix also lists several *books* that should be useful when teaching clients to use certain of these systems. Following each reference, there is a brief description of the kinds of information presented. The books listed are representative of those available.

Organizations

American Guidance Service, Minneapolis, Minnesota:
Distributes materials for the Rebus Program.
Blissymbolics Communication Institute, 862 Eglinton Avenue East, Toronto, Ontario, Canada:
Primary source of materials for teaching Blissymbolics.
Dysfunctioning Child Center, Michael Reese Medical Center, Chicago, Illinois:
Source of information relevant to teaching manual sign language to autistic children.
Gallaudet College Bookstore, Gallaudet College, Washington, D.C.:
Distributes books and other materials that are intended for teaching manual sign language (Ameslan) to deaf persons, preschool through adult. Many of these materials would be appropriate for teaching Ameslan signs to children and adults who are not deaf.

H & H Enterprises, Inc., P.O. Box 3342, Lawrence, Kansas:
   Distributes materials for the Non-SLIP Program.
Learning Resources Center, Veterans Administration Hospital, St. Louis, Missouri:
   Distributes through interlibrary loan videotaped material useful for teaching Amerind, including the *Amerind Video Dictionary*.
Trace Research and Development Center for the Severely Communicatively Handicapped, University of Wisconsin, Madison, Wisconsin:
   Distributes materials relevant to selecting and interfacing persons with gestural-assisted communication systems, both nonelectronic and electronic.

Books

KENT, L. *Language Acquisition Program for the Severely Retarded.* Champaign, Illinois: Research Press (1974).
   Program includes material for teaching a basic Ameslan vocabulary.
LAKE, S.J. *The Handbook.* Tucson, Arizona: Communication Skill Builders (1976).
   Illustrates a basic Ameslan vocabulary for mentally-retarded children through the use of photographs.
SKELLY, M. *Amer-Ind Gestural Code.* New York: Elsevier (1979).
   Illustrates by line drawings the Amerind Signs included in the *Amerind Video Dictionary*.
TOMKINS, W. *Indian Sign Language.* New York: Dover Publications (1969).
   Though not intended to be a source of Amerind Signs for speechless persons, this book illustrates (through line drawings) some American Indian Signs that could be used by this population. It does not present as useful a vocabulary for such persons, however, as does the *Amerind Video Dictionary*.
VICKER, B. *Nonoral Communication System Project 1964/1973.* Iowa City, Iowa: Campus Stores, University of Iowa (1974).
   Excellent source of information on developing and teaching the use of communication boards.
WILSON, P.S., GOODMAN, L., & WOOD, R.K. *Manual Language for the Child Without Language.* Hartford, Connecticut: Department of Mental Retardation Developmental Team, 79 Elm Street (1975).
   Outlines program for teaching Ameslan Signs to mentally retarded children.

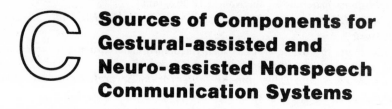

Sources of Components for Gestural-assisted and Neuro-assisted Nonspeech Communication Systems

Note

A number of organizations are listed in this appendix that manufacture or distribute components for nonspeech communication systems. The listing for each includes an address and a brief description of the types of components (or complete systems) it distributes. Further information about sources of such components (and systems) can be obtained from the Trace Research and Development Center for the Severely Communicatively Handicapped, University of Wisconsin, Madison, Wisconsin 53706.

Organizations

Bell Laboratories, Murray Hill, New Jersey
Primary source for devices intended for telephone communication by other than speech means (e.g., Morse Code).

Blissymbolics Communication Institute, 862 Eglinton Avenue East, Toronto, Ontario, Canada
Distributes Blissymbol communication boards and electronic gestural-assisted systems with Blissymbol displays.

C. N. Green, Rte 1, Box 316D, 324 Acre Avenue, Brownsburg, Ohio
Distributes several inexpensive nonelectronic gestural-assisted communication devices including a 48 page pocket-sized booklet containing labeled pictures and a basic need communication board for use in hospital and nursing home settings.

Cleo Living Aids, 3957 Mayfield Road, Cleveland, Ohio
Distributes a picture-letter communication board for use in a hospital or nursing home setting (see Figure 5.5).

Ghora-Khan Grotto, 2245 Fremont Avenue, St. Paul, Minnesota
Distributes the Hall-Roe Communication Board (see Figure 5.13).

H & H Enterprises, Inc., P.O. Box 3342, Lawrence Kansas

Distributes manipulable symbols (Non-SLIP System).

HC Electronics, Inc., 250 Camino Alto, Mill Valley, California

Distributes several portable speech synthesizers referred to as Phonic Mirror HandiVoice Systems (see Figure 5.44).

IBM, Franklin Lakes, New Jersey

IBM makes available at relatively low cost rebuilt electric typewriters that have been adapted for use by children and adults who have neuromuscular disorders affecting their upper extremities. Possible modifications include adding an armrest, a paper roll, and a keyguard (see Figure 5.23). IBM also manufactures electric typewriters that can be used as displays in electronic gestural-assisted communication systems (see Chapter 5).

Ideas, P.O. Box 741, Tempe, Arizona

Distributes the Communication Bracelet (see Figure 5.13).

Interstate Printers and Publishers, Danville, Illinois

Distributes a picture communication booklet, *Communication for the Laryngectomized,* that is intended to be used by laryngectomized adults for communicating with hospital personnel.

Prentke Romich Company, R.D. 2, Box 191, Schreve, Ohio

Distributes a variety of electronic gestural-assisted communication systems as well as switching mechanisms and other components for such systems (e.g., see Figure 5.42). They also distribute a myoswitch.

Telephone Pioneers of America, 195 Broadway, New York, New York

Local chapters fabricate electronic gestural-assisted communication devices for handicapped children and adults. Some of the devices that they have fabricated are described in a book edited by Grace Howard, entitled *Helping the Handicapped,* that was published by the Organization in 1974.

Trace Research and Development Center for the Severely Communicatively Handicapped, University of Wisconsin, Madison, Wisconsin

Distributes several electronic-gestural-assisted communication systems, including the Auto-Com Communication Board (see Figure 5.33). It also provides information regarding sources of components for other such systems.

Zygo Industries, P.O. Box 1008, Portland, Oregon

Distributes a variety of electronic gestural-assisted communication systems as well as switching mechanisms and other components for such systems.

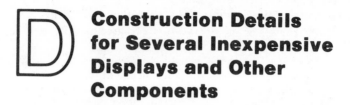

Construction Details for Several Inexpensive Displays and Other Components

Voice Operated Switch

This device can be used to control any electrical display that can be operated with a single switch, including those described in this Appendix. It will function either in a normally open or normally closed mode (i.e., a voice signal can be used either to start or stop an electrical device such as a motor) and it can be activated by almost any kind of phonation (e.g., an isolated vowel or cough). In 1977 the components were distributed in kit form by the Radio Shack Division of the Tandy Corporation for less than $7.00.

Construction details are presented in both a pictorial diagram (see Figure D.1) and a schematic diagram (see Figure D.2). Q1, Q2, and Q3 are NPN silicon transistors and Q4 is a PNP germanium transistor. One wire of the two-conductor wire that interfaces this switch with the display is connected to the terminal marked *wiper arm* (see Figure D.1) and the other wire is connected either to the terminal marked *normally open* or the one marked *normally closed* (see Figure D.1).

For a photograph of the completed unit (built on a perfbox chassis) with microphone attached, see Figure D.3. The microphone illustrated is not included in the Radio Shack Kit.

Scanning Encoding Aid Number 1

The Scanning Encoding Aid Number 1 (Figures D.4 and D.5) consists of a rotating pointer (4 rpm) that can be started and stopped by any type of switching mechanism. The source of power is two 1.5 volt "D" cells. Pictures or symbols can be attached to the 16" x 16" Plexiglass surface (the numbers in Figure D.3 are used to encode squares on a 9 x 9 matrix). The unit can be assembled from readily available components using only a hand drill, coping

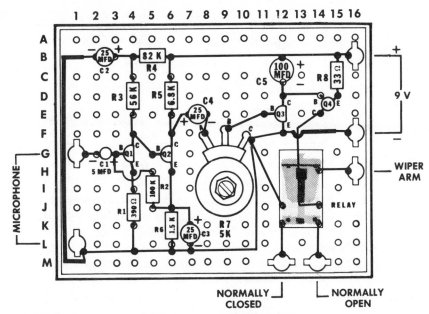

FIGURE D.1. *Pictorial diagram for voice operated switch.*
(Diagram courtesy of the Radio Shack Division of the Tandy Corporation)

saw, and screwdriver for less than $35.00 (based upon April, 1977 component prices).

Construction Details

The unit contains the following components:

Number	Description
1	⅛″ x 16¼″ x 16¼″ piece of opaque yellow Plexi-glass plastic
1	aluminum table easel (Stanrite, No. 152)
1	4 rpm, 3 volt motor (No. 3440-4R, Hankscraft Company, Reedsburg, Wisconsin)
1	screw type, two-terminal board
2	setscrew collars for ⅛″ (motor) shaft (Perfect Parts Company landing gear wheel collars)
1	¼-20 x ½″ round head machine screw and wing nut
6	4-40 x ½″ round head machine screws and nuts
1	battery holder for two type "D," 1.5 volt batteries
2	1.5 volt size "D" alkaline batteries
2 ft.	24 gage speaker wire
2 ft.	electrical insulating tape
1 pkg.	1″ self-adhesive black vinyl letters and numbers

The unit is mounted on an aluminum table easel (which can be pur-

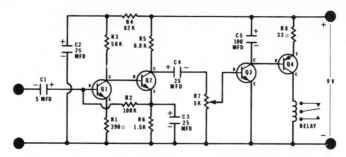

FIGURE D.2. *Schematic diagram for voice operated switch.*
(Diagram courtesy of the Radio Shack Division of the Tandy Corporation)

chased at an art supply store). The easel has a vertical extension that is intended for supporting the tops of large canvases. The rivet that attaches it to the rest of the easel is removed, and it is shortened and shaped to serve as the *pointer* (see Figure D.4).

The Plexiglass board for the unit can be purchased *cut to size* from almost any store that sells plastic in sheets (see the yellow pages of the phone book). Both sides of the Plexiglass will be covered by sheets of protective paper. Do not remove them until all holes have been drilled. Begin by drilling a hole slightly larger than ⅛″ at the center of the board for the motor shaft (which is ⅛″ in diameter). Then place the board on the easel and center it. Mark on the board the location of the center of the hole at the top of the easel (in which the rivet had been that attached the extension to the easel) and drill

FIGURE D.3. *Voice operated switch with microphone attached.*

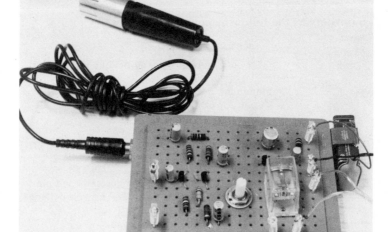

a ¼" hole in the board at this point. (A machine screw is passed through the board and easel to attach the board to the easel.) Next, drill two ¼" holes next to each other for the two terminals of the terminal strip (see Figure D.4 for the location of the terminal strip). Finally, drill six 7/64" holes in the board at the appropriate locations for attaching the motor, terminal strip, and battery holder to it (see Figures D.4 and D.5). Round the corners of the board with sandpaper; remove the protective paper; and attach the motor, terminal strip, and battery holder to the board with the 4-40 x ½" machine screws.

Form the pointer (see Figure D.4) from the piece of aluminum that served as the easel extension (it should be approximately 4½" long). Drill a ⅛" hole in it at the end opposite the point. Attach the pointer to the shaft with the two, setscrew collars (the pointer being sandwiched between them).

Run one wire from the minus terminal of the motor to the minus terminal of the battery holder. Run a second wire from the positive terminal of the motor to one terminal of the terminal strip. And run a third wire from the other terminal of the terminal strip to the positive terminal of the battery holder. (The connections do not have to be soldered, but they should be covered with insulating tape.) Insert the batteries in the battery holder. Simultaneously touch both screws in the terminal strip with the tip of a screwdriver. The pointer should rotate.

Attach the board to the easel using the ¼-20 machine screw and wing nut. The angle of the board can be increased (made closer to 90 degrees), if desired, by placing washers on the screw between the board and the easel.

If the unit is to be used for encoding, self-adhesive black vinyl numbers

FIGURE D.4. *Scanning Encoding Aid Number 1 — Front view.*

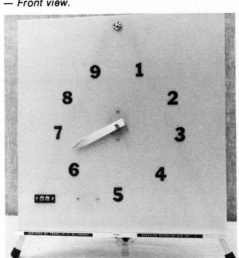

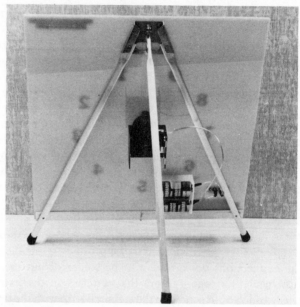

FIGURE D.5. *Scanning Encoding Aid Number 1
— Rear view.*

can be attached to the board, as in Figure D.4. Pictures can be attached to the board with tape that has adhesive on both sides.

Any switch can be attached to the terminal strip with spade tongue solderless terminals.

Scanning Encoding Aid Number 2

The Scanning Encoding Aid Number 2 (Figures D.6 and D.7) consists of a nine cell matrix display. Each cell contains a 1.5 volt miniature bulb. The bulbs are lit one after the other for approximately seven seconds in the following sequence:

1	2	3
4	5	6
7	8	9

After bulb number nine is turned off, the sequence begins again with bulb number one. Pictures or symbols can be attached to the 16¼" x 16¼" Plexiglass surface (the symbols in the illustration are Blissymbolics). The unit can be fabricated with hand tools and a soldering iron at a component cost of less than $50.00 (based on 1978 prices). It, of course, requires more skill to assemble than Scanning Encoding Aid Number 1.

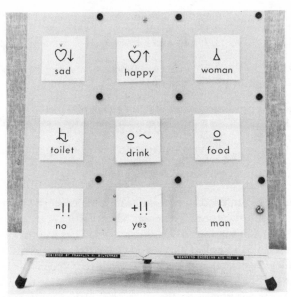

FIGURE D.6. *Scanning Encoding Aid Number 2 — Front view.*

Construction Details

The unit contains the following components:

Number	Description
1	⅛″ x 16¼″ x 16¼″ piece of opaque yellow Plexiglass plastic
1	aluminum table easel (Stanrite, No. 152)
1	1 rpm, 125 volt timing motor (International Register Company, WG-520-1)
1	setscrew collar for ⅛″ (motor) shaft (Perfect Parts Company landing gear wheel collar)
9	1.5 volt miniature bulbs with solder leads and rubber grommets to hold them in place (purchased from a Radio Shack franchise)
1	two-connector, female phone jack receptacle
1	battery holder for one size "D", 1.5 volt battery
1	1.5 volt, size "D" alkaline battery
1	3″ self-adhesive bus bar
1	9 terminal, solder-type, insulated terminal strip
1	1/16″ x 4″ x 10″ sheet of aluminum
1	2″ x 2″ circuit board
1	1/16″ x ¼″ x 1″ piece of brass (for contact rotor)
1	¾″ x 1″ x 16″ piece of wood
1	¼-20 x 1¼″ machine screw with wing nut and 12 washers

4	4-40 x ½″ machine screws and nuts
4	8-32 x 1″ machine screws and nuts
1	3/32″ diameter brass machine screw ½″ long with two brass nuts
1	3/32″ diameter compression spring ½″ long (uncompressed)
2	½″ number six wood screws
1	two-prong plug for standard outlet
15 ft.	two-conductor electrical wire (that can handle 125 volts)
50 ft.	insulated solid copper core hookup wire (that can handle 1.5 volts)
1 roll	electrical insulating tape

The unit is mounted on an aluminum table easel (which can be purchased at an art supply store). The easel has a vertical extension that is intended for supporting the tops of large canvases. The rivet that attaches it to the rest of the easel is removed and it and the extension piece are discarded. Two 3/16″ holes are drilled in the back of the ledge (which is at the bottom of the easel), one approximately two inches from each outside edge. The ¾″ x 1″ x 16″ piece of wood is placed on the ledge and pushed into contact with the back of it (so that its width is reduced by ¾″). It is held in place by the two No. 6 wood screws, but it shouldn't be attached to the easel now.

The Plexiglass board for the unit can be purchased *cut to size* at almost any store that sells plastic in sheets (see the "yellow" pages of your phone

FIGURE D.7. *Scanning Encoding Aid Number 2 — Rear view.*

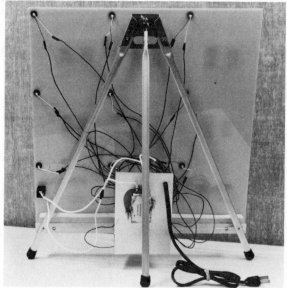

book). Both sides of the Plexiglass will be covered by sheets of protective paper. They should not be removed until all holes have been drilled. Begin by dividing the board into a 9-cell (3 x 3) matrix and draw lines defining the limits of the cells on the protective paper covering one side of the board. In the upper right-hand corner of each cell drill a hole large enough to accept the rubber grommet that holds the bulb in place (see Figure D.6). Then place the board on the easel and center it. Mark on the board the location of the center of the hole at the top of the easel (in which the rivet had been that attached the extension to the easel) and drill a ¼″ hole in the board at this point. (The ¼-20 x 1¼″ machine screw is passed through the board and easel to attach the board to the easel. The 12 washers are placed on the screw between the board and the easel to separate the two at the top.) Next, drill a ⅜″ hole for the female, two-connector phone jack receptacle on the right edge of the right-hand cell in the bottom row (see Figure D.6). Finally, drill two ⅛″ holes (one over the other) on the left edge of the middle cell in the bottom row for mounting the terminal strip and two ⅛″ holes (one over the other) on the right edge of the middle cell in the bottom row for mounting the battery holder. The edges of the board should be smoothed with sandpaper, and the corners should be rounded using a file. When these tasks have been completed, the protective paper should be removed (by pulling) from both sides of the Plexiglass and the rubber grommets (and bulbs), phone jack receptacle, terminal strip, and battery holder should be attached to the board. The 3″ self-adhesive bus bar should be attached to the rear of the board on the side of the battery holder opposite that of the terminal strip, parallel to both and approximately 2″ from the battery holder.

The next task is to construct the contact rotor assembly. The mount for this assembly is fabricated from the 4″ x 10″ sheet of aluminum (see Figure D.8). Six holes are drilled in it at the approximate locations indicated in Figure D.8. The two at the bottom in this figure (⅛″ diameter) are for attaching the mount to the rear of the easel ledge (the approximate location at which it attaches to the easel can be seen in Figure D.7). The three in the middle are for the motor: the one in the center (¼″ diameter) is for the motor shaft and the two on the sides (⅛″ diameter) are for attaching the motor to the mount (their exact location being determined by the particular motor used). And the hole at the top of the mount (¼″ diameter) is for the motor power cord (see Figure D.7). When the six holes have been drilled, two right-angle bends are made in the mount at the locations indicated in Figure D.8 by dashed lines (i.e., ¾″ and 3¾″ from the bottom). The finished mount will approximate a *J* shape, with the high part of the *J* in the back. The low (¾″) side of the *J* is centered on the rear of the easel ledge and the location of the two holes is marked on it. Two holes (⅛″ diameter) are drilled in the rear of the ledge at these points, and two 8-32 x 1″ machine screws are used to attach the mount to the rear of the easel ledge. The ¾″ x 1″ x 16″ piece of wood is now positioned on the easel ledge and attached to the rear of it by the two wood screws. (It

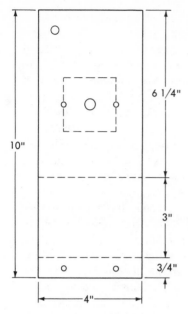

FIGURE D.8. *Mount for contact rotor assembly.*

may be necessary to cut indentations in the wood where the heads of the machine screws are located so that the wood will fit well against the rear of the ledge.) Finally, the motor is bolted to the bracket with the two 8-32 x 1″ machine screws.

The contact surface for the rotor is fabricated from a 2″ x 2″ circuit board. (A circuit board consists of a plastic insulating material that has a thin sheet of copper bonded to it.) First, mark the center of the board on the copper surface. Then, using a protractor, divide the board into nine equal segments (each would be 40 degrees) and mark the borders of each segment on the copper surface (see Figure D.9). Next, drill a ¼″ hole at the center of the board, and cut grooves through the copper coating with a triangular file at the locations marked so that the nine copper segments will be separated from each other. Finally, glue the circuit board to the mount (copper side up) at the position indicated by dotted lines in Figure D.8.

The contact rotor is fabricated from the 1/16″ x ¼″ x 1″ piece of brass. Its configuration can be seen in Figure D.10. A ⅛″ hole is drilled ¼″ from one end of it (through which it is attached to the motor shaft). A 3/32″ hole is drilled ¼″ from the other end, through which is attached the contact screw assembly. This consists of the 3/32″ diameter brass machine screw, the two nuts, and the compression spring. The machine screw is positioned so that its *head* would be in contact with the circuit board. The compression spring is placed on the machine screw so that it will be between the screw head and the hole in the contact rotor through which the screw fits. The end of the screw (with compression spring in place) is inserted in the 3/32″ hole in the contact

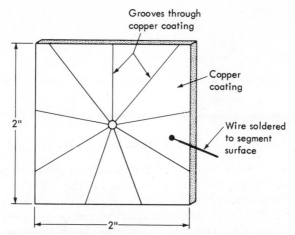

Grooves through
copy coating

Copper
coating

Wire soldered
to segment
surface

2"

2"

FIGURE D.9. *Circuit board contact surface for rotor. The hole at the center should be slightly larger in diameter than the motor shaft. The grooves in the copper coating can be cut with a triangular file.*

rotor, and the two nuts are attached to the end of the screw (see Figure D.10). These nuts are used for adjusting the length of the screw and, hence, the pressure of the screw on the contact surface. Finally, the contact rotor is slipped on to the motor shaft and held in place with the setscrew collar.

The unit should now be wired so that movement of the contact rotor will cause the lights to go on and off in the desired sequence. A schematic wiring diagram is presented in Figure D.11. The first step is to solder one end of a piece of hookup wire approximately 18″ long to the copper surface of each of the nine segments on the contact board at the locations indicated in Figure D.10. The other end of each of these wires is soldered to a terminal on the nine-terminal strip so that the segments are represented on this strip in the same order as on the contact surface. The second step is to solder one end of another piece of hookup wire approximately 18″ long to each of the terminals on the strip. The other end of each of these nine wires is soldered to one of the two leads attached to a bulb. The bulb to which each of these nine wires is soldered determines the sequence in which the bulbs will be turned on and off. The wire soldered to the terminal at the top of the strip should be soldered to a lead from the bulb in the upper left-hand cell of the matrix. That soldered to the terminal second from the top on the strip should be soldered to a lead from the bulb in the middle cell of the top row, etc. Finally, a piece of hookup wire should be soldered to each of the nine remaining bulb leads. The other ends of these pieces of wire should be soldered to the 3″ bus bar. All soldered connections to bulb leads should be covered with electrical insulating tape.

To connect the battery to the remainder of the system one end of a piece of hookup wire is soldered to the bus bar and the other end to the negative

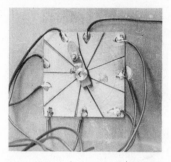

FIGURE D.10. *Contact rotor assembly.*

terminal of the battery holder. One end of another piece of hookup wire is soldered to the positive terminal of the battery holder. One inch of insulation is removed from the other end of this wire and loosely wound around the threads of one of the 8-32 machine screws that connects the motor mount to the easel. This provides an electrical connection to the contact rotor assembly. To turn the display off, the wire end is removed from the screw with which it is in contact. The battery can now be placed in the battery holder.

To wire the motor, one end of the 15 foot length of two-conductor electrical cord is inserted in the hole at the top of the motor mount. The insulation is removed from both wires at the end of the cord. A lead from the motor is

FIGURE D.11. *Schematic for Scanning-Encoding Aid Number 2. The contact rotor is turned by a 1 r.p.m. electric motor that can be started and stopped by any type of switching mechanism.*

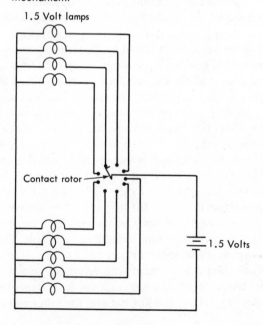

soldered to one of these wires. The other lead from the motor is soldered to one of the connectors on the phone jack receptacle, and the remaining wire from the cord is soldered to the other connector on this receptacle. A two-prong plug is attached to the other end of the electrical cord and the unit is plugged in. A switching mechanism is attached to the phone jack receptacle. When the switch is activated, the motor should turn the rotor and the bulbs should turn on and off in the desired sequence. Any switching mechanism containing a single switch that can handle 125 volts should be usable for controlling this display.

Nine symbols (that are smaller than a cell) can be attached to the Plexiglass with tape that has adhesive on both sides.

Lever Microswitch Switching Mechanism

This device can be used to control any electrical display that can be operated by a single switch. It will function in either a normally open or normally closed mode (i.e., pressure applied to the lever can be used either to start or stop an electrical device such as a motor), and it can be activated by a very light pressure. If positioned appropriately in space, it can be activated by a movement (or gesture) of almost any body part. The device consists of (1) a lever microswitch (which in 1978 cost less than $2.00), (2) a mount for positioning it in space, (3) an electrical cable for interfacing it with the control electronics or display of the communication system, and (4) a pressure surface attached to the lever.

A lever microswitch switching mechanism is illustrated in Figure D.12. The base consists of a small piece of Plexiglass plastic (plywood would work as well) to which has been glued a piece of Sculpey (a clay material that can be hardened by baking) molded to position the switch on the Plexiglass base. (If you use a material like Sculpey, *don't* place the switch in the oven when you bake it.) Black plastic electrical tape is wound around the end of the lever to serve as a pressure surface. The electrical cable attaches to the microswitch through an opening molded into the Sculpey. Spade tongue solderless terminals are attached to the two wires at the end of the cable (which would permit the device to be used to control the Scanning-Encoding Aid Number 1 described in this appendix and the Code Oscillator Alerting Device described in Chapter 5).

Etran Charts

These devices, which are used for encoding messages with an eye-pointing response mode (see Chapter 5), can be fabricated from a sheet of clear, transparent ¼ inch Plexiglass plastic 15 inches by 20 inches. (The sheet can be

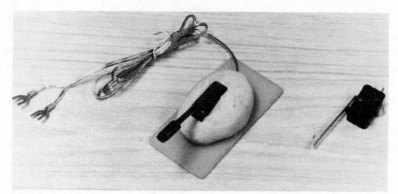

FIGURE D.12. *Lever microswitches, mounted (A) and unmounted (B).*

purchased cut to this size from a store that sells Plexiglass plastic.) There will be a sheet of protective paper attached to each side of the Plexiglass. They should not be removed before the chart has been fabricated.

A rectangular opening has to be cut in the center of the Plexiglass sheet (see Figure D.13). The outline of the opening is drawn using a ruler on the paper protecting one side of the sheet. A ¼-inch hole is then drilled in each corner of the outline of the opening. (The saw blade is inserted in these holes

FIGURE D.13. *Construction details for ETRAN Charts.*

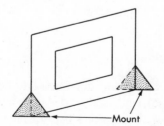

Mount

when the opening is being cut out.) A coping saw (or an electric saber saw if one is available) is used to cut the opening. The saw blade is inserted in one of the holes and a straight cut is made along a line drawn on the paper (thereby connecting that hole with another hole). This process is repeated until all four sides of the opening have been cut. The edges of the opening are smoothed and straightened with sandpaper and, if necessary, a file. The outside edges of the chart also should be smoothed, and the outside corners should be rounded using a file. When these tasks have been completed, the protective paper can be removed (by pulling) from both sides of the Plexiglass.

The next step is applying the symbols to the chart. Self-adhesive black vinyl letters and numbers one inch in height can be used for this purpose. For the ETRAN Chart they are arranged as in Figure 5.14, and for the ETRAN-N Chart they are arranged as in Figure 5.15.

The final step is fabricating a mount for the chart so that it can be positioned vertically. The piece of Plexiglass that was removed from the center of the chart can be used for this purpose. Two triangular-shaped pieces are cut from it, and one is glued at the bottom of each end of the chart perpendicular to it (see Figure D.13).

Radio Control Device for Interfacing Switching Mechanisms with Displays

It sometimes is not possible or desirable to directly connect a switching mechanism to a display through the use of a cable. The two can be interfaced in such cases by means of a miniature radio transmitter and receiver. The switching mechanism can be used to activate a small radio transmitter which sends a signal to a receiver that can activate a relay (see Chapter 6). When the relay is activated by a radio signal, it functions like a switch and activates the display with which it is interfaced.

A relatively inexpensive (less than $75.00 in 1978) radio control device which can be used for activating displays that can be controlled by a single switch can be fabricated from the transmitter and receiver of an automatic garage door opener (see Figure D.14). The transmitter and receiver can be separated by at least 50 feet. No FCC license is required to operate the device. Though the transmitter is intended to be battery-operated it can easily be adapted to a "plug in" power source by means of the type of step-down transformer designed for pocket electronic calculators that outputs the appropriate voltage.

The built-in push switch can be used to activate the transmitter or an input phone jack can be connected internally to the switch terminals so that any type of switching mechanism containing a single switch can be used to activate it. (Any electrical technician should be able to modify the transmitter in this way.) Suction cups can be attached to the bottom of the transmitter so that it can be anchored in a desired location.

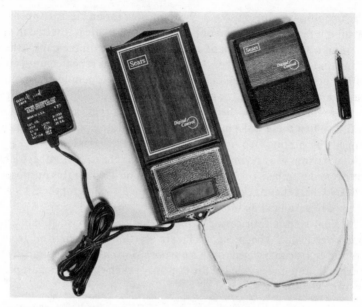

FIGURE D.14. *Radio control device for interfacing switching mechanisms with displays. The receiver is on the right and the transmitter is on the left.*

The receiver uses a 110-volt A.C. power source. One end of a two-wire cable is attached to the relay output screws on the receiver (see Figure D.14). The same type of connector is attached to the other end as would be on a switching mechanism that was compatible with the unit. This connector is plugged into the input terminal on the display intended for the switching mechanism. (Thus, the receiver is interfaced with the display unit in the same manner as a switching mechanism.)

This type of radio control device can be used with some switching mechanisms that contain more than one switch by using several transmitter-receiver combinations that operate on *different* frequencies. (The transmitter and receiver units in Figure D.14 can be adjusted internally to operate on more than 1,000 different frequencies.) One transmitter-receiver combination would be necessary for each switch in a switching mechanism.

Another approach for multiple switch, switching mechanisms would be to use the type of radio control device intended for model airplanes. These devices come with different numbers of channels. The number of channels needed would be equal to the number of switches in a switching mechanism. While both the transmitter and receiver units of such devices are more compact than multiple garage door ones, they tend to be more expensive than the latter and require an FCC license to operate. These units can be purchased at hobby shops that sell airplane models.

Device for Determining Optimal Positioning In Space for Communication Boards And Switching Mechanisms

This device will position communication boards and switching mechanisms at desired coordinates (locations) in space. It is intended to be used by a clinician when he or she is attempting to identify the most advantageous (optimal) location for a client's communication board or switching mechanism. Once this location has been determined, a permanent mount can be designed and fabricated for it. The device is made up of the following components (see Figure D.15):

1. a sturdy photographer's elevator tripod (adequate ones cost about $75.00 in 1978);
2. an aluminum bar ½″ x ½″ x 36″, at one end of which a hole has been drilled and tapped with a ¼-20 thread;
3. a c-clamp device (with a tilt head attached) designed to support a camera (which can be purchased at most large camera shops); and
4. an aluminum bar ½″ x ½″ x 18″, at the center of which a hole has been drilled and tapped with a ¼-20 thread and to each end of which a spring clamp has been bolted.

FIGURE D.15. *Device for determining optimal positioning in space for communication boards and switching mechanisms.*

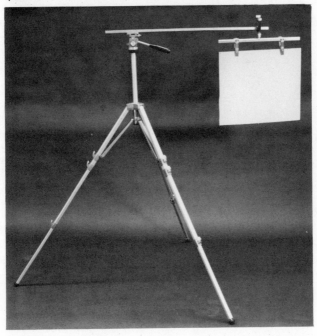

The manner in which the components are assembled is illustrated in Figure D.15. The unit can be disassembled for compact storage.

To use the unit a switching mechanism or communication board is attached to it by one or both spring clamps. The tripod is positioned so that the switching mechanism or board is *roughly* located at a point in space at which the clinician wishes to determine whether the client can use it. Exact positioning can be achieved by manipulating the adjustment controls on the tripod, the location of the C-clamp device on the bar, and the angle of the bar to which the spring clamps are attached.

Once the optimal location for a communication board or switching mechanism has been determined, it should be recorded (described) in some manner. A Polaroid photograph of the board or switching mechanism positioned appropriately in space may be helpful for this purpose.

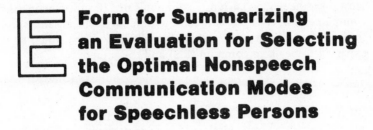

Form for Summarizing an Evaluation for Selecting the Optimal Nonspeech Communication Modes for Speechless Persons

Name _____ Sex _____ Age _____
                                                       Years   Months

Date_____ Examiner_____

Institution _____

    Address_____

    Telephone_____

    Patient's Speech Clinician _____

Condition(s) which Appear to Have Caused the Communicative Disorder

_____

_____

_____

Remarks:

Communication Status

1. How does the person currently communicate? Has the person's mode of communication changed between the time he or she became speechless (or if the person is a child, the time at which he or she would have been expected to begin to communicate) and the present?

2. What are the person's communication needs? How well does the person's current mode for transmission of messages appear to meet his or her communication needs?

3. How well does the person understand speech? Nonverbal gestural communication?

4. How well is the person able to read? Write?

5. Does the person have an intelligible, reliable method for signaling "yes" and "no"? How?

6. What messages is the person able to communicate:

    a) by speech?

    b) by gesture?

    c) by writing?

7. How "intelligible" do these messages appear to be to persons with whom he communicates:

a) by speech?

b) by gesture?

c) by writing?

8. How frequently does the person attempt to communicate:

   a) by speech?

   b) by gesture?

   c) by writing?

9. If the person is a child, how appropriate is his or her receptive-expressive communication ability developmentally?

10. How appropriate developmentally does "inner language" functioning appear to be (both verbal and nonverbal)?

Motor Status

1. Does the person have a neuromuscular disorder or an apraxia? (IF THE ANSWER TO THIS QUESTION IS NO, THERE ISN'T ANY NEED TO FURTHER EVALUATE MOTOR FUNCTIONING. IF THE ANSWER IS YES, PROCEED TO THE SECOND QUESTION.)

2. Is the motor functioning of the upper extremities adequate for:

   a) manual sign language?

   b) writing?

   c) use of a conventional typewriter?

(IF THE ANSWER TO THIS QUESTION IS YES, THERE IS NO NEED TO FURTHER EVALUATE MOTOR FUNCTIONING. IF THE ANSWER IS NO, PROCEED TO THE THIRD QUESTION.)

3. Is the motor functioning of the upper extremities adequate to reliably:

   a) indicate message components on a communication board? How?

   b) activate an electronic switching mechanism? How? What kind?

(IF THE ANSWER TO THIS QUESTION IS YES, THERE IS NO NEED TO FURTHER EVALUATE MOTOR FUNCTIONING. IF THE ANSWER IS NO, PROCEED TO THE FOURTH QUESTION.)

4. Is the motor functioning of the musculature of the face, head, and neck adequately reliable for:

   a) gestural communication?

   b) indicating message components on a communication board? How?

   c) activating an electronic switching mechanism? How? What kind?

(IF THE ANSWER TO THIS QUESTION IS YES, THERE IS NO NEED TO FURTHER EVALUATE MOTOR FUNCTIONING. IF THE ANSWER IS NO, PROCEED TO THE FIFTH QUESTION.)

5. Is the functioning of the musculature of the lower extremities or trunk adequate to reliably:

    a) indicate message components on a communication board? How?

    b) activate an electronic switching mechanism? How? What kind?

(IF THE ANSWER TO THIS QUESTION IS YES, THERE IS NO NEED TO FURTHER EVALUATE MOTOR FUNCTIONING. IF THE ANSWER IS NO, PROCEED TO THE SIXTH QUESTION.)

6. Is the functioning of any of the person's musculature adequate to reliably control a myoswitch? Which musculature?

Sensory Status

I. AUDITION

1. Does the person have a hearing loss?____If he or she has a hearing loss, how much does it interfere with speech comprehension?

2. Does the person have auditory agnosia or any other auditory perceptual or memory problem?____If he or she has such a problem, what is it and how much does it interfere with speech comprehension?

3. Does the person evince receptive aphasia?____If he or she does evince this condition, how much does it interfere with speech comprehension?

II. VISION

1. Does the person have a loss of visual acuity or a visual field problem? ___If he or she has such a problem, what is it and how much would it probably interfere with:

   a) reading?

   b) typing?

   c) indicating message components on a communication board?

   d) activating an electronic switching mechanism?

2. Does the person have visual agnosia or any other visual perceptual or memory problem?___If he or she has such a problem, what is it and how much would it probably interfere with:

   a) reading?

   b) typing?

   c) indicating message components on a communication board?

   d) activating an electronic switching mechanism?

3. Does the person evince dyslexia?___If the person does evince this condition, how much does it interfere with reading?

III. TACTILE-KINESTHETIC-PROPRIOCEPTIVE STIMULATION

1. Does the person evince any disturbance in the use of tactile, kinesthetic, or proprioceptive stimulation?___If he or she does evince such a disturbance, what is it and how much does it interfere with:

   a) manual signing?

   b) writing?

   c) typing?

   d) indicating message components on a communication board?

   e) activating electronic switching mechanisms?

Cognitive Status

1. Does the person evince mental retardation, arteriosclerosis, or any other condition that can impede cognitive functioning?___If he or she does evince such a condition, what is it and how much is is likely to interfere with:

   a) improving speech comprehension?

   b) comprehension of gestural communication?

   c) comprehension of printed or written message components?

d) improving speech?

e) improving typing or learning to type?

f) learning to use manual sign language?

g) learning to indicate message components on a communication board?

h) learning to activate an electronic switching mechanism?

i) improving writing?

Subject Index

Abstract-concrete imbalance, 88
Agglutination, 68, 71, 98
Alphaswitches, 170
American Guidance Service, 103, 104, 105, 250
American Indian Sign Language (*see* Gestural communication modes)
American Manual Alphabet, 64, 74
American Sign Language (*see* Gestural communication modes)
Amerind (*see* American Indian Sign Language)
Amerind Video Dictionary, 70, 71, 72, 224, 251
Ameslan (*see* American Sign Language)
Amyotrophic lateral sclerosis, 5, 34
Annotated Bibliography of Communication Aids, 140
Aphasia, 7–8, 14, 29, 32, 33, 37, 40, 41, 56, 60, 70, 72, 74, 76, 79, 82, 102, 107, 126, 202, 203, 212, 223
Apraxia, 6–7, 29, 33, 34, 35, 37, 40, 43, 47, 56, 60, 70, 111, 182, 183, 212, 223
Attention span, 42, 46
Attentiveness, 42, 43
Auditory agnosia, 202
Auditory functioning, 36, 199, 202
Autism, 10–11, 29, 32, 33, 35, 38, 40, 41, 42, 43, 44, 60, 66, 107, 126, 212, 223, 250
Auto-Com communication board, 32, 34, 35, 42, 43, 44, 135, 137, 154

Batteries, types of, 155
Bell Telephone Laboratories, 141, 252
Bioelectrical signals (*see* Muscle action potentials; Neuro-assisted communication modes)

Biofeedback techniques, 163, 166, 170 (*see also* Neuro-assisted communication modes)
Bizarre behaviors, 43
Blissymbolics (*see* Symbol systems for communication boards and electronic displays)
Blissymbolics Communication Institute, 94, 95, 100, 126, 250, 252
Book-page turner, 220
Braille (*see* Symbol systems for communication boards and electronic displays)
Brain waves, 163, 170 (*see also* Neuro-assisted communication modes)
Bulbar palsy, 5

Cerebellar ataxia, 5
Cerebral arteriosclerosis, 31, 204
Cerebral palsy, 5, 32, 33, 34, 35, 40, 41, 42, 43, 44, 72, 126
Chimpanzee, 107, 214
Chorea, 5
Classroom performance, 46
Cleo Living Aids, 252
Code oscillator alerting device, 140, 141
Com-Code device, 141, 152
Comhandi electronic communication system, 32
Communication:
   awareness of nature of, 212–215
   impact of nonvocal communication systems on, 30–39
Communication boards, 6, 7, 8, 11, 13, 14, 20, 30, 32, 33, 34, 35, 36, 38, 41, 47, 58, 60, 82, 94, 101, 102, 105, 111, 113–126, 189, 199, 202, 203, 215, 216, 219, 232–249, 251, 252–253

Communication boards *(cont.)*
  code oscillator alerting device for use with,
      140, 141
  examples, 88, 89, 93, 94, 114, 115, 116,
      119, 124
  factors to consider when designing, 114–
      118
  preparing instructions for using, 124–125
  strategies for indicating message compo-
      nents on, 118–124
Communication mode, selecting optimum, 12,
      13, 14
Communication orientation *(see* Speech
      pathologists)
Communication Outlook, 253
Communication potential, factors effecting:
  attitudes toward the communication mode(s)
      used, 31, 39
  cognitive status, 31
  communication mode(s) used, 31, 38–39
  desire or motivation to communicate, 31,
      37–38
  "inner" language status, 31, 37
  motor status, 31, 36
  receptive language status, 31, 37
  sensory status, 31, 36
"Communication prosthesis," 217
Computers, 156–157 *(see also* Electronic
      communication systems)
Control electronics *(see* Electronic communi-
      cation systems)
Conversation boards *(see* Communication
      boards)
Counseling clients and their families, 15, 71,
      208–210
CRT (cathode-ray tube) displays *(see* Elec-
      tronic communication systems)
Cued Speech, 64 *(see also* American Sign
      Language)

Deafness, 11, 66, 67, 181
Depression and communication, 37
Direct-selection response mode, 123–124,
      189, 199, 215
Displays *(see* Electronic communication sys-
      tems)
Disruptive behavior, 43
Drawings as symbols *(see* Symbol systems for
      communication boards and electronic
      displays)
Drawn (or written) symbols, 113, 127
Dysarthria, 4–6, 29, 32, 33, 35, 37, 60, 66, 70,
      100, 111, 212, 223
Dyslexia, 87, 113, 202, 215
Dysphonia, 8–9, 29, 32, 35, 37, 70, 212, 223

Edison Responsive Environment, 33, 40
Educational progress, 43
Electronic communication systems, 6, 7, 8,
      15, 32, 47, 127–157, 219, 220, 232–
      249, 252–253, 254–270
  construction details for components of,
      254–270
  control electronics, 59–60, 153–157
    computers, applications in, 3–4, 60, 145,
        151, 153, 154, 156–157
    functions of, 153–157
    interfacing switching mechanisms and
        displays, 154–155
    preventing switching mechanisms from
        being activated accidentally, 157
    supplying electrical power, 155
  displays, 58, 59, 101, 140–153, 175
    CRT (cathode-ray tube) displays, 140,
        144–145, 148, 149, 152, 154, 156,
        163, 168, 169, 216
    factors to consider when selecting, 152–
        153
    LCDs (liquid-crystal displays), 146, 152,
        163
    LED (light-emitting diode) displays,
        145–147, 152
    noise, light, or vibration generators,
        140–141, 152
    rectangular matrix displays, 142–144,
        149, 152, 163, 180, 215, 216, 258–
        265
    rotary scanning displays, 120, 121, 139,
        141, 152, 163, 180, 254–258
    speech generators (synthesizers), 3–4,
        111, 150–152, 156, 163
    strip printers, 144, 146–148, 152, 156,
        163, 168, 169, 216
    teletypewriters, 144, 148, 151, 152, 156,
        163, 168, 169, 170, 216
    typewriters, 59, 60, 112, 131, 144,
        148–149, 152, 163, 168, 216, 253
  switching mechanisms, 20, 36, 38, 59, 60,
        128–139, 175, 189–201, 203
    alphaswitches, 170
    factors to consider when selecting, 139
    foot trolleys, 132, 134
    functions of, 128–129
    joysticks, 132–133, 136, 144
    light-controlled (photoelectric) switches,
        59, 138–139
    magnetic proximity switches, 59
    microswitches, 59, 129–130, 141, 265,
        266
    myoswitches, 4, 165–169, 182, 199,
        249, 253
    paddles, 132, 133
    pillows, pads, and squeeze bulbs, 133
    pneumatic switches, 133, 135, 137, 139

Electronic communication systems *(cont.)*
  switching mechanisms *(cont.)*
    position (tilt) switches, 128, 130, 134,
      135, 136
    proximity switches, 134–135, 137
    push buttons, 130–131, 139
    push-plates, 130–131
    push switches, 129–134
    see-saw rocking lever, 132
    sliding handles, 132, 133
    sound-controlled (voice-activated)
      switches, 138, 139, 254–256
    touch switches, 137–138
    wobblesticks, 132, 134, 135
Encoding response mode, 120–123, 199 *(see
  also* ETRAN chart; ETRAN-N chart;
  Morse code)
Engineers, 12, 17, 19–20
English *(see* Symbol systems for communication boards and electronic displays)
ETRAN chart, 34, 115, 116, 117, 120–123,
  199, 265–267
  directions for fabricating, 265–267
  instructions for using, 122–123
ETRAN-N chart, 116, 117, 120, 121, 199,
  265–267
Expressive language, 175, 181–182
Eyepointing, 117, 120, 121, 122–123, 199
  (see also ETRAN chart; ETRAN-N
  chart)

Fingerspelling *(see* Gestural communication
  modes, American Sign Language)
Foot trolleys *(see* Electronic communication
  systems)
Frustration behavior, 42
Funding *(see* Intervention considerations)

Gallaudet College Bookstore, 67, 250
General semantics, 100
Gestural communication modes, 55–58,
  63–84, 212, 223–232
  criteria for evaluating, 63
  eye-blink encoding, 79–80, 82
  gestural Morse code, 6, 80–81, 82
  gestures for "yes" and "no", 77, 79, 82
  manual sign languages, 6, 7, 9, 10, 33, 40,
    63–79, 189, 203
    American Indian (Amerind) Sign, 33, 35,
      36, 38, 39, 40, 41, 42, 67–72, 73, 82,
      177, 181, 182, 184, 189, 251
    American Sign Language, 4, 11, 32, 33,
      34, 35, 36, 37, 40, 41, 42, 43, 44, 47,
      57, 63–67, 72, 73, 82, 102, 177, 181,
      182, 184, 250, 251

Gestural communication modes *(cont.)*
  American Sign Language *(cont.)*
    Hand Talking Chart, 76–78, 82
    Manual Self-Care Signals, 76, 77, 82
    Manual Shorthand, 74–76, 82
    Left-Hand Manual Alphabet, 74–76, 82
  pantomime (mime), 7, 8, 34, 35, 40, 41,
    42, 43, 56, 57, 67, 72–74, 82, 177,
    181
  pointing, 81, 82
  which system to use, 81–82
Gestural-assisted communication modes, 55,
  58–60, 85–161, 181, 232–249 *(see
  also* Communication boards; Electronic communication systems; Manipulatable symbols)
  criteria used for evaluating, 85–86
Ghora-Khan Grotto, 253
Glossectomy, 8, 9, 14, 29, 35, 37, 70, 111,
  212

H & H Enterprises, 251, 253
Handivoice speech synthesizers, 150–152
Hand Talking Chart (see Gestural communica-
  tion modes)
Hardware and software components of
  nonspeech communication systems,
  12, 13
HC Electronics, 253
Headpointer, 20, 123, 124, 149, 199
Headstick *(see* Headpointer)
Hearing loss, 202
Hemiplegia, 127
Homonymous hemianopsia, 202
Huntington's Chorea, 31, 204
Hyperactivity, 42, 46

IBM, 253
Ideas, Inc., 253
Ideographic symbols, 68, 95, 105 *(see also*
  American Indian Sign; Blissymbolics;
  Rebuses; LANA Lexigrams)
Illinois Test of Psycholinguistic Abilities, 182
Independence, 46
Indexing *(see* General semantics)
Inner language, 175, 180
Interstate Printers and Publishers, 253
Intervention considerations, 207–220
  assessing the impact of programs on users,
    118–119
  funding communication system compo-
    nents, 216–217
  gaining acceptance for nonvocal communi-
    cation from users and others, 208–210

Intervention considerations *(cont.)*
  gaining administrative support for
    nonspeech intervention programs, 217
  generating motivation for communication,
    210–212
  increasing awareness of the nature of com-
    munication, 212–215
  periodically reassessing communication
    needs, 215–216
  preventive maintenance for system compo-
    nents, 219
  training family members and others to inter-
    pret messages, 217–218
  utilizing electronic systems for environmen-
    tal control, 220
International languages:
  American Indian Sign as, 67–68
  Blissymbolics as, 95

Joysticks *(see* Electronic communication sys-
    tems)

Keyguard for typewriter, 131, 148–149
Kiwanis Club, 216

LANA Lexigrams *(see* Symbol systems for
    communication boards and electronic
    displays)
Laryngectomy *(see* Dysphonia)
LCDs (liquid-crystal displays) *(see* Electronic
    communication systems)
LED (light-emitting diode) displays *(see* Elec-
    tronic communication systems)
Leiter International Performance Scale, 204
Lever microswitch switching mechanism, con-
    struction details for, 265, 266
Light code-generator displays *(see* Electronic
    communication systems)
Light-controlled switches *(see* Electronic
    communication systems)
Linguistic units encoded, 58, 64, 69, 91, 95,
    98, 101, 102, 104, 105–106, 111, 151
Litigation, 176

Magnetic reed switch *(see* Proximity switches)
Manipulatable symbols 8, 10, 33, 41, 107–
    109, 113, 126–127 *(see also* Non-SLIP
    Program)
Manual alphabet for left hand *(see* Gestural
    communication modes)
Manual Self-Care Signals (see Gestural com-
    munication modes)

Manual Shorthand (see Gestural communica-
    tion modes)
Manual sign languages *(see* Gestural com-
    munication modes)
Master Chart of Communication Aids, 85
Medicaid, 216
Medicare, 216
MELDS Program, 102
Mental retardation, 9–10, 29, 31, 32, 33, 34,
    35, 37, 38, 40, 41, 42, 43, 47, 56, 60,
    66, 72, 82, 100, 102, 105, 107, 109,
    113, 126, 204, 212, 214, 223, 251
Michael Reese Medical Center, 250
Microswitches *(see* Electronic communication
    systems, switching mechanisms)
Mime *(see* Gestural communication modes)
Morse Code, 6, 38, 60 *(see also* Gestural
    communication modes; Symbol sys-
    tems for communication boards and
    electronic displays)
  oscillator for, 33, 43
Motivation, 207, 210–212
Motor functioning, assessing *(see* Selecting a
    mode)
Mouth-held writing device, 33, 127
Mouthstick, 148, 149, 199
Mr. Symbol Man, 100
Muscle action potentials, 55, 163–169 *(see
    also* Myoswitches; Neuro-assisted
    communication modes)
Muscle gestures, 58, 59, 182–201
Muscle Testing, 184, 185, 188, 189
Myocom communication device, 35
Myoswitches *(see* Electronic communication
    systems)

National Easter Seal Society, 216
Neuro-assisted communication modes, 55,
    60–61, 162–171, 181, 249 *(see also*
    Electronic communication systems)
  limitations of, 162
  use of brain wave patterns for controlling,
    170
  use of muscle action potentials for control-
    ling, 163–169
Neuromuscular disorders, 56, 102, 157, 182,
    183 *(see also* Cerebral palsy; Dysar-
    thria)
"No" signal *(see* Gestural communication
    modes)
Noise code-generator displays *(see* Electronic
    communication systems)
Nonelectronic gestural-assisted communica-
    tion systems *(see* Communication
    boards; Manipulatable symbols)
Non-SLIP Program, 41, 108, 109, 113, 251
    (see also Manipulatable symbols)

Nonspeech communication modes:
  acceptance by users and others, 46
  classification, 55-62
  conditions necessitating the use of, 4–11
  definition of, 3
  for communicating basic needs in hospitals
    and nursing homes, 74–77
  goals for intervention with, 179
  impact on communication, 30–39
  impacts on overall behavior, 42–46
  impact on speech, 39–41, 45
  intervention considerations for, 207–220
  investment required, 46–47
  long-term impact, 47
  need for, 3–28
  questions for assessing impacts of, 29–30
Nurse call systems, 220
Nurses, 12, 19–20
Nursing homes, 74–77, 179

Objective attitude, developing, 209–210
Occupational therapists, 12, 17, 19–20, 124,
    127, 177
Ontario Crippled Children's Centre, 100, 101

Paddles (*see* Electronic communication sys-
    tems)
Pads (*see* Electronic communication systems)
Pantomine (*see* Gestural communication
    modes)
Parkinsonism, 5
Parson's Language Sample, 182
Peabody Picture Vocabulary Test, 91, 180
Photo-electric switches (*see* Light-controlled
    switches)
Photographs as symbols (*see* Symbol systems
    for communciation boards and elec-
    tronic displays)
Physical therapists, 12, 19–20, 177
Pictographic symbols, 68, 86, 95, 99, 102,
    105 (*see also* American Indian Sign;
    Blissymbolics; Rebuses)
Pillows (*see* Electronic communication sys-
    tems)
Pneumatic switches (*see* Electronic communi-
    cation systems)
Porch Index of Communicative Ability, 182
Position switches (*see* Electronic communica-
    tion systems)
Positioning device for communication boards
    and switching mechanisms, 269–270
P.O.S.M. controlled typewriter, 34
Possum typewriter, 34
Premack-type plastic word symbols (*see* Sym-
    bol systems for communication boards
    and electronic displays)
Prentke Romich Company, 253

Proximity switches (*see* Electronic communci-
    ation systems)
Pseudobulbar palsy, 5
Public Law 94-142, 216
Push-buttons (*see* Electronic communication
    systems)
Push-plates (*see* Electronic communication
    systems)
Push switches (*see* Electronic communication
    systems)

Quadriplegia, 82, 113, 123, 124, 127

Radio control of displays, 154–155, 267–268
Reading, teaching of, 102
Rebuses (*see* Symbol systems for communica-
    tion systems and electronic displays)
Receptive language, 175, 178, 180–181
Rectangular scanning displays (*see* Electronic
    communication systems)
Redundancy in communication, role of, 66
Relays, 167
Rotary scanning displays (*see* Electronic
    communication systems)

Scanning Encoding Aid Number 1, 254–258
Scanning Encoding Aid Number 2, 258–265
Scanning response mode, 118–120, 142–144,
    215
  directed approach, 142, 143–144
  linear approach, 142, 143
  row-column approach, 142, 143
See-saw rocking lever (*see* Electronic com-
    munication systems)
Selecting a mode (or modes), 175–206
  assessing cognitive functioning, 182, 204
  assessing communication needs, 179
  assessing expressive language status, 181–
    182
  assessing inner language status, 180
  assessing motor functioning, 182–201
  gestures involving the face and neck,
    188, 196–198
  gestures involving the trunk and lower ex-
    tremities, 189, 200–201
  gestures involving the upper extremities,
    185–188, 190–195
  implications of motor functioning data,
    189–201
  switching mechanisms that can be acti-
    vated by particular gestures, 189–201
  assessing receptive language status, 180–
    181
  assessing sensory functioning, 182, 199,
    202–203
  audition, 202
  tactile-kinesthetic-proprioceptive func-

Selecting a mode (or modes) *(cont.)*
  assessing sensory functioning *(cont.)*
    tioning, 203
    vision, 202–203
  cost considerations, 175
  determining which it would be possible for a person to use, 182–204
  form for summarizing evaluation data, 271–278
  impact of cause of communicative disorder on, 176–177
  impact of cognitive functioning on, 176, 177, 216
  impact of emotional status on, 177, 178, 179
  impact of how person communicates on, 177–179
  impact of motor functioning on, 176, 177, 216
  impact of sensory functioning on, 176, 177, 216
  questions to be answered, 175
  selection criteria, 204–205
  worksheet for identifying optimal system or systems, 203, 204–205
Self-confidence, 42, 43, 46
Semantography *(see* Blissymbols)
Sensory functioning *(see* Selecting a mode)
Sertoma International, 216
Sign markers providing morphological and syntactic information, 65 *(see also* Signed English)
Signal detection, amplification, and shaping mechanism *(see* Neuro-assisted communication modes)
Signed English, 64–67 *(see also* American Sign Language)
Signs as symbols, 86
Sip and puff switch *(see* Pneumatic switches)
Sliding handles *(see* Electronic communication systems)
Slip-n-Slide communication board, 127
Social interaction, 42
Software *(see* Hardware and software components of nonspeech communication systems)
Solenoids:
  for activating typewriter keys, 149
  for use in myoswitches, 167
Sound-controlled switches *(see* Electronic communication systems)
Speech generators (synthesizers) *(see* Electronic communication systems)
Speech level, 39–41, 45, 177, 181, 209
Speech, machine generated *(see* Symbol systems for communication boards and electronic displays)

Speech orientation *(see* Speech pathologists)
Speech pathologists:
  communication vs. speech orientation for, 12, 15–19
  functioning as a team member, 19–20
  professional responsibilities to the communicatively handicapped, 12–15
  role in the habilitation and rehabilitation of the speechless, 11–20
Squeeze bulbs *(see* Electronic communication systems)
St. Louis Veteran's Administration Hospital, 69, 70, 71, 251
Strip printers *(see* Electronic communication systems)
Stroke, 5, 100
Suck and blow switch *(see* Pneumatic switch)
Surface electrodes, 164–165 *(see also* Neuro-assisted communication modes)
Switching mechanisms *(see* Electronic communication systems)
Symbol systems for communication boards and electronic displays, 85–113, 215
  attributes of symbols, 86
  Blissymbolics, 6, 10, 14, 34, 35, 38, 41, 43, 47, 86, 92, 94, 95–102, 105, 112, 113, 127, 180, 199, 204, 212, 215, 250
    main basic Blissymbol elements, 96
    materials for teaching, 101, 250
    representative Blissymbol communication board, 94
    strategies for vocabulary expansion, 97–100
  Braille, 86, 108, 109–111, 113, 117, 127, 142, 202
    Braille characters, 111
  criteria used for evaluating, 86–87
  criteria for selecting, 112–113
  English (or another natural language), 86, 87, 90, 91, 92–95, 98, 101, 104, 105, 107, 108, 109, 110, 111, 112, 113, 122, 127, 181, 204, 212
  machine-generated speech, 86, 111–112
  Morse Code, 80, 86, 112, 113, 131, 139, 140, 142, 145, 151, 152, 153, 156, 168, 169, 170, 178
  photographs and drawings, 38, 86, 87–92, 112, 113, 204, 212
    degree of ambiguity, 90
    degree of complexity, 89–90
    level of abstraction, 87–89
    set size, 90
    suggestions for picture symbols, 91–92
  Premack-type plastic word symbols, 86, 107–109, 113, 126, 142, 212
    Non-SLIP Program, 108, 109, 212–214

Symbol systems for communication boards
and electronic displays *(cont.)*
Premack-type plastic word symbols *(cont.)*
representative shapes, 109
rebuses, 86, 102–105, 113, 250
dictionary-like compilations of, 103, 105
morphological variations, 102, 104
representative examples, 103
Yerkish Language (LANA Lexigrams), 86,
105–107, 113
design elements, 106

Tactile-kinesthetic-proprioceptive function-
ing, 36, 199, 202, 203
Tactile symbols *(see* Braille; Premack-type
plastic word symbols)
"Talking Broach" communication aid, 140,
146, 147
"Talking Hand" system, 74–76
Teachers, classroom, 12, 19–20
Telephone communication, 111–112, 113,
151, 152, 179
Telephone dialer, 220
Telephone Pioneers of America, 216, 253
Teletypewriters *(see* Electronic communica-
tion systems)
Television sets, 220
Temper tantrums, 42, 45–46
Thermostat, 220
Tilt switches *(see* Position switches)
Total communication, 11, 32, 33, 34, 40, 41,
42, 43, 56, 66
Touch switches *(see* Electronic communica-
tion systems)

Trace Research and Development Center for
the Severely Communicatively Handicapped, 85, 126, 140, 251, 253
"Twenty questions", 77
Typewriters *(see* Electronic communication
systems)
Typing ability, 178, 203

United Cerebral Palsy, 216

Verbal output *(see* Speech level)
Vibration code-generator displays *(see* Elec-
tronic communication systems)
Visual agnosia, 202
Visual functioning, 36, 109–111, 199
Vocational Rehabilitation Commission, 216
Voice switches, 254 *(see also* Sound-
controlled switches)

Wheelchair mounting for communication
board, 116
Wobblesticks *(see* Electronic communication
systems)
Writing, 127, 177–178, 179, 182, 203

Yerkes Regional Research Center, 105
Yerkish Language *(see* Symbol systems for
communication boards and electronic
displays)
"Yes" signal *(see* Gestural communication
modes)

Zygo Industries, 253

Author Index

Abelson, C., 232
Abrams, P., 223
Adams, M. R., 6, 21, 79, 80, 82, 232
Allen, J. B., 232
Anderson, K., 224, 232
Andrews, L. M., 166, 170, 171
Anthony, G. M., 6, 22, 33, 48, 226
Archer, L., 95, 157, 232
Aronson, A. E., 5, 6, 22, 182, 184, 206
Arthur, G., 204, 205
Assal, G., 224

Bady, J. A., 71, 83, 218, 220, 224, 231, 245
Bailey, P., 237
Baker, E., 8, 23, 126, 158, 236
Baletsa, G., 236
Balick, S., 9, 21, 40, 42, 48, 72, 73, 74, 83, 224
Barnes, S., 224
Baron, N., 224
Bartak, L., 224
Basmajian, J. V., 165, 171
Battison, D., 240
Battison, R., 224
Beckett, J. W., 10, 27, 231
Beesley, M., 233
Bell, C. L., 105, 161
Bell, D. J., 224
Benaroya, S., 224
Bennett, D. N., 7, 8, 27, 245
Bergman, J. S., 235
Berry, T., 8, 23, 126, 158, 236
Beynon, J. D. E., 242
Bicker, D. D., 9, 21, 224
Bliss, C. K., 95, 98, 100, 101, 157, 233
Bobby, B., 233

Bonvillian, J. D., 10, 21, 32, 48, 224
Boone, D. R., 8, 21
Bornstein, H., 58, 61, 64, 65, 83, 225, 227
Bour, J. S., 242
Bralley, R. C., 233
Bridgman, P. W., 3, 21
Brink, J., 6, 23, 33, 43, 49, 236
Brookner, S. P., 9, 21, 32, 40, 42, 48, 225
Brown, J. R., 5, 6, 22, 182, 184, 206
Brown, J. V., 105, 161
Brown, W. P., 6, 28, 35, 51, 100, 161, 225, 233, 246, 247
Brumfitt, P. J., 147, 160, 242
Brunn, G., 233
Buelow, D., 129, 139, 159, 238
Bullock, A., 6, 21, 32, 42, 48, 233
Burnside, S., 6, 21
Butler, O., 6, 21, 233
Buttet, J., 224

Calculator, S. N., 233
Cameron, H., 7, 8, 23, 33, 49, 74, 76, 78, 83, 227
Campagna, J., 24, 49, 238
Capozzi, M., 235
Carlson, F. L., 6, 21, 32, 48, 101, 157, 225, 233
Carpenter, C., 241
Carrier, Jr., J. K., 10, 21, 22, 41, 51, 107, 108, 109, 126, 157, 158, 212, 213, 214, 220, 228, 233, 234, 238, 244
Certo, N., 245
Charbonneau, J. R., 6, 22, 32, 48, 234, 244
Chen, L. Y., 6, 7, 8, 22, 32, 48, 74, 75, 76, 83, 225
Chester, S. L., 225

Christinoz, D., 234
Churchill, T., 240
Chusid, J. G., 164, 170
Clappe, C., 6, 22, 32, 48, 234
Clark, C. R., 102, 103, 104, 105, 158, 161, 234
Clark, T. A., 225
Clarkson, D. C., 6, 25, 241
Clement, M., 234
Cohen, L. K., 6, 7, 8, 22, 225, 234
Cohen, M., 71
Colby, K. M., 234
Collins, D. W., 139, 158, 234
Colucci, S., 235
Combs, R. G., 4, 6, 22, 35, 51, 163, 169, 170, 171, 243, 249
Copeland, K., 6, 7, 8, 22, 149, 158, 220, 234
Cote, C., 6, 22, 32, 48, 234
Cox, A., 224
Creedon, M. P., 10, 22, 32, 40, 48, 225
Critcher, C. G., 234
Crochetiere, J. W., 235, 236
Culatta, B., 235
Curry, B., 235

Dalrymple, G. F., 6, 21, 32, 42, 48, 233, 244
Danca, J. M., 6, 21, 32, 42, 48, 233
Daniels, L., 184, 185, 188, 189, 205
Darley, F. L., 5, 6, 22, 182, 184, 206
Davies, C. O., 102, 103, 104, 105, 158, 161, 234
Davis, A., 224
Davis, G. A., 235
Davis, L., 226
Dean, M. B., 11, 25, 34, 44, 50, 229
DeLamore, K., 227
DePape, D. J., 235, 237
DeVilliers, J. G., 225
Dewan, E. M., 163, 169, 170, 171, 249
DiCarrado, C., 72, 83, 230
Dixon, C., 235
Donaldson, R., 8, 9, 27, 35, 51, 69, 71, 84, 231
Drinker, P., 244
Duffy, J. R., 7, 22, 56, 61, 181, 206, 225
Duffy, R. J., 7, 22, 56, 61, 181, 206, 225
Duncan, J. L., 33, 40, 42, 48, 70, 71, 83, 225
Dunn, L. M., 91, 158, 180, 206

Eagleson, H. M., 7, 8, 22, 33, 40, 48, 74, 76, 77, 83, 226
Egan, J. J., 6, 22, 33, 48, 226
Egerton, S. W., 235
Egolf, D. B., 225

Ehrlich, M. D., 111, 158, 235
Eichler, J. H., 6, 24, 34, 50, 121, 158, 239
Eisenson, J., 7, 22
Elder, P. S., 235
Ellsworth, S., 33, 40, 49, 226
Englehart, T. W., 235
English, S. T., 226
Evans, C. R., 170, 171
Evans, M. A., 11, 28, 52, 232
Eylenberg, J. B., 111, 160, 243

Farmer, A., 9, 24, 34, 50, 227
Feallock, B., 33, 49, 118, 158, 226, 235
Fenn, G., 6, 23, 33, 49, 226
Fenton, J., 6, 23, 33, 49, 118, 158, 236
Fischer, H., 11, 24, 50, 228
Fish, K., 236
Flanagan, K., 244
Fletcher, E. C., 226
Foldi, N., 226
Foster, R. E., 230
Fothergill, J., 236, 247
Fouldes, J., 6, 21, 233
Foulds, R. A., 235, 236
Fouts, R. S., 10, 23, 33, 40, 42, 43, 49, 226
Freiman, R., 226
Fristoe, M., 226
Fulwiler, R. L., 10, 23, 33, 40, 42, 49, 226
Fust, R. S., 7, 8, 27, 35, 51, 69, 71, 84, 231

Gaddis, W., 236
Gannon, R., 245
Gardner, B., 214, 220
Gardner, H., 8, 23, 126, 158, 226, 236
Gardner, J. O., 229
Gardner, R., 214, 220
Gazzaniga, M. S., 8, 23, 49, 107, 126, 158, 236
Geffner, D. S., 72, 83, 228, 230
Geisler, C. D., 6, 28, 237, 247, 248
Gertenrich, R. L., 33, 49, 127, 158, 236
Gitlis, K. R., 33, 40, 49, 226
Glass, A. V., 8, 23, 33, 49, 107, 126, 158, 236
Goehl, H., 10, 27, 231
Goldberg, H. R., 6, 23, 33, 49, 118, 158, 236
Goldojarb, M. F., 7, 8, 23, 226
Goldstein, H., 7, 8, 23, 33, 49, 74, 76, 78, 83, 227
Goodman, L., 10, 28, 227, 232, 251
Goodwin, M., 33, 40, 49, 236
Goodwin, T. C., 33, 40, 49, 236
Gordon, J., 236, 245
Gordon, K. C., 227

Gosling, T., 240
Graham, L. W., 227, 236
Grahm, S., 234
Grant, M., 22, 32, 48, 234
Grecco, R., 9, 23, 227
Greco, J. A., 234
Green, C. N., 236, 252
Green, L. C., 9, 23, 227
Greene, G., 9, 21, 40, 42, 48, 72, 73, 74, 83, 224
Griffin, J., 8, 9, 27, 35, 51, 69, 71, 84, 231
Grilley, K., 118, 123, 161, 247
Grimmel, M., 227

Hagen, C., 6, 23, 33, 43, 49, 236
Haight, C., 10, 23, 227
Hall, S. M., 227
Hammond, J., 237
Hammond, P. H., 249
Hannah, E. P., 229
Hanson, W. R., 7, 8, 23, 227
Hardiman, C. J., 238
Harding, P. J. R., 237
Harmon, G. M., 6, 23
Harper, B., 230
Harris, C. A., 225
Harris-Vanderheiden, D., 6, 10, 23, 34, 35, 43, 44, 49, 52, 100, 158, 233, 235, 237, 238, 247
Hartley, N., 6, 24, 238
Havemeyer, S., 226
Hayes, H. T. P., 227
Hazard, G., 22, 32, 48, 234
Head, H., 7, 24
Heber, R., 9, 27
Hehner, B., 238
Helfrich, K. R., 7, 24, 34, 43, 49, 227
Henkle, J. E., 238
Hill, S. D., 6, 24, 34, 49, 238
Hoffmeister, R. J., 9, 24, 34, 50, 227
Holbrook, A., 238
Hollander, F. M., 10, 24, 227
Hollis, J. H., 228, 238
Holmland, B. A., 238, 239
Holt, C., 129, 139, 159, 236, 238, 243, 247
Honke, L. E., 6, 22, 33, 48, 226
Hossain, K. S., 242
Howard, G., 216, 220, 239
Hughes, J., 228
Hyta, M. B., 227

Iles, G. H., 239
Irwin, D. L., 228
Isensee, L., 224
Israel, B. L., 239

Jarkler, B., 233
Jarrow, J. E., 231
Jefcoate, R., 239
Jenkins, R., 34, 50, 239
Johnston, H. B., 239
Jones, M. V., 239
Juhrs, P. D., 11, 24, 227

Kafafian, H., 239
Kahn, J. V., 228
Karlins, M., 166, 170, 171
Kates, B., 6, 24, 34, 41, 43, 50, 95, 101, 159, 160, 239, 241, 245
Kavanagh, R. N., 238, 239
Keirnan, C., 239
Kelso, D., 245, 247
Kent, L., 9, 24, 215, 220, 228, 251
Kiernan, C., 228
Kiesow, J., 228
Kimble, S. L., 9, 24, 34, 41, 43, 50, 228
Kingman, V. J., 237
Kirk, S., 182, 206
Kirk, W., 182, 206
Kirschner, A. E., 228
Kladde, A. G., 6, 24, 34, 41, 50, 240
Klein, L. S., 224
Klinger, J. L., 240
Knudson, A. B., 8, 22, 33, 40, 48, 74, 76, 77, 83, 226
Koller, J. J., 228
Kollinzas, G., 11, 27, 51, 230
Kolstoe, B. J., 240
Konstantareas, M., 11, 24, 34, 41, 43, 50, 228
Kop, P. F. M., 243
Kopchick, Jr., G. A., 9, 10, 25, 228
Korzybski, A., 100, 159
Koselka, M. J., 229
Kotkin, R., 33, 40, 49, 226
Kozak, A. J., 237
Krause, A. E., 239
Kuchar, E., 11, 28, 52, 232
Kuntz, J. B., 240

La Croix, Z. E., 234
Lake, S. J., 9, 25, 66, 83, 229, 251
Lamers, D. F., 6, 28, 247
Lang, J., 22, 32, 48, 234
Lappin, J. S., 239
Larson, T., 10, 25, 229
Lavoy, R. W., 6, 25, 240
Lebeis, R. F., 10, 25, 34, 41, 50, 229
Lebeis, S., 10, 25, 34, 41, 50, 229
Leibel, J., 11, 25, 229

Levett, L. M., 9, 25, 34, 41, 43, 50, 72, 73, 74, 83, 229
Linville, S. E., 41, 50, 229
Lippert, J. C., 237
Lippke, B., 227
Lloyd, L. L., 9, 25, 226, 228, 229, 240
Long, D., 24, 49, 238
Lovejoy, K. M., 230
Lowe, H., 240
Lowman, E. W., 240
Lucas, E. V., 11, 25, 34, 44, 50, 229
Luitse, W. J., 245
Lunteren, A. V., 245
Luster, M. J., 236, 240, 247
Lykos, C. M., 64, 83
Lywood, D. W., 6, 28, 240, 248

McCarthy, J., 182, 206
McDonald, E. T., 6, 25, 34, 50, 118, 159, 237, 240, 241
McDonald, J. J., 164, 170
McDowell, P., 11, 27, 51, 230
MacKenzie, P., 6, 10, 28, 35, 51, 100, 161, 246
McNaughton, S., 6, 10, 25, 26, 34, 41, 43, 50, 95, 100, 101, 159, 160, 237, 239, 241
McPherson, H., 11, 28, 52, 232
Maling, R. G., 6, 25, 241
Manning, R. P., 239
Mansell, M., 248
Markowicz, H., 224
Marquis, J., 6, 28, 35, 52, 249
Mayberry, R., 107, 159, 229
Meaney, M., 224
Meek, C. L., 145, 160
Melrose, J., 6, 27, 245
Menyuk, P., 11, 26, 229
Miller, A., 11, 26, 34, 41, 50, 229
Miller, E. E., 11, 26, 34, 41, 50, 229
Miller, J., 241
Miller, K., 11, 24, 50, 228
Montgomery, J., 241
Moogk-Soulis, C. A., 241
Moore, M. V., 242
Moores, D. F., 11, 26, 229
Mulholland, T., 170, 171
Munch, J., 24, 49, 238
Murphy, N. O., 9, 21, 32, 40, 42, 48, 225
Musil, A., 11, 27, 51, 230
Myklebust, H. R., 10, 26, 37, 51, 56, 61, 180, 206

Nabaui, C. D., 242
Naecher, S., 24, 49, 238
Naughton, J. M., 225

Nelson, K. E., 10, 21, 32, 48, 224
Nelson, P. J., 242
Neuman, S., 224
Newell, A. F., 147, 160, 242
Nicol, E., 34, 51, 242
Nuffer, P. S., 7, 8, 26, 242
Nugent, C. L., 242

Offir, C. W., 11, 26, 34, 41, 51, 230
Ogilvie, H., 224
Olson, T., 67, 83, 101, 160, 230, 242
Ormond, T. F., 233
Owens, M., 230
Oxman, J., 11, 24, 50, 228

Padden, C., 224
Parish, G., 242
Parkel, D. A., 105, 160, 242
Parsons, S. D., 41, 51, 244
Peak, T., 10, 22, 107, 108, 109, 126, 158, 212, 213, 214, 220, 234
Pearson, K. L., 7, 22, 56, 61, 181, 206, 225
Pei, M., 67–68, 83
Penfield, W., 7, 26
Perron, J. V., 6, 7, 8, 26, 243
Peters, L., 6, 10, 26, 230
Pettet, A., 11, 25, 229
Pfeiffer, D., 232
Porch, B., 182, 206
Porter, W., 6, 23, 33, 43, 49, 236
Premack, A. J., 10, 26, 107, 126, 160, 214, 220, 243
Premack, D., 8, 10, 23, 26, 49, 107, 126, 158, 160, 214, 220, 236, 243
Prince, S., 243
Prior, M. R., 230
Prutting, C. A., 226

Rahimi, M. A., 111, 160, 243
Raitzer, G. A., 238, 243, 247
Ralston, A., 145, 160
Ransay, D. A., 243
Ratusnik, C. M., 11, 26, 35, 51, 243
Ratusnik, D. L., 11, 26, 35, 51, 243
Reagan, W., 229
Reinen, S., 6, 10, 28, 35, 51, 100, 161, 246
Reuter, D. B., 111, 160
Rice, O. M., 35, 51, 163, 169, 171, 243, 249
Richardson, T., 10, 26, 35, 51, 230
Ricks, D. M., 11, 26, 230
Rinard, G., 243
Ring, N., 244
Robbins, N., 230

Robenault, I. P., 244
Roberts, L., 7, 26
Romack, D. W., 10, 25, 228
Rosen, M., 244
Rosenberg, G., 244
Ross, A., 244
Routh, D. K., 230
Rowe, J. A., 6, 23, 33, 49, 226
Roy, O. Z., 6, 22, 32, 48, 234, 244
Rumbaugh, D. M., 214, 220, 244
Rutter, M., 224

Saarnio, I., 244
Salvin, A., 230
Sampson, D., 244
Sanders, D. A., 230, 244
Sarno, J., 230
Sarno, M., 230
Sayre, J. M., 6, 26, 118, 160, 244
Schaeffer, B., 11, 27, 35, 41, 51, 230
Scheibel, C., 6, 10, 28, 35, 51, 100, 161, 246
Schiefelbusch, R. L., 230, 244
Schinsky, L., 7, 8, 9, 27, 35, 51, 69, 71, 84, 231
Schlanger, B. B., 231
Schlanger, P. H., 7, 8, 27, 35, 41, 51, 72, 73, 74, 83, 226, 228, 230, 231
Schmidt, A., 235
Schmidt, M. J., 41, 51, 244
Schultz, A. R., 6, 25, 34, 50, 118, 159, 241
Schurman, J. A., 117, 160, 245
Seligman, J., 245
Shaffer, T. R., 10, 27, 231
Shane, H., 6, 27, 245
Shannon, C. E., 66, 84
Shipley, K. G., 231
Shwedyk, E., 245
Silverman, E.-M., 95, 160
Silverman, F. H., 29, 30, 33, 40, 42, 47, 48, 51, 70, 71, 83, 95, 160, 218, 219, 220, 224, 225, 231, 245
Silverman, H., 95, 160, 239, 245
Skelly, M., 6, 7, 8, 9, 27, 35, 41, 51, 69, 71, 84, 231, 251
Sklar, M., 7, 8, 27, 245
Sloman, L., 11, 28, 52, 232
Smilovitz, R., 10, 25, 228
Smith, C. H., 11, 27, 231
Smith, J., 245
Smith, R. W., 7, 8, 9, 27, 35, 51, 69, 71, 84, 230
Smorto, M. P., 165, 171
Snapper, A. G., 243
Soede, M., 245
Sontag, E., 245
Spas, D. L., 231

Speilman, M., 237
Speldt, P., 233
Spiegel, D., 9, 21, 40, 42, 48, 72, 73, 74, 83, 224
Spradlin, J., 182, 206, 228, 238
Sprague, M. J., 6, 28, 35, 52, 249
Stassen, H. G., 245
Steele, D., 245
Stein, J., 72, 84
Sterne, R. G., 235
Stevens, H. A., 9, 27
Stohr, P. G., 10, 28, 232
Stromore, K. A., 237
Sutherland, D., 245
Sutherland, G. F., 10, 27, 231
Swisher, L., 230

Talkington, L. W., 227
Tatman, T., 11, 27, 231
Tenenbaum, D., 231
Tolstrup, I. M., 246
Tomkins, W., 67, 68, 69, 70, 84, 231, 251
Tomlinson, R., 22, 32, 48, 234
Topper, S. T., 10, 27, 35, 51, 231
Torok, Z., 20, 27, 163, 169, 171, 249
Traub, D. A., 246
Traynor, C. D., 246

Vail, J. L., 231
Valley, V., 237
VanBiervliet, A., 232
Vanderheiden, D. H., 6, 10, 28, 35, 51, 100, 161, 225, 246 (*see also* Harris-Vanderheiden, D.)
Vanderheiden, G. C., 6, 28, 35, 44, 52, 117, 118, 119, 120, 123, 124, 127, 129, 139, 159, 161, 225, 233, 235, 236, 237, 238, 240, 243, 246, 247, 248
Vaneldik, J. F., 237
VanHook, K. E., 10, 28, 232
Vasa, J. J., 6, 28, 240, 248
Vaughn, G. R., 8, 22, 33, 40, 48, 74, 76, 77, 83, 226
Vicker, B., 6, 28, 35, 52, 118, 161, 248, 251
Volk, A. M., 6, 28, 247, 248
VonGlasersfeld, E., 105, 106, 161

Waldo, L. J., 248
Wardell, R., 248
Warner, H., 105, 160, 161, 242
Warrick, A., 249
Weaver, W., 66, 84

Weber, S. C., 180, 206
Webster, C. D., 11, 24, 25, 27, 28, 35, 44, 50, 52, 228, 229, 231, 232
Wendt, E., 6, 28, 35, 52, 249
Wepman, J. M., 88, 161
Wesley, S., 224
White, R. A., 105, 160, 242
White, S. D., 6, 28, 249
Wilber, R. B., 58, 62, 232
Wilson, M. S., 245
Wilson, P. S., 10, 28, 35, 41, 52, 227, 232, 251
Wing, L., 11, 26, 230
Wood, R. K., 10, 28, 232, 251

Woodcock, R. W., 102, 103, 104, 105, 158, 161, 234
Worthingham, C., 184, 185, 188, 189, 205

Yoder, D. E., 237

Ziskind, A., 249
Ziskind, R., 249
Zurif, E. B., 8, 23, 126, 158, 226, 236
Zweiban, S. T., 232